OXFORD MEDICAL PUBLICATIONS

THE CLASSIFICATION AND DIAGNOSIS OF HEADACHE DISORDERS

FRONTIERS IN HEADACHE RESEARCH SERIES

Published by Lippincott-Raven:

Published by Oxford University Press:

The Classification of Headache Disorders

EDITED BY

Jes Olesen

Department of Neurology, Glostrup Hospital,
University of Copenhagen, Denmark

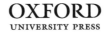

This book has been printed digitally and produced in a standard specification
in order to ensure its continuing availability

OXFORD
UNIVERSITY PRESS

Great Clarendon Street, Oxford OX2 6DP

Oxford University Press is a department of the University of Oxford.
It furthers the University's objective of excellence in research, scholarship,
and education by publishing worldwide in

Oxford New York

Auckland Cape Town Dar es Salaam Hong Kong Karachi
Kuala Lumpur Madrid Melbourne Mexico City Nairobi
New Delhi Shanghai Taipei Toronto
With offices in
Argentina Austria Brazil Chile Czech Republic France Greece
Guatemala Hungary Italy Japan South Korea Poland Portugal
Singapore Switzerland Thailand Turkey Ukraine Vietnam

Oxford is a registered trade mark of Oxford University Press
in the UK and in certain other countries

Published in the United States
by Oxford University Press Inc., New York

ISBN 978-0-19-856590-1

Printed and bound in Great Britain by CPI Antony Rowe, Chippenham and Eastbourne

Preface

Disease classification has developed into a distinct branch of medical science over the last couple of decades. It has been gradually accepted that, without a valid and reliable classification and associated explicit diagnostic criteria, other disease-related research is difficult or impossible. Headache is a good example of this development. Until the first edition of the International Classification of Headache Disorders published in 1988, headache disorders were very poorly classified and no explicit diagnostic criteria existed. During that period of time, headache research progressed slowly and interesting results were often disregarded because the type of patients included in the study could always be disputed. The epidemiology of headache disorders was likewise not well-described and socio-economic consequences of the disorders were unknown.

The first edition of the International Classification of Headache Disorders (ICHD-1) represented a huge step forward and actually placed the headache disorders among the best classified and defined neurological disorders. This led to a surge of epidemiological and mechanism-oriented studies. The first edition was of such quality that a need for revision did not arise until almost 15 years later, when the Second International Headache Classification Committee started its work. The resulting revision: International Classification of Headache Disorders Second Edition (ICHD-2) was published in January 2004.

ICHD-2 forms the background of the present publication, which does not repeat the classification, but focuses on its application in research and clinical practice. Special emphasis is on new entities in ICHD-2 and on new ways of separating primary and secondary headaches. Also extensively covered are research possibilities presented by ICHD-2. While ICHD-2 is very condensed and difficult to read, the present volume is more user friendly. Hopefully, it will be useful and interesting reading for all those caring for headache patients as well as for researchers in headache, and others with a general interest in disease classification.

Jes Olesen
September 2004

Contents

Session II The primary headaches: Part I—the migraines

Session III The primary headaches: Part II

Session IV The secondary headaches: Part I

Session V The secondary headaches: Part II

Session VI Practical implementation and research

Contributors

Aamodt, A.H.	Norwegian National Headache Centre, Trondheim University Hospital, Norwegian University of Science and Technology, Norway
Alarcón, F.	On behalf of the Latin American Migraine Study Group
Alberti, Andrea	Neuroscience Department, University of Perugia, Italy
Aranaga, N.	On behalf of the Latin American Migraine Study Group
Ashina, Messoud	Danish Headache Center and Department of Neurology, Glostrup Hospital, University of Copenhagen, DK-2600 Glostrup, Copenhagen, Denmark
Ashina, Sait	Danish Headache Center and Department of Neurology, Glostrup Hospital, University of Copenhagen, DK-2600 Glostrup, Copenhagen, Denmark
Aulet, S.	On behalf of the Latin American Migraine Study Group
Autret, A.	On behalf of the Société Francaise d'Etudes Des Migraines et Céphalées (SFEMC)
Baudesson, G.	On behalf of the Société Francaise d'Etudes Des Migraines et Céphalées (SFEMC)
Beghi, E.	Mario Negri Institute and Neurological Clinic, University of Milano-Bicocca, Milan, Italy
Bendtsen, Lars	The Danish Headache Center, Department of Neurology, University of Copenhagen, Glostrup Hospital, 2600 Glostrup, Denmark
Bigal, Marcelo E.	Department of Neurology, Epidemiology, and Population Health, Albert Einstein College of Medicine, Bronx, NY. Montefiore headache Clinic, Bronx, NY; The New England Center for Headache, Stamford, CT, USA
Bousser, Marie-Germaine	Service de neurologie, Hôpital Lariboisière, 2, rue Ambroise Paré, 75475 Paris Cedex 10, France
Burstein, Rami	Department of Anesthesia and Critical Care, Harvard Institutes of Medicine, Room 830, 77 Avenue Louis Pasteur, Boston, MA 02115, USA
Capocchi, Giuseppe	Neurologic Clinic, Department of neuroscience, University of Perugia, Italy
Cecchini, Alberto P.	University Centre for Adaptive Disorders and Headache, IRCCS "C Mondino" Foundation, Pavia
Chapman, E.	On behalf of the Latin American Migraine Study Group

Chautard, M.H.	Astra Zeneca, France
Conterno, L.	On behalf of the Latin American Migraine Study Group
Corigliano, Donatella	Department of neurology and Otholaringology, University of Rome "La Sapienza", Italy
Couch, J.	University of Oklahoma Health Sciences Center, Oklahoma City, OK, USA
Creach', C.	On behalf of the Société Francaise d'Etudes Des Migraines et Céphalées (SFEMC)
Dodick, D.	Mayo Clinic , Scottsdale, AZ, USA
Donnet, A.	On behalf of the Société Francaise d'Etudes Des Migraines et Céphalées (SFEMC)
Dousset, V.	On behalf of the Société Francaise d'Etudes Des Migraines et Céphalées (SFEMC)
Eriksen, Malene K.	Danish Headache Center, University of Copenhagen, Department of Neurology, Glostrup University Hospital, Nordre Ringvej 57, 2600 Glostrup, Denmark
Estévez, E.	On behalf of the Latin American Migraine Study Group
Fabre, N.	On behalf of the Société Francaise d'Etudes Des Migraines et Céphalées (SFEMC)
Ferrari, Michel D.	Department of neurology, K5Q-95, Leiden University Medical Center, P.O. Box 9600, 2300 RC Leiden, The Netherlands
First, Michael B.	Columbia University College of Physicians and Surgeons, 1051Riverside Drive – Unit 60, New York, N.Y. 10032, USA
Fortini, Daniela	IRCCS S Lucia, Rome
Garcia-Pedroza, F.	On behalf of the Latin American Migraine Study Group
Garrido, J.	On behalf of the Latin American Migraine Study Group
Géraud, G.	On behalf of the Société Francaise d'Etudes Des Migraines et Céphalées (SFEMC)
Gessner, U.	Bayer Vital GmbH, Consumer-Care, D-51149 Cologne, Germany
Ghiotto, Natascia	University Centre for Adaptive Disorders and Headache, IRCCS "C Mondino" Foundation, Pavia
Giacomini, Patrizia	Department of neurology and Otholaringology, University of Rome "La Sapienza", Italy
Gil, Rosario	Department of Nerology, Hospital Clinico Universitario, University of Valencia, Spain
Giraud, G.	On behalf of the Société Francaise d'Etudes Des Migraines et Céphalées (SFEMC)
Girot, M.	Department of Neurology, Lille University Hospital, France
Goadsby, Peter J.	Headache Group, Institute of Neurology, Queen Square, London WC1N 3 BG, United Kingdom
Grazia, Sances	University Centre for Adaptive Disorders and Headache, IRCCS "C Mondino" Foundation, Pavia

Guaschino, E.	University Centre for Adaptive Disorders and Headache, IRCCS "C Mondino" Foundation, Pavia
Guégan-Massardier, E.	On behalf of the Société Francaise d'Etudes Des Migraines et Céphalées (SFEMC)
Guy, N.	On behalf of the Société Francaise d'Etudes Des Migraines et Céphalées (SFEMC)
Göbel, Hartmut	Kiel Pain Clinic, Heikendorfer Weg 9-27, 24149 Kiel, Germany
Heinze, Axel	Kiel Pain Clinic, Heikendorfer Weg 9-27, 24149 Kiel, Germany
Heinze-Kuhn, Katja	Kiel Pain Clinic, Heikendorfer Weg 9-27, 24149 Kiel, Germany
Hénon, H.	Department of Neurology, Lille University Hospital, France
Hettiarachchi, J.	Pfizer Inc, 235 East 42nd St. 235/10/10, New York, NY 10017, USA
Jakubowski, Moshe	Department of Anesthesia and Critical Care, Harvard Medical School, Boston, MA 02115 USA
Jensen, Rigmor	The Danish Headache Center, Department of Neurology, University of Copenhagen, Glostrup Hospital, 2600 Glostrup, Denmark
Kolodner, K.	IMR, a Division of AdvancePCA, Hunt Valley, MD, USA
Kubisch, Christian	Institute of Human Genetics, University of Bonn
Kunickas, R.	Traumatology Emergency Ward, Red Cross Hospital, Kaunas Lithuania
Láinez, Miguel, J.A.	Department of Nerology, Hospital Clinico Universitario, Department of Neurology Hospital Clínico Universitario, Avda. Blasco Ibàñez, 17, 46110 Valencia, Spain
Lance, James W.	Lance, James W, Institute of Neurological Sciences, Prince of Wales Hospital Suite 5A, 54 Queen St, Woollahra, NSW 2025, Australia
Lanteri-Minet, M.	Department of Evaluation and Treatment of Pain, Hopital Pasteur, 30, Voi Romaine, 06002 Nice Cedex 1, France
Leston, J.	On behalf of the Latin American Migraine Study Group
Leys, D.	Department of Neurology, Lille University Hospital, France
Lipton, Richard B.	Departments of Neurology, Epidemiology and Social Medicine Albert Einstein College of Medicine 1165 Morris Park Ave Rm 332 Bronx, New York 10461, USA
Lucas, C.	Department of Neurology, Lille University Hospital, Clinique Neurologique, Hôpital Salengro, C.H.R.U., 59037 –Lille, France
Macias-Islas, M.	On behalf of the Latin American Migraine Study Group
Mackowiak, M.A.	Department of Neurology, Lille University Hospital, France

Manzoni, G.C.	Headache Center, Section of Neurology, Department of Neuroscience, University of Parma, Parma Italy
Marchione, Pasquale	Department of Neurology and Otholaringology, University of Rome "La Sapienza", Viale dell'Universitá 30, 00185 Rome, Italy
Massiou, H.	On behalf of the Société Francaise d'Etudes Des Migraines et Céphalées (SFEMC)
Mazzotta, Giovanni	Neuroscience Department, University of Perugia, Italy
Mick, G.	On behalf of the Société Francaise d'Etudes Des Migraines et Céphalées (SFEMC)
Mickeviciene, D.	Department of Neurology, Red Cross Hospital, Kaunas Lithuania and Department of Neurology, Medical University Clinic, Kaunas Lithuania
Monzillo, P.	On behalf of the Latin American Migraine Study Group
Morillo, L.E.	Javeriana University, Bogotá, Colombia (On behalf of the Latin American Migraine Study Group)
Nappi, Giuseppe	University Centre for Adaptive Disorders and Headache, IRCCS "C Mondino" Foundation, Via Ferrata 6, 27100 Pavia and Department of Neurology and Otolaryngology, University "La Sapienza", Rome, Italy
Navez, M.	On behalf of the Société Francaise d'Etudes Des Migraines et Céphalées (SFEMC)
Núnez, L.	On behalf of the Latin American Migraine Study Group
Obelieniene, D.	Department of Neurology, Medical University Clinic, Kaunas, Lithuania
Olesen, Jes	Department of Neurology Glostrup Hospital, University of Copenhagen, Ndr. Ringvej 57, 2600 Glostrup, Denmark
Pascual, Ana M.	Department of Nerology, Hospital Clinico Universitario, University of Valencia, Spain
Pedini, Mauro	Computer Science Educational Laboratory, Faculty of Medicine, Neurologic Clinic, University of Perugia, Italy
Perez, A.	On behalf of the Latin American Migraine Study Group
Petersen-Braun, M.	Bayer Vital GmbH, Consumer-Care, D-51149 Cologne, Germany
Plascencia, N.	On behalf of the Latin American Migraine Study Group
Pradalier, A.	On behalf of the Société Francaise d'Etudes Des Migraines et Céphalées (SFEMC)
Radat, F.	On behalf of the Société Francaise d'Etudes Des Migraines et Céphalées (SFEMC)
Rodriguez, C.	On behalf of the Latin American Migraine Study Group
Sakai, Fumihiko	Kitasato University Hospital, 1-15-1 Kitasato, Sagamihara Kanagawa, 228-8555 Japan
Salvador, Antonio	Department of Nerology, Hospital Clinico Universitario, University of Valencia, Spain

Samá, Domenico	Department of Neurology and Otholaringology, University of Rome "La Sapienza", Italy
Sand, T.	Norwegian National Headache Center, Trondheim University Hospital, Faculty of medicine, Norwegian University of Science and Technology , Trondheim, Norway
Sandrini, Giorgio	University Centre for Adaptive Disorders and Headache, IRCCS "C Mondino" Foundation, Pavia
Sanin, L.C.	On behalf of the Latin American Migraine Study Group
Sarchielli, Paola	Neurologic Clinic, Neuroscience Department, University of Perugia, Italy
Schrader, H.	Norwegian National Headache Center, Trondheim University Hospital, Faculty of medicine, Norwegian University of Science and Technology , Trondheim, Norway
Silberstein, Stephen	Director, Jefferson Headache Center and Professor of Neurology, Thomas Jefferson University Hospital, Philadelphia, Pennsylvania, USA
Silva, F.	On behalf of the Latin American Migraine Study Group
Simonovis, N.	On behalf of the Latin American Migraine Study Group
Steiner, Timothy J.	Division of Neuroscience, Faculty of Medicine, Imperial College London, Charing Cross Campus, St. Dunstan's Road, London W6 8RP, United Kingdom
Stovner, L.J.	Norwegian National Headache Center, Trondheim University Hospital, Faculty of medicine, Norwegian University of Science and Technology , Trondheim, Norway
Surkiene, D.	Department of Neurology, Medical University Clinic, Kaunas, Lithuania
Takeuchi, Y.	On behalf of the Latin American Migraine Study Group
Tassorelli, Cristina	University Centre for Adaptive Disorders and Headache, IRCCS "C Mondino" Foundation, Pavia
Thomsen, Lise Lykke	Danish Headache Center, University of Copenhagen, Department of Neurology, Glostrup University Hospital, Nordre Ringvej 57, 2600 Glostrup, Denmark
Todt, Unda	Institute of Human Genetics, University of Bonn
Torelli, P.	Headache Center, Section of Neurology, Department of Neuroscience, University of Parma, Parma Italy
Valade, D.	On behalf of the Société Francaise d'Etudes Des Migraines et Céphalées (SFEMC)
Vento, Claudio	Department of Neurology and Otholaringology, University of Rome "La Sapienza", Italy
Viallet, M.	Department of Neurology, Lille University Hospital, France
Weingärtner, U.	Bayer Vital GmbH, Consumer-Care, D-51149 Cologne, Germany

Wiendels, Natalie J.   Department of Neurology, Leiden University Medical Center, Leiden, The Netherlands

Waage, A.   Department of Medicine, Section for Hematology, Trondheim University Hospital, Norwegian University of Science and Technology, Norway

Session
1

Principles and tools

1 Migraine with and without allodynia: new sub-classification of migraine

R. Burstein and M. Jakubowski

The prevalance of cutaneous allodynia

We have recently shown using quantitative sensory testing technique, that migraine headache may be associated with high incidence (about 75%) of ipsilateral cutaneous allodynia, particularly in periorbital and temporal skin areas, and proposed that this is the very reason why patients feel that during migraine, their skin hurts in response to otherwise innocuous activities such as combing hair or wearing it in a pony tail, shaving, taking a shower, brushing their upper teeth, wearing glasses or earrings, or resting their head on the migraine side.[1]

Although not termed as such, several important papers described cutaneous allodynia in migraine patients. In 1873, Edward Living[2] quoted Tissot in his seminal book 'on Megrim' as saying "So painful is this hyperaesthesia in a certain stage of the seizure with some people that, he [the patient] could not bear anything to touch his head". In 1953, Harold Wolff[3] performed the first quantitative study on extracranial hypersensitivity during migraine. He measured 'deep pain threshold' in migraine patients first when pain-free, and then during migraine using the Hardy deep pain dolorimeter. He found that in cranial tissue, deep pain thresholds were high during headache-free period and low during the headache. The zone of low threshold expanded to include areas on the non-painful side of the head and deep pain threshold began to decrease several hours after the onset of headache. This hypersensitivity outlasted the headache for hours and even days. Wolff interpreted the extracranial hypersensitivity as 'resulting from secondary involvement of the extracranial vessels' (i.e. hematomas and tissue damage). In 1960, James Lance[4] found that the majority of migraine patients he studied experienced scalp tenderness during migraine attacks. In his meticulous documentation, he wrote: "Tenderness of the scalp during or after the headache was experienced by some 2/3 [317/500] of our patients. This may be so severe as to prevent the patient from lying on the affected side, or described only as abnormal sensitivity when combing or brushing the hair. This tenderness may involve any part of the scalp, face, or nuchal region ...". Like Wolff, seven years before him, Lance proposed that scalp tenderness is a result of "wide spread distension of extracranial blood vessels or spasm of sub-occipital and scalp muscles". Between 1981 and 1994, Tfelt-Hansen, Olesen, Lous, and Jensen[5–10] found high prevalence of pericranial tenderness of myofacial tissue in common migraine, and proposed that axonal reflexes between extracranial arteries and neighboring myofacial tissue may account for the observed tenderness. In 1985, Waelkens[11] stated that a number of his patients were afraid of physical contact during migraine (he called it haptephobia). In 1987, Drummond[12] studied scalp tenderness and sensitivity to pain in migraine patients and reported that scalp tissues were more tender in migraine patients than in controls, both during migraine and for several days after the migraine had subsided, and that although the tenderness was greatest at the site of migraine, other areas of the scalp and neck were also more sensitive. That year, Blau[13] wrote "Occasionally men state that they cannot bear their shirt collar closed because the tightness is irritating during a migraine". In 1998, Carl Dahlof[14] studied safety aspects of triptan therapy and noted that *haptephobia*, a dislike of being touched, can begin before the injection of sumatriptan. Collectively, these studies gave rise to the notion that the origin of migraine headache involves extracranial blood vessels, and muscles and tendons.

In a series of preclinical and clinical studies that started in 1996, we proposed an alternative interpretation to scalp tenderness during migraine. We proposed that sensitization of spinal trigeminovascular neurons (i.e. central sensitization) mediates the development of cutaneous allodynia and muscle tenderness (Fig. 1.1).

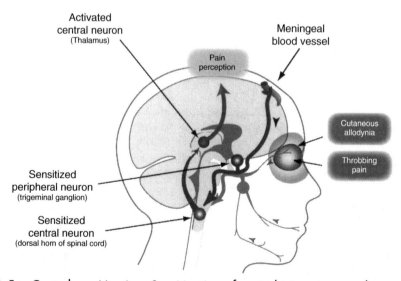

Fig. 1.1 Central sensitization. Sensitization of central trigeminovascular neurons in nucleus caudalis mediates cutaneous allodynia.

Critical to understanding this proposal are the remarkable similarities between the temporal changes in the development of peripheral and central sensitization in the rat, and their corresponding clinical manifestations during the course of migraine. The induction of peripheral sensitization in the rat occurs rapidly within 5–20 min after applying inflammatory soup (IS) onto the dura,[15,16] whereas central sensitization develops over 20–120 min and becomes firmly established only 120–240 min after IS.[17] Similarly in patients, throbbing transpires some 5–20 min after the onset of headache, whereas cutaneous allodynia starts between 20 and 120 min, and becomes firmly established only 120–240 min after the onset of headache.[18] According to our scenario, meningeal nociceptors become sensitized a few minutes after their initial activation. The continued barrage of impulses arriving from sensitized meningeal nociceptors gradually stimulates the development of central sensitization in spinal trigeminovascular neurons. Eventually, central trigeminovascular neurons change their physiological properties and remain inveterately sensitized, independent of incoming impulses from meningeal nociceptors.

Therapeutic implications: defeating migraine pain with triptans is a race against the development of cutaneous allodynia

To test whether central sensitization, as manifested by cutaneous allodynia, presents an obstacle to migraine therapy, we studied migraine patients repeatedly on three visits to the clinic: in the absence of migraine (baseline); before and after *early* triptan treatment (initiated within the first hour of one attack; before the establishment of central sensitization); and before and after *late* triptan treatment (initiated 4 h from onset of another attack; after the establishment of central sensitization). We found that the success rate of rendering a migraine patient pain-free is tightly associated with the absence or presence of cutaneous allodynia at the time of triptan therapy.[1] Patients who developed allodynia during the course of an attack were by far more likely to be rendered pain-free when triptan therapy was administered before rather than after the establishment of cutaneous allodynia (Fig. 1.2B), and those who never developed allodynia were highly likely to be rendered pain-free at any time after the onset of pain (Fig. 1.2A). In the presence of allodynia, triptan treatment brought about a complete pain relief in only 5/34 (15%) attacks. In the other 29 attacks (85%), triptan treatment reduced the pain level by about 40%. Pain thresholds for heat, cold, and mechanical stimuli of the periorbital skin shifted significantly ($p < 0.0001$) from normal values at baseline into the allodynic zone at the pre-treatment time point of the attack and remained there after treatment: pain thresholds dropped from 45.6 ± 0.6°C to 40.1 ± 0.6°C for heat; increased from 12.7 ± 1.2 to 20.7 ± 1.5°C for cold; and dropped from 112.6 ± 6.6 to 29.8 ± 6.6 g for mechanical skin stimulation. Notwithstanding the partial pain relief, triptan treatment did terminate the throbbing in 70% of the attacks and reduced throbbing intensity by more than half in an additional 19% of these attacks. In contrast, in the absence of allodynia (Fig. 1.2), triptan treatment effectively eliminated the pain

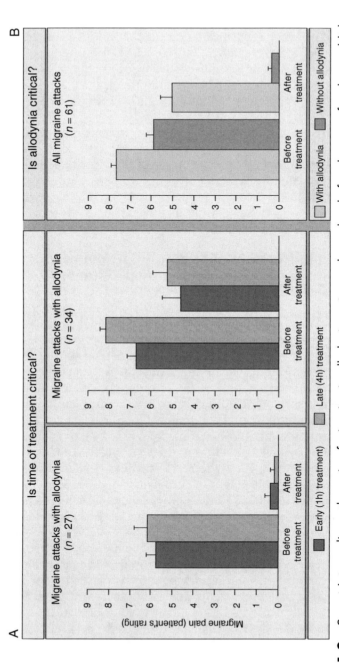

Fig. 1.2 Sumatriptan relieves the pain of migraine in allodynic patients when taken before but not after the establishment of allodynia (adapted from Burstein *et al.*, 2004).

in 25/27 (93%) attacks, and abolished throbbing. In these attacks, pain thresholds for heat, cold, and mechanical stimuli of the periorbital skin remained well outside the allodynic zone throughout the attacks and unchanged from baseline (i.e. between attacks): heat pain thresholds remained above 46°C; cold pain thresholds remained below 13°C; mechanical pain threshold remained above 100 g.

These results have led us to propose a new guideline for triptan treatment: (a) patients with allodynia should take triptans as early as possible into the attack before the emergence of any sign of allodynia; (b) after the onset of allodynia, patients may still use triptans if they find significant benefits in partial pain relief; (c) allodynia-free patients can expect excellent results from triptans at any time during the attack.

More support to this proposal could be found in clinical studies in which early treatment of migraine attacks with triptans resulted in significantly higher incidence of pain-free status.[19–22]

The race against the development of cutaneous allodynia is actually a race against the establishment of central sensitization

Since cutaneous allodynia of migraine is a manifestation of sensitization of central trigeminovascular neurons, we used our rat model for cutaneous allodynia induced by intracranial pain to examine whether *early* sumatriptan administration can *prevent* the development of central sensitization, and whether *late* sumatriptan administration can *reverse* inveterate central sensitization. We found that the effects of sumatriptan on spinal trigeminovascular neurons depends on whether the drug is given before or after the establishment of central sensitization and cutaneous allodynia.[23] Early sumatriptan intervention effectively prevented the induction of central sensitization, whereas late sumatriptan intervention could not reverse an already established central sensitization.

Late sumatriptan intervention effectively counteracted neuronal measures of central sensitization that depend on peripheral input from the meninges: dural receptive fields, which initially expanded by IS, shrunk back to their original size after treatment (Fig. 1.3); neuronal response threshold to dural indentation (g), which initially decreased after IS, increased significantly after sumatriptan. On the other hand, late sumatriptan intervention did not reverse aspects of central sensitization that reflect intrinsic activity: spontaneous firing rate (spikes/s), which initially increased after S, remained elevated after sumatriptan (Fig. 1.4); neuronal response magnitude to skin brushing, which initially increased after IS, remained elevated after sumatriptan; and neuronal response threshold to heating of the skin, which initially dropped after IS, remained low after sumatriptan. Early sumatriptan intervention effectively blocked the development of all aspects of central sensitization expected to be induced by IS 2 h later: dural receptive fields did not expand; neuronal response threshold to dural indentation did not decrease; spontaneous firing rate did not increase; and neuronal response thresholds to skin stimuli remained unchanged.

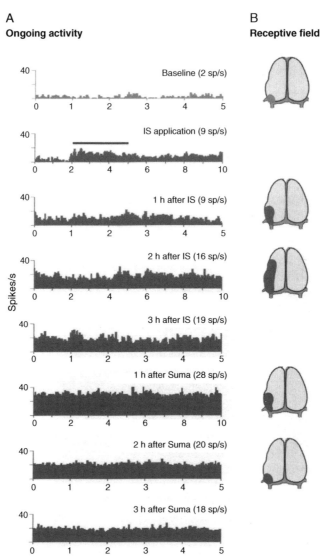

Fig. 1.3 *Late* sumatriptan treatment cannot reverse IS-induced increase in spontaneous activity but can effectively reverse expansion of dural receptive field (adapted from Burstein and Jakubowski, 2004).

Based on our studies[1,23] and studies by Longmore,[24] Riad[25], and Potrebic[26] we concluded that triptans act peripherally to block the transmission of pain signals from the dura, but do not act directly on the central neurons in spinal trigeminal nucleus. Such peripheral action of triptans can explain our observations that these drugs are highly effective, *whether given early or late*, in terminating throbbing in patients, and

A
Ongoing activity

B
Receptive field

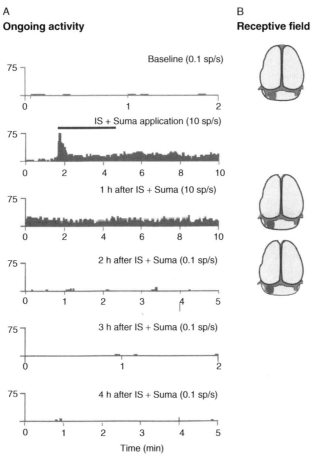

Fig. 1.4 *Early* sumatriptan treatment effectively prevents IS-induced increase in spontaneous activity and expansion of dural receptive field (adapted from Burstein and Jakubowski, 2004).

reversing hypersensitivity to mechanical stimulation of the dura in central trigeminovascular neurons. This peripheral action also explains why *early* triptan intervention is effective in terminating migraine pain and blocking the development of cutaneous allodynia, as it disrupts the input necessary for the development of central sensitization. There is evidence that the peripheral action of triptans cannot counteract the inveterate. Ongoing sensitization in the central trigeminovascular neurons can explain the failure of *late* triptan intervention to terminate migraine pain or reverse the exaggerated skin sensitivity in attacks already associated with allodynia, and triptans' inability to abolish the increased spontaneous activity and hypersensitivity to mechanical and thermal stimulation of the skin in central trigeminovascular neurons.

The relatively high incidence of cutaneous allodynia in migraine patients and the benefits of timing triptan therapy to precede allodynia call for adding a new classification to the diagnosis of migraine: migraine with and without allodynia.

Acknowledgments

This work has been supported by NIH grants DE-10904 (National Institutes of Dental and Craniofacial Research) and NS-35611 (National Institutes of Neurological Disorder and Stroke), and by a grant from GlaxoSmithKline.

References

1. Burstein R, Jakubowski M, Collins B. Defeating migraine pain with triptans: a race against the development of cutaneous allodynia. *Ann Neurol* 2004; **55**: 19–26.
2. Liveing E. On megrim, sick headache. Nijmegen: Arts & Boeve Publishers, 1873.
3. Wolff HG, Tunis MM, Goodell H. Studies on migraine. *Arch Int Med* 1953; **92**: 478–84.
4. Selby G, Lance JW. Observations on 500 cases of migraine and allied vascular headache. *J Neurol Neurosurg Psychiat* 1960; 23–32.
5. Tfelt-Hansen P, Lous I, Olesen J. Prevalence and significance of muscle tenderness during common migraine attacks. *Headache* 1981; **21**: 49–54.
6. Lous I, Olesen J. Evaluation of pericranial tenderness and oral function in patients with common migraine, muscle contraction headache and 'combination headache'. *Pain* 1982; **12**: 385–93.
7. Jensen K, Tuxen C, Olesen J. Pericranial muscle tenderness and pressure-pain threshold in the temporal region during common migraine. *Pain* 1988; **35**: 65–70.
8. Gobel H, Ernst M, Jeschke J, *et al.* Acetylsalicylic acid activates antinociceptive brain-stem reflex activity in headache patients and in healthy subjects. *Pain* 1992; **48**: 187–95.
9. Jensen R, Rasmussen BK, Pedersen B, *et al.* Prevalence of oromandibular dysfunction in a general population. *J Orofacial Pain* 1993; **7**: 175–82.
10. Jensen K. Extracranial blood flow, pain and tenderness in migraine. Clinical and experimental studies. *Acta Neurol Scand Suppl* 1993; **147**: 1–27.
11. Waelkens J. Warning symptoms in migraine: characteristics and therapeutic implications. *Cephalalgia* 1985; **5**: 223–8.
12. Drummond PD. Scalp tenderness and sensitivity to pain in migraine and tension headache. *Headache* 1987; **27**: 45–50.
13. Blau JN. Adult migraine: the patient observed. In: *Migraine—clinical, therapeutic, conceptual and research aspects* (ed. Blau JN). Cambridge: Chapman and Hall Ltd, 1987: p. 3–30.
14. Dahlof CG, Mathew N. Cardiovascular safety of 5HT1B/1D agonists–is there a cause for concern? *Cephalalgia* 1998; **18**: 539–45.
15. Strassman AM, Raymond SA, Burstein R. Sensitization of meningeal sensory neurons and the origin of headaches. *Nature* 1996; **384**: 560–4.
16. Levy D, Strassman AM. Distinct sensitizing effects of the cAMP-PKA second messenger cascade on rat dural mechanonociceptors. *J Physiol* 2002; **538**: 483–93.
17. Burstein R, Yamamura H, Malick A, *et al.* Chemical stimulation of the intracranial dura induces enhanced responses to facial stimulation in brain stem trigeminal neurons. *J Neurophysiol* 1998; **79**: 964–82.
18. Burstein R, Cutrer FM, Yarnitsky D. The development of cutaneous allodynia during a migraine attack: clinical evidence for the sequential recruitment of spinal and supraspinal nociceptive neurons in migraine. *Brain* 2000; **123**: 1703–9.

19. Pascual J, Cabarrocas X. Within-patient early versus delayed treatment of migraine attacks with almotriptan: the sooner the better. *Headache* 2002; **42**: 28–31.
20. Cady RK, Sheftell F, Lipton RB, *et al.* Effect of early intervention with sumatriptan on migraine pain: retrospective analyses of data from three clinical trials. *Clin Ther* 2000; **22**: 1035–48.
21. Mathew NT. Early intervention with almotriptan improves sustained pain-free response in acute migraine. *Headache* 2003; **43**: 1075–9.
22. Nett R, Landy S, Shackelford S, *et al.* Pain-free efficacy after treatment with sumatriptan in the mild pain phase of menstrually associated migraine. *Obstet Gynecol* 2003; **102**: 835–42.
23. Burstein R, Jakubowski M. Analgesic triptan action in an animal model of intracranial pain: a race against the development of central sensitization. *Ann Neurol* 2004; **55**: 27–36.
24. Longmore J, Shaw D, Smith D, *et al.* Differential distribution of 5HT1D- and 5HT1B-immunoreactivity within the human trigemino-cerebrovascular system: implications for the discovery of new antimigraine drugs. *Cephalalgia* 1997; **17**: 833–42.
25. Riad M, Tong XK, el Mestikawy S, *et al.* Endothelial expression of the 5-hydroxytryptamine1B antimigraine drug receptor in rat and human brain microvessels. *Neuroscience* 1998; **86**: 1031–5.
26. Potrebic S, Ahn AH, Skinner K, *et al.* Peptidergic nociceptors of both trigeminal and dorsal root ganglia express serotonin 1D receptors: implications for the selective anti-migraine action of triptans. *J Neurosci* 2003; **23**: 10988–97.

2 The International Classification of Headache Disorders (ICHD)*

J. Olesen

Undoubtedly, most physicians consider disease classification to be boring, impossible to learn by heart, and clinically not very useful. This may be true in the sense that practicing physicians do not know classifications or diagnostic criteria by heart and do not even have time to look the criteria up except in special cases. However, we are all working on the basis of some sort of classification and use some sort of diagnostic criteria, often without knowing it. In the first instance, a new classification system is mostly important for research, but after it has been used for some years, all new research results in the particular field have been gathered using that system. Therefore, all new information which the practicing physician uses for treatment decisions has its origin in an internationally accepted classification system and its diagnostic criteria. In this way, new classification systems alter clinical practice. Classification systems also have more direct effects. For example, the explicit diagnostic criteria for migraine without aura[1] request knowledge only about duration of attack, severity of pain, unilaterality, pulsating or no pulsating quality, and aggravation or no aggravation of pain by physical activity as well as knowledge about the associated symptoms like nausea, vomiting, photo- and phonophobia. This serves as a clear guideline to the clinical interview and makes it unnecessary, in most cases, to ask many questions that physicians used in the past to characterize a headache.

The Headache field has enjoyed a systematic hierarchical classification system and associated explicit (previously called operational), diagnostic criteria for more than 15 years after the publication of the first edition at the Classification of the

---

*The International Classification of Headache Disorders. 2nd edition (ICHD-2) and the 10th International Classification of Diseases, neurological adaptation (ICD-10 NA) classification of headache disorders.

International Headache Society (IHS) (ICHD-1) in 1988.[2] Building on ICHD-1, the second edition of the International Classification of Headache Disorders (ICHD-2) has recently been published.[1] Like its predecessor, it will have a dominating influence on research and clinical practice for at least the next decade.

General principles of disease classification and diagnostic criteria

To classify disease means to decide how many different entities that should be recognized and to order them in a logical system. There are two tendencies in classification: lumping and splitting. Lumping headache disorders leads in the extreme to one category: headache. To physicians interested in headache, this sounds as a highly theoretical option, but it is the way many general physicians and the general population classify headache disorders. If they are a little bit more sophisticated, they recognize the difference between migraine and other headaches. When professionals talk about headache disorders, lay persons often believe that it does not include migraine and it is often useful toward politicians and other decision makers to talk about 'migraine and other headaches'. For extreme splitters, it is possible to diagnose an almost endless variety of headaches. Taken to the extreme, this leads to the attitude that: 'There are no diseases only patients'. Each patient has special characteristics and therefore would merit his or her own category of subdiagnosis. The whole idea of classification is, however, to identify groups of patients, who largely have a similar symptomatology and/or etiology, thus, facilitating the study and treatment of a number of similar patients. A good disease classification represents a compromise between lumping and splitting. In deciding the number of categories and their interrelationship, it is possible to include any evidence regarding the particular disease. Even sophisticated studies of brain blood flow, biochemistry, or genetics can be taken into account when constructing the classification system. Diagnostic criteria should, on the other hand, include only parameters that are available to the physician when diagnosing patients.

It is often suggested that there should be two different classifications: One for research that can be detailed and another for clinical practice, that should be simple and very easy to apply. It is absolutely hopeless, however, to have different classifications for research and clinical practice because research results obtained with one kind of classification are not applicable to patients diagnosed according to another system. The solution to this problem is a hierarchical classification[1,2] not only where patients can be diagnosed in the same large groups but also where the diagnosis can be done in subgroups and subgroups of subgroups. With such a system, patients can be diagnosed according to the first or second digit in general practice, while special clinics and researchers may diagnose to the third or fourth digit. Ideally, a classification system should be based on etiology, but very often the etiology is not known. The classification system then has to use clinical features and the results of laboratory tests, and thus is based on phenomenology. The latter applies to the primary headaches while etiology is used to classify the secondary headaches in ICHD-2.

The history of headache classification

The first attempt at creating a headache classification was made by an ad hoc committee of the National Institute of Health in America. It published a paper entitled: 'Classification of Headache' in 1962.[3] This classification became quite widely used in North America and parts of Europe but never gained true international acceptance or broad use. It recognized only a few headache disorders and its so-called definitions of different headache disorders were wide open for individual interpretation. Migraine, for example, was defined as "recurrent attacks of headache, widely varied in intensity, frequency, and duration. The attacks are commonly unilateral in onset; are usually associated with anorexia, and sometimes with nausea and vomiting; and some are proceeded by, or associated with, conspicuous sensory, motor, and mood disturbances; and are often familial." Some attempts were made to operationalize the diagnostic criteria for migraine.[4,5] These criteria were never internationally accepted, but formed a valuable basis for the subsequent classification work. In 1985, the International Headache Society (IHS) formed a headache classification committee, which in 1988 published the First International Classification of Headache Disorders (ICHD-1).[2] It contained operational (now called explicit) diagnostic criteria for all headache disorders. The system was endorsed by all national headache societies that were members of the IHS and by the World Federation of Neurology. The classification was translated into more than 20 different languages and has been used throughout the world as the only internationally accepted headache classification system. The World Health Organization accepted the major principles of ICHD-1. After 15 years of service, the ICHD-1 has now been replaced by ICHD-2 published in January 2004 following more than 4 years of intense preparations by a new international headache classification committee. The classification is available on the IHS website.[6] A slide kit is also available for downloading. A short version of the classification has been developed and is available on the IHS website and as a printed pocket folder.[7]

ICHD-2 classification and terminology

Like its predecessor, ICHD-2 is hierarchical using up to four digits to code for all varieties of headache disorders. These are now organized in 14 major groups. Groups 1–4 cover the primary headaches (Table 2.1), groups 4–12 the secondary headaches, group 13 the cranial neuralgias, and facial pain, and group 14 other headaches, cranial neuralgias or primary facial pain (Table 2.2). New groups in ICHD-2 are group 10 Headache attributed to disorder of homeostasis and group 13 Headache attributed to psychiatric disorder. Also new is the subdivision of group 14 into headache not elsewhere classified and headache where insufficient information is available to classify. New entities have been included within most groups but particularly so in Chapter 4, which was previously called miscellaneous primary headaches and now 'other primary headaches'. Major reorganization has also taken place within the chapter on headache attributed to substance use, especially the clear recognition of medication

Table 2.1 Classification of primary headaches (first level, with selected disorders at second and third levels)

ICHD-II code	ICD-10NA code	Diagnosis
1.	**[G43]**	**Migraine**
1.1	[G43.0]	Migraine without aura
1.2	[G43.1]	Migraine with aura
1.5.1	[G43.3]	Chronic migraine
2.	**[G44.2]**	**Tension-type headache (TTH)**
2.1	[G44.2]	Infrequent episodic tension-type headache
2.2	[G44.2]	Frequent episodic tension-type headache
2.3	[G44.2]	Chronic tension-type headache
3.	**[G44.0]**	**Cluster headache and other trigeminal autonomic cephalalgias**
3.1	[G44.0]	Cluster headache
3.2	[G44.03]	Paroxysmal hemicrania
4.	**[G44.80]**	**Other primary headaches**
4.5	[G44.80]	Hypnic headache
4.6	[G44.80]	Primary thunderclap headache
4.7	[G44.80]	Hemicrania continua
4.8	[G44.2]	New daily-persistent headache (NDPH)

overuse headache. An appendix has been added, which includes research criteria for new types of headache not yet sufficiently validated.

The taxonomy of headache disorders was quite markedly changed in ICHD-1, notably by the introduction of the terms migraine with aura and migraine without aura to replace common and classical migraine as well as tension-type headache replacing tension headache or muscle contraction headache. This change of taxonomy has largely been successful. Therefore, few changes have been made to the taxonomy of ICHD-2. Previously used terms are presented whenever such terms have existed just like in ICHD-1.

ICHD-2 diagnostic criteria

The obvious difficulty in constructing diagnostic criteria for headache disorders is the lack of biochemical or other diagnostic markers. ICHD-1 criteria were therefore constructed using clinical features and easily available results of laboratory investigations. ICHD-2 has continued this tradition. The diagnostic criteria previously called operational are now called explicit diagnostic criteria. This means that terms such as sometimes, usually, often etc. are avoided and instead numerical figures are given. Sometimes criteria are monothetic, requiring the presence or absence of a single characteristic. At other times, the criteria are polythetic requiring, for example, two out of four characteristics. These kinds of criteria allow the use of characteristics that occur in, for example 50% of the patients, such as the pain criteria of migraine without aura. The basic system from DSM-4[8] used in ICHD-1 is still used in ICHD-2.

Table 2.2 Classification of secondary headaches (first level, with selected disorders at second and third levels)

ICHD-II code	ICD-10NA code	Diagnosis [and aetiological ICD-10 code]
5.	**[G44.88]**	**Headache attributed to head and/or neck trauma**
5.1	[G44.880]	Acute post-traumatic headache
5.2	[G44.3]	Chronic post-traumatic headache
5.3	[G44.841]	Acute headache attributed to whiplash injury [S13.4]
5.4	[G44.841]	Chronic headache attributed to whiplash injury [S13.4]
6.	**[G44.81]**	**Headache attributed to cranial or cervical vascular disorder**
6.2.2	[G44.810]	Headache attributed to subarachnoid haemorrhage (SAH) [I60]
6.4.1	[G44.812]	Headache attributed to giant cell arteritis (GCA) [M31.6]
7.	**[G44.82]**	**Headache attributed to non-vascular intracranial disorder**
7.1.1	[G44.820]	Headache attributed to idiopathic intracranial hypertension (IIH) [G93.2]
7.2.1	[G44.820]	Post-dural puncture headache [G97.0]
7.4	[G44.822]	Headache attributed to intracranial neoplasm [C00-D48]
7.6.2	[G44.82]	Post-seizure (post-ictal) headache [G40.x or G41.x to specify seizure type]
8.	**[G44.4 or G44.83]**	**Headache attributed to a substance or its withdrawal**
8.2	[G44.41 or G44.83]	Medication-overuse headache (MOH)
9.		**Headache attributed to infection**
9.1.1	[G44.821]	Headache attributed to bacterial meningitis [G00.9]
9.4.1	[G44.821]	Chronic post-bacterial meningitis headache [G00.9]
10.	**[G44.882]**	**Headache attributed to disorder of homoeostasis**
11.	**[G44.84]**	**Headache or facial pain attributed to disorder of cranium, neck, eyes, ears, nose, sinuses, teeth, mouth or other facial or cranial structures**
11.2.1	[G44.841]	Cervicogenic headache [M99]
12.	**[R51]**	**Headache attributed to psychiatric disorder**
12.1	[R51]	Headache attributed to somatization disorder [F45.0]
12.2	[R51]	Headache attributed to psychotic disorder [code to specify aetiology]
13.	**[G44.847, G44.848, or G44.85]**	**Cranial neuralgias and central causes of facial pain**
13.1	[G44.847]	Trigeminal neuralgia
14.	**[R51]**	**Other headache, cranial neuralgia, central or primary facial pain**
14.1	[R51]	Headache not elsewhere classified
14.2	[R51]	Headache unspecified

Thus, the criteria contain several letter headings: A, B, C and each letter heading has to be fulfilled in order to get a diagnosis.

ICHD-2 and WHO classification

The International classification of diseases, ninth edition (ICD-9) contained only a few headache entities and very important syndromes such as tension-type headache were not included under neurology. However, the much more detailed classification and the diagnostic criteria of ICHD-1 were largely accepted by the WHO and included in ICD-10.[9] This meant that all primary headache syndromes were now grouped under neurology. Unfortunately, the United States of America has not yet adopted ICD-10, which has greatly hampered a reasonable reimbursement of headache experts and therefore, also the development of services to headache patients. From ICD-10, a so-called neurological adaptation (ICD-10 NA) was developed[10] which is more detailed and includes most of the headache disorders classified in ICHD-1. A further document: *ICD-10 guide for headaches* was published to provide a crossway between ICD-10[11] NA and ICHD-1. In ICHD-2, it was decided to include both the IHS and ICD-10 NA code numbers. The latter system is less detailed. Different ICHD diagnoses may therefore often receive the same ICD-10 NA diagnosis. Table 2.1 gives ICHD-2 codes and diagnoses as well as ICD-10 NA codes.

Scientific evaluation of ICHD classifications

Classifications have to be measured against some kind of standard. For headache disorders, no gold standard exists and the scientific evaluation and improvement must be an iterative process with advances taken in many small steps. The criteria for migraine without aura of ICHD-1 and ICHD-2 have been validated by the advent of the triptans. When these drugs are given by injection, the response rate is approximately 80–90%[12,13] indicating that the criteria delineate a fairly homogenous group of patients. Unfortunately, there are no biochemical or imaging parameters that can serve as external validators for the headache classification. Likewise, the sensitivity and specificity of the diagnostic criteria of ICHD-1 could only be compared to the diagnosis of expert physicians,[14] but not to an objective external standard. Since the first edition has now been in use for more than 15 years and has worked well, ICHD-2 diagnosis can be compared to ICHD-1 diagnoses of the same patients.[15,16]

An important feature of a classification system is that it should be generalizable, i.e. applicable in diverse clinical settings ranging from general practice to highly specialized headache centers. The classification should also be exhaustive, which means that there should be a diagnosis for every patient and it should be reliable with a low interrater diagnostic variability. Several studies in the general population have shown ICHD-1 to be exhaustive[17,18] and also the reliability and validity of the ICHD-1 have been fairly good.[19–21] ICHD-2 is so young that there have still not been studies on its reliability, validity, and exhaustiveness.

Research opportunities offered by ICHD-2

Like its predecessor, ICHD-2 is eminently suitable for scientific studies. Because the diagnostic criteria are so explicit, they can be tested in a variety of clinical settings. This is a good example of low technology research, which can be done in almost any department that has a significant flow of patients. The secondary headaches are the least studied of all. It remains largely unknown how the characteristics are of the different types of secondary headache. For almost each of them, any large series with a careful prospective clinical description of the headache would be valuable. Also criterion d, which specifies that headache gets better or disappears after treatment of the cause of the headache, is virtually unstudied. Is it really true that headache caused by a meningioma disappears after successful removal of it, or do a significant number of patients continue to have the headache? In the latter case, a diagnosis of chronic post-meningeoma headache would be documented. The same question can be asked for a large number of secondary headaches. Is it true that headache can be caused by depression? Or are migraine and depression just comorbid disorders? The number of questions that can be asked is almost endless. Finally, as the genetics of migraine and other headache disorders becomes better understood and genotype–phenotype correlation studies appear, that may lead to significant changes in our concepts and to future revisions of the classification.

References

1. IHS. The International Classification of Headache Disorders: 2nd edition. *Cephalalgia* 2004; **24** (Suppl 1): 9–160.
2. IHS. Headache Classification Committee of the International Headache Society. Classification and diagnostic criteria for headache disorders, cranial neuralgias and facial pain. *Cephalalgia* 1988; **8** (7): 1–96.
3. Ad Hoc. Committee on Classification of Headache. Classification of Headache. *JAMA* 1962; **179**: 717–18.
4. Olesen J, Krabbe AA, Tfelt-Hansen P. Methodological aspects of prophylactic drug trials in migraine. *Cephalalgia* 1981; **1** (3): 127–41.
5. Tfelt-Hansen P, Olesen J. Methodological aspects of drug trials in migraine. *Neuroepidemiology* 1985; **4** (4): 204–26.
6. IHS. IHS web-site: www.i-h-s.org. In: International Headache Society.
7. IHS. ICHD-II Abbreviated Pocket version. *Cephalalgia* 2004; **24** (Suppl 1): 1–160.
8. Diagnostic and Statistical Manual of Mental Disorders (DSM) IV. Washington DC: American Psychiatric Association; 1995.
9. WHO. World Health Organization. The International Statistical Classification of Diseases and Related Health Problems. 10th rev. Geneva: World Health Organization; 1992–1994.
10. WHO. World Health Organization. Application of the International Classification of Diseases to Neurology. 2nd ed. Geneva: World Health Organization; 1997.
11. ICD-10 Guide for Headaches. International Headache Classification Committee. *Cephalalgia* 1997; **17** (Suppl 19): 1–82.
12. Cady RK, Wendt JK, Kirchner JR, *et al*. Treatment of acute migraine with subcutaneous sumatriptan. *JAMA* 1991; **265** (21): 2831–5.

13. Treatment of migraine attacks with sumatriptan. The Subcutaneous Sumatriptan International Study Group. *N Engl J Med* 1991; **325** (5): 316–21.
14. Iversen HK, Langemark M, Andersson PG, *et al*. Clinical characteristics of migraine and episodic tension-type headache in relation to old and new diagnostic criteria. *Headache* 1990; **30** (8): 514–9.
15. Eriksen M, Thomsen L, Andersen I, *et al*. Clinical characteristics of 362 patients with familial migraine with aura. *Cephalalgia* 2004; **24** (7): 564–75.
16. Eriksen MK, Thomsen LL, Russell MB. Prognosis of migraine with aura. *Cephalalgia* 2004; **24** (1): 18–22.
17. Rasmussen BK, Jensen R, Olesen J. A population-based analysis of the diagnostic criteria of the International Headache Society. *Cephalalgia* 1991; **11** (3): 129–34.
18. Russell MB, Rasmussen BK, Thorvaldsen P, *et al*. Prevalence and sex-ratio of the subtypes of migraine. *Int J Epidemiol* 1995; **24** (3): 612–8.
19. Leone M, Filippini G, D'Amico D, *et al*. Assessment of International Headache Society diagnostic criteria: a reliability study. *Cephalalgia* 1994; **14** (4): 280–4.
20. Michel P, Dartigues JF, Henry P, *et al*. Validity of the International Headache Society criteria for migraine. GRIM. Groupe de Recherche Interdisciplinaire sur la Migraine. *Neuroepidemiol* 1993; **12** (1): 51–7.
21. Merikangas KR, Whitaker AE, Angst J. Validation of diagnostic criteria for migraine in the Zurich longitudinal cohort study. *Cephalalgia* 1993; **13** (Suppl 12): 47–53.

3
Principles and tools: questionnaires, structured interviews, diaries, and calendars

R. Jensen and L. Bendtsen

Headache is mainly a subjective phenomenon and we urgently need a biological marker, both in the diagnostic process and in the long-term follow-up guiding the physicians in the treatment strategy. In headache, we have to rely on the history of the patients and on a negative workup, where other diseases are excluded. In clinical practice, the efficiency of taking the history can be greatly augmented by the use of various instruments because headache patients, like most other pain patients, tend to report the most recent and the most severe headaches. In this chapter, we aim to discuss which instruments are the best to use for the diagnosis and treatment of headache and suggest future areas for research.

Epidemiology

Questionnaires are widely used in epidemiology as screening tools because they are easy to apply to large populations at reasonably low costs. Calculations of results and statistics are also fairly easy as the standardizations of questions and modern technology can provide the results within a fairly short period of time. Before 1988, epidemiological research in headache was sparse and rather hazardous but after the introduction of the first version of IHS classification system in 1988 (ICHD-1)[1], very large epidemiological studies in headache disorders have been conducted. Most of the studies have been based on self-administered questionnaires and very useful and fairly congruent information about prevalence and socioeconomic impact have been provided.[2–4] Are the questionnaires valid and do they provide us with the correct information? What is the correct answer, what is the gold standard for the questionnaires? Usually the clinical interview is considered as the gold standard but even here there is not complete agreement between different clinicians, so the answer is not as simple as it seems.

The most simple question: 'Have you ever have had a headache?' appears to be specific but in the first epidemiological study from 1989 based on ICHD-1, the absolute agreement rate between the questionnaire and the clinical interview was 96%.[5] Four percent of the population appeared to have experienced some headaches during early life although they had reported no headache in the questionnaire, whereas none reported headache in the questionnaire and denied it at the interview.[5] With respect to more detailed information about other primary headaches, the agreement rate declines considerably especially with respect to coexisting headaches within the same subject and their frequency.[5,6]

Most large epidemiological studies have only focused on the presence or absence of headache or on the prevalence of migraine versus non-migrainous headaches.[6–10] Gervil et al. created a simple questionnaire with only four questions as they aimed to identify migraineurs from a large twin-register consisting of 5360 persons and verified the diagnosis by a structured telephone interview by a physician trained in headache.[7] With this simple questionnaire they were able to identify 91% of all migraineurs and with a combination of two of the four questions they could also identify 93% of patients with migraine with aura and 74% of those with migraine without aura.[7] Likewise two more recent studies had presented very simple self-administered screening tool for migraine, where they were able to identify more than 90% of migraineurs referred to a headache specialist.[9,10] In The Danish Epidemiological Study from 1989, the diagnosis of migraine and tension-type headache were compared between a self-administered, very detailed questionnaire and a clinical interview by a specialized neurologist.[5,11] The sensitivity was as low as 0.51 for migraine and 0.43 for episodic tension-type headache, whereas the specificity was fairly high – 0.92 and 0.96 respectively. It was concluded that the questionnaire was not satisfactory for a precise IHS-diagnosis.[5] Except for epidemiological studies of chronic daily headache,[12] which is not included in either of the ICHD classification systems,[1,13] only few studies have focused on other primary or secondary headaches, and the present instruments are only rarely designed for these purposes.

In conclusion, simple self-administered questionnaires are fairly useful for screening purposes and for identification of migraine versus non-migraine, whereas more detailed information is needed for specific IHS diagnoses or epidemiological purposes.

Structured interviews

Semistructured or structured interviews are very popular in headache research, and the quality of the obtained information is usually considered to be reliable and useful. Structured interviews by telephone can nevertheless be rather time demanding and very often lay persons are hired specifically for these purposes. However, it is necessary to be aware of the observer bias in such interviews. Thus, the diagnoses obtained by lay persons differed considerably from those obtained by specialized headache doctors in an elderly French population.[14] The prevalence of migraine was 5.5% when the lay persons had interviewed the population, whereas the prevalence increased to 11.1% after the specialists' interview.[14] The main discrepancies were caused by an underestimation of the frequency of headache and/or the accompanying symptoms by the lay persons. The sensitivity of such structured interviews are reasonably high, which means that those subjects that report headaches are true positive headache sufferers, whereas the specificity is somewhat lower in such interviews. In epidemiology and clinical research, it is always a compromise between sensitivity and specificity. Lay persons' interviews will therefore result in somewhat lower prevalence rates and a loss of some subjects with infrequent and probably also insignificant headaches, whereas those subjects with more frequent and clinically relevant headaches will be identified. It is therefore important to be absolutely aware of the principal aim of an epidemiological study and to choose a lay person interviewer if the purpose is a screening process for the clinically affected persons. Epidemiological studies, where more detailed information about all headaches including the infrequent, mild ones are required, should be performed by a specialist in headache. Such important methodological variations may to some extent explain the variations between prior epidemiological studies. To our knowledge, no comparative studies between telephone interviews and clinical interviews have been conducted.

Clinical interviews

When different epidemiological instruments are compared, a high agreement between questionnaire and clinical interview with respect to diagnosis is usually obtained, whereas the agreement with respect to frequency of headache is generally low.[15] In Swedish schoolchildren, the diagnosis of both migraine and tension-type headache was fairly congruent when a self-administered questionnaire was compared to a clinical interview, whereas the frequency of headache was greatly underestimated at the interview compared to a subsequent diary recording for at least 3 weeks.[15] Likewise, when a diagnostic diary based on the ICHD-1 criteria was introduced (Fig. 3.1), a comparative study between a clinical interview and a subsequent 4 weeks' diary was performed.[16] There was a quite good agreement in the diagnosis of migraine (82%), whereas the diary revealed a considerable underestimation (60%) of episodic tension-type headache and a significant overestimation (78%) of chronic tension-type headache at the interview.[16] The diagnostic agreement between two different observers blinded for each other's diagnoses was 100% and the diagnostic diary was introduced as a very reliable and useful instrument.

Diagnostic diaries

Where should diaries be used and where is there a need for development of new instruments? The diagnostic diary is used on a daily basis, in which detailed information of the headache is recorded every night, on a day with headache. Detailed questions about start time of the headache, any aura symptoms, quality, location and intensity of pain, aggravation of pain by physical activity and accompanying symptoms are recorded for at least 4 weeks (Fig. 3.1). Furthermore, the patients

After each question put one X in the box which is most appropriate.
Name: Birthday:

19	Date:	/	/	/	/	/	/	/
When did the headache begin?	Indicate nearest hour:							
Just before the headache began, was there any disturbance of	vision:	☐	☐	☐	☐	☐	☐	☐
	other senses:	☐	☐	☐	☐	☐	☐	☐
Was the headache	rightsided:	☐	☐	☐	☐	☐	☐	☐
	leftsided:	☐	☐	☐	☐	☐	☐	☐
	both sides:	☐	☐	☐	☐	☐	☐	☐
Was the headache	pulsating/throbbing:	☐	☐	☐	☐	☐	☐	☐
	pressing/tightening:	☐	☐	☐	☐	☐	☐	☐
Was the headache* See below	mild:	☐	☐	☐	☐	☐	☐	☐
	moderate:	☐	☐	☐	☐	☐	☐	☐
	severe:	☐	☐	☐	☐	☐	☐	☐
Did the headache change with physical activity such as walking stairs	worse:	☐	☐	☐	☐	☐	☐	☐
	unchanged:	☐	☐	☐	☐	☐	☐	☐
	better:	☐	☐	☐	☐	☐	☐	☐
Did you suffer from nausea?	no:	☐	☐	☐	☐	☐	☐	☐
	mild:	☐	☐	☐	☐	☐	☐	☐
	moderate:	☐	☐	☐	☐	☐	☐	☐
	severe:	☐	☐	☐	☐	☐	☐	☐
Were you bothered by light?	no:	☐	☐	☐	☐	☐	☐	☐
	mildly:	☐	☐	☐	☐	☐	☐	☐
	moderately:	☐	☐	☐	☐	☐	☐	☐
	severely:	☐	☐	☐	☐	☐	☐	☐
Were you bothered by sounds?	no:	☐	☐	☐	☐	☐	☐	☐
	mildly:	☐	☐	☐	☐	☐	☐	☐
	moderately:	☐	☐	☐	☐	☐	☐	☐
	severely:	☐	☐	☐	☐	☐	☐	☐
When did the headache disappear?	Indicate nearest hour:							
Did anything provoke this attack?	specify:							
Did you take any medicine? Mention each different compound, how much you took, and when you took it (nearest hour).	name:							
	how much:							
	time:							
	name:							
	how much:							
	time:							

*Mild: Does not inhibit work performance or other activities
Moderate: Inhibits, but does not prohibit work performance and other activities
Severe: Prohibits work and other activities
Copyright: Foundation for Migraine Research c/o Jes Olesen, Copenhagen, Denmark.

Fig. 3.1 Diagnostic headache diary.

are requested to record all drugs (including simple painkillers) and precise time of intake on the diary. This is a highly important information both for the doctor and for the patient as they usually are surprised over the medication intake and usually tend to underestimate this (especially of OTC drugs) during the interview. Use of the diary results in finding more episodic tension-type headaches, fewer patients have chronic headaches than by the history and several headache diagnoses within the same patient can also be identified. The diagnostic diaries may also provide very valuable information about possible trigger factors and patient compliance because the patients are kept responsible for a systematic, daily recording during at least a 4-week period and are requested to bring them to all consultations and to discuss the obtained information with their physician. In specialized headache centres, diaries are therefore very important instruments for both diagnostic and treatment purposes.

To increase the precision, we send a detailed questionnaire and a diagnostic headache diary to all patients referred to the Danish Headache Center at least 4 weeks before their very first consultation. A detailed instruction is included in a covering letter and patients are asked to complete the diary in the following period and bring the information with them at the first consultation. This strategy gives the patients time to think and obtain important information about their previous admissions, headache evolution, their former and present treatment, and most important to record their headaches and their drug intake in a prospective, daily manner. Having this information saves valuable time, improves the diagnostic process, and facilitates the treatment planning considerably. Finally, such baseline information together with the information at discharge is mandatory in the evaluation of treatment. The drawbacks are that diaries have to be kept on a daily basis, are not always simple to survey, and may be time demanding for the general practitioners and other colleagues without specific interest in headache. In specialized headache clinics, where patients usually suffer from severe and frequent headaches, diagnostic diaries have proven their value but their general acceptance is still limited.

It can be concluded that in relation to the distinction between episodic and chronic tension-type headache and especially so with the new definition of chronic migraine and medication overuse in the ICHD-2,[13] it is extremely important that diagnostic diaries are used and kept for several weeks before a precise diagnosis is applied to the patients. For implementation of ICHD-2 criteria in general practice and other medical specialities, development of more simple diagnostic instruments are warranted.

Headache calendars

Once the diagnostic diary is correctly filled in for a sufficient period of time and the first consultation is completed, it is possible to switch to the headache calendar (Fig. 3.2). Once patients have learned to distinguish between tension-type headache and migraine or other headaches, they are generally able to fill in the calendar correctly.

For your **migraine attacks** indicate the severity as:

1, mild   2, medium   3, severe

1)   A mild attack does not inhibit work or other activities.

2)   A medium attack inhibits but does not prohibit work or other activities.

3)   A severe attack prohibits work and/or other activities.

For your **tension-type headache** use one or more crosses to indicate severity as defined above:

x, mild   xx, medium   xxx, severe

For attacks of **cluster headache** use letters a, b, and c for severity as defined above

a, mild   b, medium   c, severe

HEADACHE CALENDAR
The year 20__

The headache calendar is used to record all episodes of headache during an entire year. This information will greatly assist your doctor in selecting the best treatment, and it may help yourself to identify factors in your life, which worsen or improve your headache condition.
Bring this calendar to each consultation with your doctor.

Name:

Social Security No.:

Address.

Telephone:

The owner of this card is being treated for headache/migraine by Dr.:

	Jan.	Feb.	Mar.	Apr.	May	June	July	Aug.	Sept.	Oct.	Nov.	Dec.	
1													1
2													2
3													3
4													4
5													5
6													6
7													7
8													8
9													9
10													10
11													11
12													12
13													13
14													14
15													15
16													16
17													17
18													18
19													19
20													20
21													21
22													22
23													23
24													24
25													25
26													26
27													27
28													28
29													29
30													30
31													31

Fig. 3.2 Headache calendar.

Table 3.1 Problematic areas in the registration of headache

- Several headache diagnoses within the same patient
- Secondary headaches
- Registration of medication intake
- Cluster headaches and other short-lasting attacks
- Migraine aura
- Implementation of diagnostic diaries in general practice
- Acceptance and correct use of ICHD-2 criteria

As with epilepsy and other periodic disorders, the use of such a calendar is invaluable in the long-term adjustment for the prophylactic strategy. The calendar is much easier to keep for the patient than the diary and can be carried in a notebook. It contains information from a whole year in one card and the evolution over time and the response to prophylactic treatment or cessation of daily intake of analgesics can easily be assessed. It is also a very important tool in the direct dialogue with the patients with respect to annual variations, treatment, and evolution. Many patients continue in fact with the calendar after discharge from the clinics. In the future, computerized systems will probably be the preferred tools and have already been introduced in clinical trials with great success. The online systems facilitate recording, reliability and data processing but are yet also more costly and complicated. To our knowledge, systematic comparisons between electronic and paper diaries have not yet been published. In the ICHD-2 classification system, there are problematic areas where new instruments should be developed (Table 3.1) and systematic clinical research can thus be highly encouraged.

In conclusion, headache calendars are easy to use and very useful for the long-term survey of headache evolution and treatment response.

Finally, it is important that the various instruments are used for their specific purposes, which is summarized in Table 3.2. Furthermore, it can strongly be recommended that they are validated against the gold standard in headache diagnosis, namely a clinical interview by a headache expert. Because of the unambiguous

Table 3.2 Recommendations for instruments in the diagnosis and treatment of headache

	Screening	Epidemiol	Diagnosis	Treatment	QoL
Self-admin Q	√	√			
Structured interview	√	√	√		
Diagnostic diary			√	√	
Calendar				√	
Specific Q					√

nature of the IHS-classification system and the hierarchical structure, new diaries and calendars can hopefully help us to develop simple decision trees for the classification of various headaches. Such instruments will probably also aid the implementation of the ICHD-2 classification system and increase the general knowledge of and interest in headache disorders. New diagnostic instruments must be kept simple and very clear as experiences from other medical fields clearly indicate that acceptance and diagnostic processing are closely related to simplicity.

References

1. Headache Classification Committee of the International Society. Classification and diagnostic criteria for headache disorders, cranial neuralgias and facial pain. *Cephalalgia* 1988; **8** (Suppl 7): 1–98.
2. Stewart WF, Lipton RB, Celentano DD, *et al*. Prevalence of migraine headache in the United States. Relation to age, sex, race and other sociodemographic factors. *JAMA* 1992; **267**: 64–69.
3. Goebel H, Petersen-Braun M, Soyka D. The epidemiology of headache in Germany: a nationwide survey of a representative sample on the basis of the headache classification of the International Headache Society. *Cephalalgia* 1994; **14**: 97–106.
4. Henry P, Michel P, Brochet B, *et al*. A nationwide survey of migraine in France: prevalence and clinical feures in adult. *Cephalalgia* 1992; **12**: 229–37.
5. Rasmussen BK, Jensen R, Olesen J. Questionnaire versus clinical interview in the diagnosis of headache. *Headache* 1991; **31**: 290–5.
6. Hagen K, Zwart JA, Vatten I, *et al*. Head-Hunt validity and reliability of a headache questionnaire in a large populations based study in Norway. *Cephalalgia* 2000; **20**: 244–51.
7. Gervil M, Ulrich V, Olesen J, *et al*. Screening for migraine in the general population: validation of a simple questionnaire. *Cephalalgia* 1998; **18**: 342–8.
8. Tom T, Brody M, Valabhji A, *et al*. Validation of a new instrument for determining migraine prevalence: the USCD migraine Questionnaire. *Neurology* 1994; **44**: 925–8.
9. Pryse-Philips W, Aube M, Gawel M, *et al*. A headache diagnosis project. *Headache* 2002; **42**: 728–37.
10. Lipton RB, Dodick D, Kolodner K, *et al*. Patterns of health care utilisation for migraine in England and in the United States. *Neurology* 2004; **60**: 441–8.
11. Rasmussen BK, Jensen R, Schroll M, *et al*. Epidemiology of headache in a general population – A prevalence study. *J Clin Epidemiol* 1991; **44**: 1147–57.
12. Castillio J, Murioz P, Guitera V, *et al*. Epidemiology of chronic daily headache in the general population. Headache 1999; **39**: 190–6.
13. The International Classification of headache disorders, 2nd edition. *Cephalalgia* 2004; **24** (Suppl 1): 1–160.
14. Tzouria C, Gagniere, B Amrani M El, *et al*. Lay versus expert interviewers for the diagnosis of headache in a large sample of elderly people. *J Neurol Neurosurg Psych* 2003; **74**: 238–41.
15. Laurell K, Larsson B, Eeg-Olufson O. Headache in school children: agreement between different sources of information. *Cephalalgia* 2003; **23**: 420–8.
16. Russell M, Rasmussen BK, Brennum J, *et al*. Presentation of a new instrument. The diagnostic headache diary. *Cephalalgia* 1992; **12**: 369–74.

4

Comparison of a pharmacy-based observational study with GCP-conform clinical studies with effervescent acetylsalicylic acid in migraine

M. Petersen-Braun, U. Weingärtner, U. Gessner, and H. Göbel

Introduction

Approximately half of the patients suffering from migraine headache treat themselves by using OTC drugs. Despite the common usage of acetylsalicylic acid (ASA) for self-treatment of acute migraine attacks, data about the usage, efficacy, and safety under real-life conditions in self-medication are lacking. Data about the drug use in self-medication under the terms of the patients' management in everyday life can only be derived directly from the patients. In order to specifically target patients with self-medication, a pharmacy-based observational approach has been used. In this context, the reliability and reproducibility of patient-reported data have been evaluated.

Objectives

This study aims to assess whether a pharmacy-based observational study (PHOBS) investigating the OTC usage of effervescent acetylsalicylic acid (Aspirin® Migräne) in the treatment of acute migraine attacks yields results comparable to those of three GCP-conform clinical trials with the same drug. The validity of this new tool in post-marketing drug research was also assessed.

Methods

Efficacy, safety, and tolerability of effervescent acetylsalicylic acid (Aspirin® Migräne) in self-medication and information about the drug usage and the characteristics of self-treated migraine attacks were investigated in a pharmacy-based observational study, conducted from October 2001 to October 2002 in Germany. Two hundred and ninety-six patients with migraine headache recruited in 156 pharmacies treated their acute migraine attacks with Aspirin® Migräne. Each patient had the opportunity to document up to three different migraine attacks. The questionnaire consisted of 36 questions including an anamnestic part, questions about the drug usage, efficacy, and safety. In order to investigate the patient's ability for self-diagnosis, a shortened version of the 'Kieler Headache Questionnaire'[1] was included, which is validated to differentiate between migraine and tension-type headache. The course of headache severity and migraine-associated symptoms were self-assessed by the patients over a period of 2 h after tablet intake. To assess the influence of wording in the questionnaire on the incidence of adverse events, two different methods were used: One half of the patients described adverse events by answering an open-end question. The other half recorded adverse events by means of a closed-end question in check-list type consisting of 11 known side effects of acetylsalicylic acid (e.g. nausea, stomach pain, gastro-intestinal complaints) and one item unlikely to be related to the drug (fatigue).

The results of the PHOBS about the efficacy and safety were compared to those of three randomized, double-blind, placebo-controlled multicenter studies investigating the effect of 1000 mg effervescent acetylsalicylic acid (2×500 mg; Aspirin® Migräne) on the treatment of acute migraine attacks.[2-4] The parameters for assessing the efficacy in the PHOBS were the same as in the three controlled clinical trials: reduction in severity from moderate or severe headache to mild or none 2 h after intake, pain-free at 2 h, headache recurrence at 2–24 h, remission of associated migraine symptoms at 2 h, use of escape medication, and global assessment of efficacy. Additionally, the incidence of adverse events were compared.

Results

Patients enrolled in the controlled clinical trials suffered from migraine with or without aura according to the classification of the International Headache Society (IHS). In the PHOBS, proper self-diagnosis of migraine was assessed by using the Kieler Headache Questionnaire. In 92.7% of the documented attacks, the criteria of the IHS were fulfilled demonstrating the patients' ability to self-diagnose migrainous headache correctly. Table 4.1 displays the baseline characteristics of the different study populations.

Table 4.1 Baseline characteristics

	Study I [2] (N=296)	Study II [3] (N=374)	Study III [4] (N=356)	PHOBS (N=433)
No. of documented attacks (ASA)	169	222	146	578
Severe headache at baseline (%)	58.6	45.5	69.2	66.3
Male/female (%)	16.6/83.4	17.6/82.4	11.6/88.4	24.3/75.0*
Age (years)	42.2 ± 11.7	38.3 ± 12.2	41.8 ± 11.8	41.6 ± 13.6
Height (cm)	167.2 ± 7.9	167.2 ± 7.4	167.0 ± 7.6	170.1 ± 8.7
Weight (kg)	69.4 ± 14.3	64.8 ± 12.0	68.0 ± 11.9	69.4 ± 13.3

*0.7% missing.

The number of documented attacks treated with ASA was highest in the PHOBS due to the fact that up to three attacks could be reported, whereas in the controlled clinical trials only one ASA-treated attack was included, respectively. Patients in the PHOBS tended to report more severe headache at baseline compared to the study population in the clinical trials (66.3% vs. 45.5%–69.2%). The demographic data were comparable between the different study populations.

The headache response rate 2 h post-dose (reduction from moderate or severe headache to mild or none) was 72.7% in the PHOBS compared to 49.3–55.0% in the controlled trials. Within the PHOBS, the response rate was reproducible over the three documented attacks (72.0–73.7%). Furthermore, the proportion of patients, pain free at 2 h after intake, was remarkably lower in the three controlled trials (25.3–29.0%) compared to the PHOBS (45.8%). Accordingly, the proportion of patients assessing the efficacy to be very good or good in PHOBS was higher (76.8%) compared to that of the clinical trials (32.5–45.6%). Headache recurrence 2–24 h post-dose varied between 15.4% and 33.6% in the controlled studies and was highest in the PHOBS with 45.0% while the use of escape medication was comparable in all studies (38.5–45.0%). The incidence of accompanying symptoms such as nausea, photo- and phonophobia was also evaluated at baseline and after 2 h of drug intake. The remission rates for the different associated migraine symptoms did not vary significantly within the respective study. The remission rates between the studies lay almost within the same range with exception of study I revealing slightly lower rates.

In the PHOBS, non-serious adverse events were reported in 12.6% of all 578 acute migraine attacks. Total adverse event rates in the clinical studies occurred with a similar frequency (8.3–16.2%); however, the frequency of adverse events classified by the physicians to be drug related was noticeably lower (0.6–4.7%). The incidence of adverse events in the PHOBS was markedly influenced by the method of documenting in the questionnaire. In the group recording adverse events by means of a closed-end question (302 attacks), the incidence of patient-reported adverse events was twofold higher compared to the group with the open-end

Table 4.2 Efficacy parameters and adverse events

Objective	Study I [2]	Study II [3]	Study III [4]	PHOBS
Mild/no pain at 2 h	55.0%	52.5%	49.3%	72.7%*
Pain free at 2 h	29.0%	27.1%	25.3%	45.8%*
Headache recurrence 2–24 h	15.4%	17.6%	33.6%	45.0%
Use of escape medication	38.5%	45.0%	42.5%	36.9%
remission (at 2 h) of				
◆ nausea	48.4%	63.6%	65.8%	70.8%*
◆ photophobia	49.0%	61.6%	58.9%	66.7%*
◆ phonophobia	52.2%	63.8%	63.0%	63.8%*
Global assessment	45.6%	32.5%	39.8%	76.8%
(very good/good)				
Adverse events total	8.3%	16.2%	12.9 %	12.6%
Drug-related adverse events	0.6%	4.1%	4.7%	–

*Last observation carried forward (LOCF).

question (276 attacks) (16.6% vs. 8.3%). Independent of the type of question, the most frequently reported adverse event was stomach pain (5.4% open-end question; 6.3% closed-end question), which is in accordance with the known side effects of the drug. The open-end question did not cause the documentation of events likely related to the substance (Table 4.2).

Discussion

In the PHOBS, Aspirin® Migräne was rated noticeably better in terms of response at 2 h, pain free at 2 h, and global assessment compared to the results of the controlled clinical studies. The partially better efficacy results are in accordance with meta-analyses of clinical trials showing higher efficacy rates in trials without placebo-control.[5] This effect may be triggered by the patients' and clinicians' anticipation of a possible placebo treatment, which they expect to be less powerful leading to lower responder rates compared to non-placebo-controlled trials. Furthermore, more than half of the patients in the PHOBS already used the investigated product in the past. Hence it can be assumed that new purchases were based on former positive experiences with the drug (treatment success, good tolerability). Thus a positive patient selection cannot be ruled out. Nevertheless, the PHOBS delivered reproducible efficacy data. The response rate derived from treatment of three different attacks lay in the same range demonstrating the consistency and validity of the patient-reported data.

In all studies, the incidence of total adverse events were comparable. However, in the controlled trials, the frequency of adverse events classified by the physicians to be drug related was markedly lower compared to the patient-reported events in the PHOBS in which no physicians' assessment is possible. Therefore, it can be assumed that the rate of drug-related adverse events (side effects) in the PHOBS also may be lower.

In the PHOBS, the type of question influences the incidence of patient-reported adverse events. The closed-end question in checklist form leads to higher rates of adverse events compared to the open-end questions, which is in accordance with other findings.[6] The higher incidence of adverse events in the closed-end question group may be triggered by the list of potentially occurring side effects influencing the patients' perception. This assumption is supported by the incidence of 'fatigue', an adverse event not known to be related to the drug, which ranked second in the closed-end question group (5.6%). Furthermore, patients may not always distinguish between symptoms of the disease itself and adverse events caused by the medication, which also may increase the incidence of adverse events (e.g. nausea, vomiting).

Conclusions

Results from three clinical studies with Aspirin® Migräne could be confirmed in a pharmacy-based observational study in OTC usage. In comparison to controlled clinical trials, the non-placebo-controlled approach of the PHOBS leads partially to higher efficacy rates but was consistent over three documented attacks. The incidence of patient-reported adverse events in PHOBS tends to be higher compared to the *drug-related side effect rate* evaluated by physicians in controlled clinical trials. The consistency and reproducibility of the results demonstrate that pharmacy-based observational studies deliver valid and meaningful findings about the usage, efficacy, and safety under real-life conditions, which complement the results from controlled clinical studies.

References

1. Göbel H, ed. *Schmerzmessung: Theorie, Methodik, Anwendungen bei Kopfschmerzen*. pp 285–7. Gustav Fischer Verlag, Stuttgart, Jena, New York; 1992.
2. Lange R, Schwarz JA, Hohn M. Acetylsalicylic acid effervescent 1000 mg (Aspirin®) in acute migraine attacks; a multicentre, randomized, double-blind, single-dose, placebo-controlled parallel group study. *Cephalalgia* 2000; **20**: 663–7.
3. The EMSASI Study Group. Placebo-controlled Comparison of Effervesent Acetylsalicylic Acid, Sumatriptan and Ibuprofen in the Treatment of Migraine Attacks. *Cephalalgia* (in press) 2004.
4. Diener HC, Eikermann A, Gessner U *et al*. Efficacy of 1000 mg effervescent acetylsalicylic acid and sumatriptan in treating associated migraine symptoms. *Eur Neurol* 2004; (submitted).
5. Eikermann A, Diener HC. Effect of active treatment is lower when using placebo control in clinical trials on acute therapy of migraine. *Cephalalgia* 2003; **23**: 344–7.
6. Fisher S, Bryant SG, Kent TA, *et al*. Patient drug attributions and postmarketing surveillance. *Pharmacotherapy* 1994; **14** (2): 202–9.

5 Diagnostic criteria for primary headaches of ICHD 2nd edition 2004[*]

M. Pedini, A. Alberti, G. Mazzolla, and P. Sarchielli

Introduction

The first version of the software, based on the diagnostic criteria of the IHS classification for primary headaches 1988,[1] was developed in 2000 to evaluate the applicability of the diagnostic criteria by specialized headache centers. The analysis of over 500 clinical charts from nine Italian headache centers always gave unambiguous diagnoses. But for various reasons, a concordance between the clinical diagnosis and that derived from the software was found only in 69% of the cases, in which the u error for the total number of charts analyzed did not exceed 2.2%.[2] During 2004, the software was rewritten to make it more compatible with the new diagnostic criteria of the ICHD 2nd edition 2004.[3] In the course of the first screenings of hundreds of clinical charts performed by us, a certain discrepancy was noted, as in the case of the first version, between the diagnoses elaborated by the software and those reported by the clinician (a detailed analysis of the results is in progress); moreover, with the introduction of the concept of 'probability', unlike what was found with the criteria of the first edition, it was shown that a single set of clinical data can yield multiple diagnoses.

Materials and methods

The software was developed using CA DBfast® ver. 2.0 int. for Windows® (Computer Associates International, Inc., New York), an extended version of dBase

[*]Diagnostic criteria for primary headaches of ICHD 2nd edition 2004: Electronic Clinical Sheets Ver. INT.W.2.0®

language for Windows®; the software was tested under Microsoft Windows® OS ver. 95 – XP. The use of dBASE archives (DBF) allows the direct transfer of the data to the major software (i.e. Microsoft Excel®, SPSS®) making the statistical analysis easy and versatile. The IHS Diagnostic Criteria for Primary Headaches 2.0 is available in International and Italian versions.

Minimum requirements to install and run

IBM PC or compatible, Microsoft Windows® OS ver. 95 – XP, CPU 166 MHz (INTEL Celeron® not recommended), 32–128 MB of RAM dependent on the version of the Operating System, 2 MB of free hard disk space, 256-bit colour display at 800×600 resolution, CD-ROM drive (for installation), audio support not required. The software works in a network or stand-alone environment.

Discussion

The software, in version 1.0 based on the diagnostic criteria of the IHS classification for primary headaches 1988[1] and in version 2.0 based on the criteria of the ICHD 2nd edition 2004,[3] is divided into four parts:

1. management of the patient's personal data;
2. management of the patient's clinical data (divided into two sheets: one contains the input data necessary for the clinician to obtain the diagnosis or diagnoses according to the criteria of the ICHD 2nd edition 2004,[3] and the second contains useful, but not essential data, for the diagnostic elaboration by the software);
3. analysis of the clinical data introduced (formulation of the diagnosis or diagnoses);
4. useful programs (automatic creation of research indices, creation of a backup copy of the programs and data, restoration of programs and data from a backup copy).

Part (1), relative to the patient's personal data, has remained unchanged in the two versions of the software, whereas part (2), relative to the patient's clinical data, has been appropriately modified in order to incorporate variations and introduction of data essential for a correct processing of the parameters needed for the diagnosis or diagnoses according to the criteria of the ICHD 2nd edition 2004.[3] The two sheets relative to the latest version of the software are shown in Figs. 5.1 and 5.2.

Part (3), relative to the analysis of the clinical data, has undergone a profound transformation. In version 1.0, in fact, one exited a precise route of data analysis once the correct diagnosis was found, whereas in version 2.0, because of the introduction of the qualifier 'probability' in the ICHD 2nd edition 2004,[3] it is necessary to go through the entire data analysis routine, which almost always results in multiple possible diagnoses. In Fig. 5.3, the analytical algorithms of the clinical data in versions 1.0 and 2.0 of the software are presented.

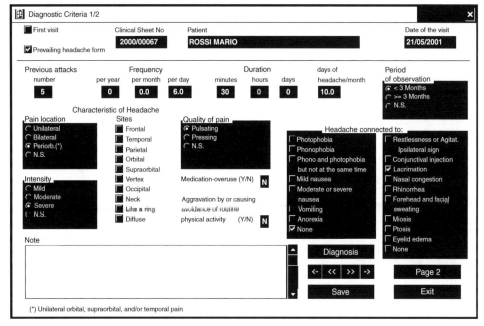

Fig. 5.1

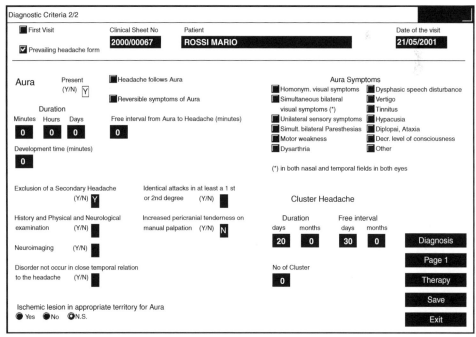

Fig. 5.2

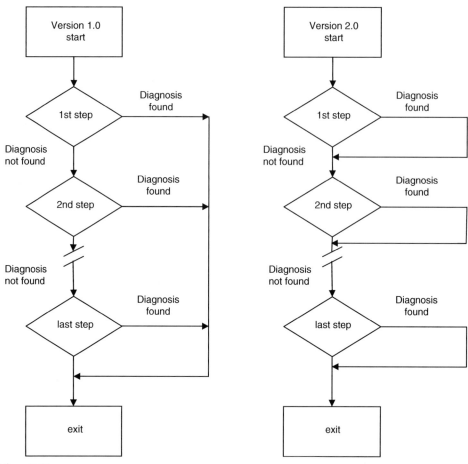

Fig. 5.3

The dramatic impact due to the variations introduced in the ICHD 2nd edition 2004[3] is evidenced in the examples provided, in which the analysis of the same set of clinical data with the software of versions 1.0 and 2.0 yields truly impressive results.

EXAMPLE 5.1

	IHS diagnostic criteria for primary headaches ver. 1.0	IHS diagnostic criteria for primary headaches ver. 2.0
No. of previous attacks	>200	>200
Frequency of attacks	30/month	30/month
Duration of attacks	1 day	1 day
Days of headache/month	30	30

Continued

EXAMPLE 5.1—Cont'd

	IHS diagnostic criteria for primary headaches ver. 1.0	IHS diagnostic criteria for primary headaaches ver. 2.0
Period of observation	≥6 months	≥3 months
Pain location	Unilateral	Unilateral
Intensity	Moderate	Moderate
Quality of pain	Pressing	Pressing
Accompanying symptoms	Nausea	Mild nausea
Associated signs	None	None
Medication overuse	Not present	No
Aggravation by or causing avoidance of routine physical activity	Yes	Yes
Aura	No	No
Exclusion of a secondary headache	Yes	Yes
Increased pericranial tenderness on manual palpation	No	No
Diagnosis	1.1.0.0 Migraine without aura	1.1.0.0 Migraine without aura 1.5.1.0 Chronic miraine 2.3.2.0 Chronic tension-type headache not associated with pericranial tenderness

EXAMPLE 5.2

	IHS diagnostic criteria for primary headaches ver. 1.0	IHS diagnostic criteria for primary headaches ver. 2.0
No. of previous attacks	>200	>200
Frequency of attacks	30/month	30/month
Duration of attacks	1 day	1 day
Days of headache/month	30	30
Period of observation	≥6 months	≥3 months
Pain location	Bilateral	Bilateral
Intensity	Severe	Severe
Quality of pain	Pulsating	Pulsating
Accompanying symptoms	None	None
Associated signs	None	None
Medication overuse	Not present	No
Aggravation by or causing avoidance of routine physical activity	No	No

Continued

EXAMPLE 5.2—Cont'd

	IHS diagnostic criteria for primary headaches ver. 1.0	IHS diagnostic criteria for primary headaches ver. 2.0
Aura	No	No
Exclusion of a secondary headache	Yes	Yes
Increased pericranial tenderness on manual palpation	No	No
Diagnosis	2.2.2.0 Chronic tension-type headache not associated with pericranial tenderness	1.6.0.1 Probable migraine without aura 2.4.1.0 Probable infrequent episodic tension-type headache 2.4.2.0 Probable frequent episodic tension-type headache 2.3.2.0 Chronic tension-type headache not associated with pericranial tenderness

Conclusions

By using the software version 1.0, it was particularly evident how one-third of the diagnoses elaborated by the program were discordant, for various reasons, with those formulated by the clinician. The use of the present version has dramatically shown how the variations in the diagnostic criteria reported in the ICHD 2nd edition 2004[3] lead to an increase of diagnoses containing 'probable forms'. To this end, our group has conducted a specific study of tension-type headache and has proposed some possible changes to the diagnostic criteria in order to limit the possibility of having more 'probable forms' in the formulation of the diagnosis concerning primary headaches.[4] The software, in the present version, allows the diagnoses of migraine with and without aura (for both young and adult patients) to the second diagnostic digit and to the third digit for chronic migraine. The diagnosis of tension-type headache and cluster headache is allowed to the third diagnostic digit. Soon, the software will be able to formulate a diagnosis for all the forms of headache with aura to the third digit and routines will then be implemented for the evaluation of all primary headaches.

References

1. Headache Classification Committee of the International Headache Society. Classification and diagnostic criteria for headache disorders, cranial neuralgias and facial pain. *Cephalalgia* 1988; **8** (Suppl 7): 1–96.
2. Gallai V, Sarchielli P, Alberti A, *et al*. Application of the 1988 International Headache Society Diagnostic Criteria in Nine Italian Headache Centers using a Computerized Structured Record. *Headache* 2002; **42**: 1016–24.
3. Headache Classification Subcommittee of the International Headache Society. The International Classification of Headache Disorders: 2nd edition. *Cephalalgia* 2004; **24** (Suppl 1): 9–160.
4. Gallai V, Sarchielli P, Alberti A, *et al*. ICHD 2nd Edition: Some considerations on the application of criteria for primary headaches. (In press in *Cephalalgia*) 2004.

6
Prevalence of migraine in the primary care setting

J. Couch and J. Hettiarachchi

Introduction

According to general population surveys, migraine is a prevalent and debilitating disorder, affecting 13% of the adult population (18% of women and 7% of men), in the United States.[1] Patients with migraine utilize healthcare resources to a greater extent,[1,2] although migraine may not be the primary reason for the visit to the healthcare provider.[2] The prevalence of migraine in patients seeking medical care is unknown, but may be higher than that in the general population. This study has been performed to determine the prevalence of migraine in an unrestricted population of patients visiting a primary care office for any reason.

Methods

The study was conducted at 28 primary care provider (PCP) sites in 13 states. Each PCP site was linked geographically to one of the 13 headache expert sites (neurologist or internist specializing in headache). Men and women, aged ≥18 years, who visited the office of a PCP for any reason were asked by the office staff whether they had experienced a headache during the past 3 months. Patients reporting at least one headache during the past 3 months were asked to complete two written questionnaires, which were labeled with preprinted patient identification numbers: the Migraine Assessment in Primary Care (MAP) and the Pfizer Migraine Survey (PMS). The MAP included two questions based on International Headache Society (IHS) diagnostic criteria for migraine[3] to screen patients for migraine (Table 6.1). Patients were designated MAP-positive (MAP-P) if they had any two pain characteristics plus one associated symptom on the questionnaire (Table 6.1). Patients not meeting this criterion were designated MAP-negative (MAP-N), and those whose questionnaires did not contain enough information to classify the patients as positive or negative were termed MAP-inconclusive (MAP-I). All patients who were

Table 6.1   Questions based on IHS criteria utilized for the MAP screener

	Never	Rarely	Less than half the time	Half the time or more
6. During the *last 3 months*, how often did you have the following with your headaches?				
a. The pain was worse on just one side				
b. The pain was pounding, pulsing, or throbbing				
c. The pain was moderate or severe				
d. The pain was made worse by activities such as walking or climbing stairs				
7. During the *last 3 months*, how often did you have the following with your headaches?				
a. You felt nauseated or sick to your stomach				
b. You saw spots, stars, zigzags, lines or gray areas continuously for several minutes or more before or during your headaches				
c. Light bothered you (a lot more than when you didn't have headaches)				
d. Sound bothered you (a lot more than when you didn't have headaches)				

A MAP-P screen for migraine is defined as an answer of 'less than half the time' or 'half the time or more' on two or more of question 6, and one or more of question 7.

MAP-P, as well as a sampling of MAP-N and MAP-I patients (the next consecutive MAP-N or MAP-I patient after a MAP-P patient was identified) were given the opportunity to visit a headache expert for a diagnostic evaluation, including a structured diagnostic interview and clinical examination. It was assumed that fewer patients scoring negative or inconclusive would choose to visit the expert, compared with those scoring positive.

During the headache expert visit, patients were given a structured diagnostic interview for migraine and physical and neurological examinations, completed additional questionnaires and were assigned one of five diagnoses: (1) migraine without aura; (2) migraine with aura; (3) other migraine; (4) any combination of the above; or (5) no migraine. The population prevalence was calculated based on the proportion of patients in the initial population with and without headaches, and on the proportion of patients with headache who had migraines, adjusted for the positive

Table 6.2 Calculation of estimated 3-month prevalence of migraine

Prevalence calculation	All patients	Men	Women
Crude prevalence of migraine:	43%	34%	47%
$$\dfrac{\text{Patients positive on migraine screener (2594)}}{\text{Patients with headaches in last 3 months (6013)}}$$			
Adjusted prevalence, based on PPV and NPV on the MAP screener:	61%	49%	68%
$0.43 + [(1 - 0.43)(1 - NPV) - 0.43\,(1 - PPV)]$			
Primary care population prevalence:	29%	17%	37%
$0.61 \times \dfrac{\text{Patients with headaches in last 3 months (6013)}}{\text{Patients in primary care population (12,714)}} \times 100$			

predictive value (PPV) and negative predictive value (NPV) of the MAP compared with the diagnosis by the headache expert.

The PMS questionnaire covered migraine headache experience, associated symptoms, disability and treatments; it was not used to calculate prevalence.

Results

Of 12,714 patients screened, 6013 (47%) had at least one headache in the past 3 months. A total of 4700 patients filled out the MAP; only 10% of patients (432/4123)

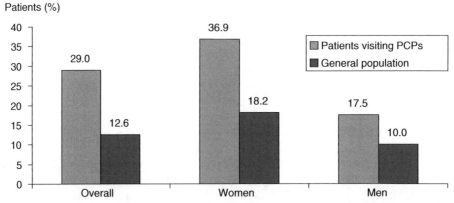

Fig. 6.1 Prevalence of migraine in this study for patients visiting PCPs compared with a large general population survey.[1]

identified headache as the reason for the medical visit. Of the 4700 patients completing the MAP, 2594 (55%) were MAP-P, 1703 (36%) were MAP-N and 403 (9%) were MAP-I. A total of 1464 patients accepted referrals to the headache experts, and 773 (53%) visited the expert. Of those who visited the expert and received a diagnosis, 481/588 MAP-P patients were diagnosed with migraine (yielding a PPV of 0.82) while 84/155 MAP-N patients received a nonmigraine diagnosis (yielding an NPV of 0.54). The overall prevalence of migraine during the 3 months prior to the study in this unselected population of patients visiting a PCP was estimated to be 29% (37% in women and 17% in men) (Table 6.2), higher than that in the general population[1] (Fig. 6.1). Based on the PMS questionnaire, 197 (36%) of the 552 patients diagnosed with migraine were previously unaware that they had migraine.

Conclusions

The 3-month prevalence of migraine in patients presenting for primary care in this study (29%) was higher than the 1-year prevalence reported in the general population (13%).[1] Of the migraineurs diagnosed by the experts, 36% were unaware that they had migraine. Only 10% of those diagnosed with migraine by the expert were seeing their PCP for headache. Migraine appears to be much more common than has been recognized previously among patients who seek medical care from primary care offices.

References

1. Lipton RB, Stewart WF, Diamond S, *et al.* Prevalence and burden of migraine in the United States: data from the American Migraine Study II. *Headache* 2001; **41**: 646–57.
2. Clouse JC, Osterhaus JT. Healthcare resource use and costs associated with migraine in a managed healthcare setting. *Ann Pharmacother* 1994; **28**: 659–64.
3. Headache Classification Committee of the International Headache Society. Classification and diagnostic criteria for headache disorders, cranial neuralgias and facial pain. *Cephalalgia* 1988; **8** (Suppl 7): 1–96.

7
Prevalence, clinical characteristics, and medication of migraine in Latin America: a population-based survey

L. E. Morillo, L. C. Sanin, F. Alarcón, N. Aranaga,
S. Aulet, E. Chapman, L. Conterno, E. Estévez,
F. Garcia-Pedroza, J. Garrido, J. Leston,
M. Macias-Islas, P. Monzillo, L. Núñez, A. Perez,
N. Plascencia, C. Rodríguez, F. Silva,
N. Simonovis, Y. Takeuchi, and J. Hettiarachchi

Migraine is a common disease worldwide, ranked among the 20 leading causes of disability by the World Health Organization.[1] Although the prevalence of migraine varies among surveyed populations,[2] the prevalence in Latin America has not been established by large-scale population studies. Also, the symptoms and disability associated with migraine, as well as the pattern of medication use by migraineurs, have not been well-documented in Latin American regions.[3–6] The objectives of this study were to determine the 1-year point prevalence and clinical characteristics of migraine among residents aged ≥15 years in Latin American urban communities and to document their medical consultation preferences and patterns of medication use.

Methods

This was a cross-sectional study of two urban communities from each of the six participating countries (Argentina, Brazil, Colombia, Ecuador, Mexico, and Venezuela).

Random households were selected by identifying sampling units, and male and female residents aged ≥15 years were invited to participate. Subjects were screened for past headaches that were unrelated to head trauma, systemic disease, or alcohol use; those with any mental or neurological disorder likely to invalidate their ability to comply with interview requirements were excluded from the study. In each country, research teams consisted of an experienced clinical neurologist, an epidemiologist, and statisticians. A previously validated, face-to-face interview questionnaire, based on International Headache Society (IHS) criteria[7] for migraine with or without aura and tension-type headache, was completed for all headache sufferers. The questionnaire included 49 questions about symptoms and migraine-related disability,[8] the use of health resources, and the frequency of use and choice of medications in the acute treatment of migraine. With the exception of local language differences, the questionnaire was identical in each of the six participating countries. Interviewed subjects were asked explicitly about headache of most concern. The time frame of the questions regarding headache was limited to a one-year period prior to the day of the interview.

Results

Survey results reported are only for migraine with and without aura; results exclude tension-type headaches. Of 8618 people available for screening, 3575 were screen-positive for headaches. Of these eligible subjects, 2637 (73.8%) agreed to participate and completed interview questionnaires. Of the respondents, 1916 (73%) were women and 721 (27%) were men. The most predominant age group was 20–29 years (23%). A total of 798 subjects (647 women, 151 men) met the strict IHS criteria for migraine with and without aura. Using borderline migraine criteria, an additional 314 cases of migraine were identified (233 women, 81 men).

Age-adjusted one-year point prevalence of migraine with or without aura for each country was as follows (women/men): Argentina, 6.1%/3.8%; Brazil,17.4%/7.8%; Colombia, 13.8%/4.8%; Ecuador, 13.5%/2.9%; Mexico, 12.1%/3.9%; and Venezuela, 12.2%/4.7% (Table 7.1). In all countries except Argentina, a distinct peak prevalence for migraine was observed in women between the ages of 30 and 50 years. No distinct age-specific peak was observed in men with migraine. No previous diagnosis of migraine was reported by 65% of headache sufferers.

Only 18% of subjects reported migraine frequency of >1 per month; 15% reported having >15 migraine headaches per month; and 59% of subjects reported experiencing 1–8 headaches per month. Moderate to severe pain was reported by 94.2% of the migraineurs. Associated symptoms of nausea or vomiting, photophobia, phonophobia, and osmophobia were 'almost always' present during migraine attacks for 30.3%, 76.4%, 85.1%, and 47.7% of subjects, respectively.

Overall, 59% of migraineurs reported that they had not consulted any medical professional for their headache in the year prior to the interview. The percentages varied among participating countries, ranging from a high of 72% in Brazil to a low of 48% in Mexico (Table 7.2). Overall, 14% of migraineurs had visited a general

Table 7.1 Crude and age-adjusted one-year point prevalence of migraine with or without aura

Migraine* (%)	Argentina	Brazil	Colombia	Ecuador	Mexico	Venezuela
Females	5.6 (4.1–7.1)†	16.7 (14.2–19.1)	14.2 (11.9–16.5)	13.8 (11.1–16.4)	12.4 (10.1–14.6)	12.2 (10.1–14.2)
Female cases/n	51/907	149/890	129/905	92/667	102/821	124/1015
Males	3.5 (2.1–4.9)	7.3 (5.0–9.6)	5.0 (3.4–6.6)	2.9 (1.5–4.3)	3.6 (2.1–5.1)	4.8 (2.9–6.7)
Male cases/n	22/633	36/496	34/686	16/558	20/559	23/481
Age adjusted‡						
Females	6.1 (5.4–6.7)	17.4 (13.4–18.4)	13.8 (12.9–14.8)	13.5 (12.6–14.4)	12.1 (11.2–12.9)	12.2 (11.3–13.1)
Males	3.8 (3.2–4.5)	7.8 (6.9–8.7)	4.8 (4.1–5.5)	2.9 (2–3.5)	3.9 (3.3–4.6)	4.7 (3.9–5.4)

*Strict IHS criteria codes 1.1, 1.2.
†95% confidence interval.
‡Age-adjusted estimates—direct method.

Table 7.2 Medical professional consultation by migraineurs in Latin America in the previous year

Consultations (%)	Argentina	Brazil	Colombia	Ecuador	Mexico	Venezuela
General practitioner	8.2	8.7	25.8	15.7	17.2	6.1
Neurologist	8.2	4.3	4.9	5.6	8.2	2.0
Other specialist	15.1	5.9	4.3	10.2	4.9	13.6
Alternative practitioner	4.1	1.1	3.7	4.6	13.9	1.4
Emergency department	10.9	7.6	10.4	0	8.2	19.7
Did not consult	53.4	72.4	50.9	63.9	47.5	57.1
n =	73	185	163	108	122	14/

practitioner; this percentage ranged from 26% in Colombia to 6% in Venezuela. Overall, 5% of migraineurs reported consulting a neurologist, and 8% reported visiting other specialists. The percentage of migraineurs using the emergency department ranged from nearly 20% in Venezuela to 0% in Ecuador. Of all subjects with migraine surveyed, 3% needed hospital admission for fewer than 3 days.

The use of headache medications at some time in the previous year was reported by 88% of migraineurs; 62% said that they had used headache medication 'more than half of the time' or 'almost always' when they had a migraine, 29% reported 'never' or 'almost never' using medication, 19% took medication once a week, 17% took medication 2–3 times per week, 6% used medication 4–6 times a week, and 7% took medication every day.

Paracetamol and salicylates were the most widely used agents. In all countries except Brazil (1.1%) and Argentina (0%), 16–26% of migraineurs used paracetamol. Salicylates were used by 15–38% of subjects in all countries except Venezuela (2.7%). Use of nonsteroidal anti-inflammatory drugs was reported by 30% of migraineurs in Colombia and 20% in Venezuela. Dypirone (metamizol), a nonnarcotic analgesic, was used by 51% of migraineurs in Brazil and by 23% in Venezuela. Ergot derivatives were used by 26% and 31% of subjects in Argentina and Ecuador, respectively. Use of triptans, which require a prescription, and therefore would be unavailable to those who did not consult a medical practitioner, was very limited— even among subjects diagnosed with migraine. No migraineurs in Brazil, Colombia, and Venezuela used triptans.

Conclusions

Migraine is a common disorder in Latin American urban communities, affecting approximately 6–17% of women and 3–8% of men. Migraine predominantly affects women aged 30–50 years, most of whom experience moderate to severe pain. The low use of migraine-specific triptans and the common use of nonprescription medications by Latin American migraineurs are notable.

References

1. World Health Organization. *The World Health Report 2001. Mental Health: New Understanding, New Hope.* Available at: www.who.int/whr2001. Accessed March 25, 2004.
2. Stewart WF, Simon D, Shechter A, *et al.* Population variation in migraine prevalence: a meta-analysis. *J Clin Epidemiol* 1995; **48**: 269–80.
3. Sachs H, Sevilla F, Barberis P, *et al.* Headache in the rural village of Quiroga, Ecuador. *Headache* 1985; **25**: 190–3.
4. Garcia-Pedroza F, Chandra V, Ziegler DK, *et al.* Prevalence survey of headache in a rural Mexican village. *Neuroepidemiology* 1991; **10**: 86–92.
5. Lavados PM, Tenhamm E. Epidemiology of migraine headache in Santiago, Chile: a prevalence study. *Cephalalgia* 1997; **17**: 770–7.
6. Lavados PM, Tenhamm E. Consulting behaviour in migraine and tension-type headache sufferers: a population survey in Santiago, Chile. *Cephalalgia* 2001; **21**: 733–7.
7. Headache Classification Committee of the International Headache Society. Classification and diagnostic criteria for headache disorders, cranial neuralgias and facial pain. *Cephalalgia* 1988; **8** (Suppl 7): 1–96.
8. Stewart WF, Lipton RB, Kolodner K, *et al.* Reliability of the migraine disability assessment score in a population-based sample of headache sufferers. *Cephalalgia* 1999; **19**: 107–14.

8
Discussion summary, allodynia: principles and tools

B. Richard and M. D. Lipton

The discussion began with a focus on allodynia. Prof. Lars Stovner asked if the superior treatment response to triptans prior to the development of allodynia could be an artifact of attack selection; he suggested that attacks treated prior to the development of allodynia may be unusually mild or easy to treat. Dr Burstein replied that the presence or absence of allodynia, not the intensity of pain at the time of treatment, predicts treatment response; patients with severe pain and no allodynia respond well to triptans while patients with mild pain and allodynia do not. This suggests that the treatment benefits of treating prior to allodynia are not a consequence of attack selection.

Prof. Stovner was also concerned that early treatment might lead to more days of treatment and an increased risk of medication-overuse headache. Dr Burstein pointed out that early triptan treatment was needed for patients who develop allodynia but treatment was effective at any point for those who do not develop allodynia. Early treatment reduces headache recurrence and re-treatment, decreasing the average number of treatments per attack. Prof. Olesen recommended firm dose limits to minimize the risk of medication-overuse headache. Dr Limroth suggested that diaries should be used to monitor treatment pattern and identify individuals at risk for dose escalation and overuse headache.

Dr Burstein's proposal to include allodynia in the next version of the ICHD was controversial. He argued that allodynia should be included in the classification of migraine as it is an important part of the biology, predicts treatment response, and may predict the development of headache escalation. Several counter arguments were raised. First, Prof. Goadsby pointed out that allodynia is not specific to migraine; it occurs in other headaches including the trigeminal autonomic cephalgias. Prof. Jensen noted that allodynia is also prominent in trigeminal neuralgia. Dr Burstein argued that allodynia in migraine and allodynia in cluster headache or trigeminal neuralgia may have different mechanisms. Prof. Silberstein noted that specificity is not a requirement for every feature used in classification. For example, nausea occurs both in migraine, cluster, and secondary headaches yet remains useful as a defining feature of migraine.

Prof. James Lance suggested that allodynia should not be part of the classification because allodynia does not occur consistently within a patient from attack-to-attack. Dr Burstein disagreed. In his research, if attacks go untreated for 4 h, allodynia consistently develops or fails to develop as a stable within-person characteristic. The exception is the occasional patient who did not have allodynia develops it during long-term follow-up. Prof. Lipton noted that in migraine, nausea, aura, photophobia, and phonophobia are variably present within a person from attack to attack.

Finally, if allodynia is to be used in classification, there must be simple, reliable, and valid ways of defining it in clinical practice. Dr Burstein's research methods require hours of work examining patients during attacks using specialized equipment and are therefore unsuitable for application in clinical practice. One simple approach for identifying allodynia at the bedside is the use of a questionnaire. Dr Burstein has developed and is validating such a questionnaire. An alternative approach is to look for mechanical (or brush) allodynia at the bedside. During the poster session, Ashkenazi *et al.* reported on bedside testing for mechanical allodynia by applying a gauze pad over the skin of the forehead. They found brush allodynia in 60% of episodic migraine sufferers tested during attacks and in 9% tested interictally. Prof. Silberstein indicated that these methods are specific but not sensitive. Dr Burstein concurred and suggested that this method may miss the migraine sufferers who have heat or cold but not mechanical allodynia.

There was some discussion on diaries and other diagnostic tools. Prof. Jensen was asked about the interpretation of diagnostic diaries when patients treat early. She indicated that diaries are the optimal method for capturing symptoms of a particular attack; if treatment attenuates the symptoms, the diary may be difficult to interpret. Prof. Olesen suggested that in a migraine sufferer treated with a triptan, triptan response might be useful to define aborted migraine.

Dr Limroth was asked about the effect of medication overuse on the effects of prophylactic medication. He indicated that there is a strong clinical impression, but sparse systematic data, that preventive medications do not work in the setting of medication overuse. He speculated that overuse and withdrawal may be very robust migraine triggers.

Session

11

The primary headaches:
Part I – the migraines

9 The classification of migraine

R. B. Lipton and M. E. Bigal

Migraine is a chronic neurological disorder characterized by episodic attacks of headache and associated symptoms. It is characterized by recurrent attacks of pain and associated symptoms, typically lasting from 4 to 72 h. The disability of migraine can be severe and imposes a considerable burden on the sufferer and the society.

Before 1988, the headache classification systems that were available did not have clear operational rules, and nomenclature varied widely. In 1988, the International Headache Society (IHS) instituted a classification system that has become the standard for headache diagnosis, particularly for clinical research, the International Classification for Headache Disorders-I (ICHD-I).[6] The second edition of the revision of this system was released in 2004 (ICHD-II). Herein, we review the migraine classification under ICHD-II.

The classification of migraine

Migraine is classified into five major categories, the two most important of which are *Migraine without aura* (1.1) and *Migraine with aura* (1.2) (Table 9.1). This is unchanged from 1988 but, in comparison with the ICHD-I, there is a restructuring of the criteria for migraine with aura. *Chronic migraine* (1.5.1) has been added. Ophthalmoplegic 'migraine', now considered a cranial neuralgia, has been moved to item 13 (*Cranial neuralgias, and central causes of facial pain*). When a patient fulfills criteria for more than one type of migraine, each type should be diagnosed and coded. Since chronic migraine usually develops from episodic migraine, a patient coded 1.5.1 will usually have an additional code for the antecedent disorder (usually 1.1).

In the following sections, we detail the classification of the migraine subtypes.

Migraine without aura (Table 9.3)

Migraine without aura is a clinical syndrome characterized by headache features and associated symptoms (Table 9.2). According to the ICHD-II, if a patient fulfills criteria for more than one type of migraine, each type should be diagnosed. Criteria for migraine without aura can be met by various combinations of features.

Table 9.1 The ICHD-II classification of migraine

1.1 Migraine without aura
1.2 Migraine with aura
    1.2.1 Typical aura with migraine headache
    1.2.2 Typical aura with non-migraine headache
    1.2.3 Typical aura without headache
    1.2.4 Familial hemiplegic migraine (FHM)
    1.2.5 Sporadic hemiplegic migraine
    1.2.6 Basilar-type migraine
1.3 Childhood periodic syndromes that are commonly precursors of migraine
    1.3.1 Cyclical vomiting
    1.3.2 Abdominal migraine
    1.3.3 Benign paroxysmal vertigo of childhood
1.4 Retinal migraine
1.5 Complications of migraine
    1.5.1 Chronic migraine
    1.5.2 Status migrainosus
    1.5.3 Persistent aura without infarction
    1.5.4 Migrainous infarction
    1.5.5 Migraine-triggered seizures
1.6 Probable migraine
    1.6.1 Probable migraine without aura
    1.6.2 Probable migraine with aura

No single feature is required. Since two of the four pain features are required, a patient with unilateral, throbbing pain may meet the criteria but so does a patient with bilateral, pressure pain, if the pain is moderate, and aggravated by physical activity. Similarly, only one of the two possible associated symptom combinations is required. Patients with nausea but not photophobia or phonophobia fill the

Table 9.2 ICHD-II diagnostic criteria for 1.1 *Migraine without aura*

A. At least five attacks fulfilling criteria B–D
B. Headache attacks lasting 4–72 h (untreated or unsuccessfully treated)
C. Headache has at least two of the following characteristics:
    1. unilateral location
    2. pulsating quality
    3. moderate or severe pain intensity
    4. aggravation by or causing avoidance of routine physical activity (e.g. walking or climbing stairs)
D. During headache at least one of the following:
    1. nausea and/or vomiting
    2. photophobia and phonophobia
E. Not attributed to another disorder

Table 9.3 ICHD-II diagnostic criteria for 1.2.1 *Typical aura with migraine headache*

A. At least two attacks fulfilling criteria B–D
B. Aura consisting of at least one of the following, but no
    motor weakness:
    1. fully reversible visual symptoms including positive features
        (e.g. flickering lights, spots, or lines) and/or negative features
        (i.e. loss of vision)
    2. fully reversible sensory symptoms including positive features
        (i.e. pins and needles) and/or negative features (i.e. numbness)
    3. fully reversible dysphasic speech disturbance
C. At least two of the following:
    1. homonymous visual symptoms and/or unilateral sensory
        symptoms
    2. at least one aura symptom develops gradually over ≥5 min
        and/or different aura symptoms occur in succession over ≥5 min
    3. each symptom lasts ≥5 and ≤60 min
D. Headache fulfilling criteria B–D for 1.1 *Migraine without aura* begins
    during the aura or follows aura within 60 min
E. Not attributed to another disorder

requirements as do patients without nausea or vomit, but with photophobia and phonophobia.

For migraine without aura, the ICHD-II requires at least five lifetime attacks, which last from 4 to 72 h. If the patient falls asleep during migraine and wakes up without it, duration of the attack is until time of awakening. In children, attacks may last 1–72 h and in young children, photophobia and phonophobia may be inferred from behavior. If attack frequency ≥15 days/month, the IHS establishes coding 1.5.1 chronic migraine.

Migraine with aura and its subtypes

The aura of migraine is characterized by focal neurological phenomena that usually proceed, but may accompany or occur in the absence of headache. Table 9.3 presents the features of typical aura according to the IHS. Most aura symptoms develop over 5–20 min, last 20 min on average, but rarely more than 60 min. Visual aura is the most common form. The aura often has a hemianoptic distribution in the shape of a crescent with a bright, ragged edge, which scintillates. Scotoma, photopsia, or phosphenes, fortification spectra and other visual manifestations may occur. Visual distortions, such as metamorphopsia, micropsia, or macropsia are more common in children.

Sensory symptoms are the second most common aura and occur in about one-third of the migraine with aura patients. They usually consist of numbness (negative symptom) and tingling or paresthesia (positive symptoms). The distribution is often cheiro-oral (face and hand) but can be hemisensory. Hemimotor weakness, dysphasia, and incoordination with other signs of brain stem dysfunctions can occur, being by far less common. Rarely, changes in level of consciousness are present.

Migraine with typical aura is the most common form of migraine with aura. The aura's duration is no less than 4 min but no longer than 60 min (and usually around 20 min).[9] If more than one aura symptom is present (e.g. visual and sensory symptoms), the accepted duration is proportionally increased (Table 9.3).

A number of nonmigrainous headaches, including cluster headache, chronic paroxysmal hemicrania, and hemicrania continua have been described to be unusually associated with aura.[18–20] The 2003 criteria classify such headaches under the code *Typical aura with nonmigraine headache* (1.2.2). In those cases, the aura occurs in close association with a headache that does not meet the criteria for migraine without aura (1.1).

Some subjects present otherwise typical aura not associated with headache. The IHS codes this phenomenon as *Typical aura without headache* (1.2.3), a disorder which often occurs in middle-aged men.[24] Within the same patient, some auras may occur without headache and others with headache. The distinction between this entity and transient ischemic attacks may require investigation, especially if aura begins after age 40, if negative features are predominant (i.e. hemianopia), or if the aura is prolonged or very short, other causes should be ruled out.[25]

A rare form of migraine with aura, *Familial hemiplegic migraine* (1.2.4), is an autosomal dominant disorder. This is the first migraine syndrome to be linked to a specific genetic set of polymorphisms. The ICHD-II criteria for FHM include the following: 1 – The presentation fulfills criteria for migraine with aura; 2 – The aura includes some degree of hemiparesis and may be prolonged; 3 – At least one first-degree relative has identical attacks. Cerebellar ataxia may occur in 20% of the FHM sufferers.

A new subtype of migraine with aura is presented in the 2003 classification, *Sporadic hemiplegic migraine* (1.2.5). These patients have migraine with aura including motor weakness but do not have an affected first or second degree relative.

Basilar-type migraine (1.2.6) is mostly seen in young adults. Patients with familial hemiplegic migraine have basilar-type symptoms in 60% of cases. Therefore, basilar-type migraine should only be diagnosed when no motor weakness is present. A distinguishing feature of basilar-type migraine is a symptom profile, which suggests posterior fossa involvement. Symptoms are often bilateral. To be classified as basilar according to the IHS, two or more fully reversible aura symptoms of the following types must be documented: dysarthria, vertigo, tinnitus, decreased hearing, double vision, ataxia, decreased level of consciousness, simultaneous bilateral visual symptoms in both the temporal and nasal field of both eyes, simultaneous bilateral paresthesias. The headache meets criteria for migraine without aura.

Childhood periodic syndromes that are commonly precursors of migraine

Childhood periodic syndromes that are commonly precursors of migraine (1.3) include the cyclic vomiting syndrome (1.3.1), abdominal migraine (1.3.2), and benign paroxysmal vertigo (1.3.3).

Cyclic vomiting syndrome (1.3.1) was reported to affect 2–2.5% of schoolchildren in some studies. It is characterized by recurrent episodes of unexplained nausea and vomiting. The attacks usually last few hours and are characterized by episodic attacks of vomiting and intense nausea, stereotypical in the individual patient, in a child who is symptom-free between attacks. Vomiting occurs at least 4 times/h for at least 1 h and no signs of gastrointestinal disease can be found.

Abdominal migraine (1.3.2) is a common disorder that may affect 8%–12% of all schoolchildren, characterized by recurrent attacks of abdominal pain associated with anorexia, nausea, and sometimes vomiting. The abdominal pain has all of the following characteristics: a. Midline location, periumbilical or poorly localized; b. Dull or 'just sore' quality; c. Moderate or severe pain intensity. During abdominal pain, there are at least two of the following: a. Anorexia; b. Nausea; c. Vomiting; d. Pallor. No abnormalities can be elicited on physical or subsidiary examination.

About 20% of schoolchildren between 5 and 15 years of age reported suffering from episodes of vertigo over a year. The most important cause of this presentation is *Benign Paroxysmal Vertigo* (1.3.3), a disorder characterized by transient episodes of vertigo. Children with this disorder develop full-blown migraine later in life. Criteria required for diagnoses are: A. At least five attacks and duration from minutes to hours; B. Unilateral throbbing headache may be associated with some attacks; C. Multiple episodes of severe vertigo, and often nystagmus or vomiting without warning, resolving spontaneously; D. Normal neurological examination; audiometric and vestibular functions normal between attacks; E. Normal electroencephalogram.

Retinal migraine (1.4)

Retinal migraine is characterized by repeated attacks of monocular scotoma or blindness lasting less than 1 h. Episodes of transient monocular visual loss may not be temporally related to the patient's headache. Patients are usually less than 44 years old and often have a history of other manifestations of migraine. Retinal TIA must be ruled out by appropriate investigation, as the most likely differential diagnosis. The IHS diagnostic criteria require at least two attacks of: 1 – Fully reversible monocular positive visual phenomena, scotomata, or blindness confirmed by examination during attack or (after proper instruction) by patient's drawing of monocular field defect during an attack; 2 – Headache that meets criteria for migraine without aura (1.1), begins during or following the visual symptoms within 60 min; 3 – Normal ophthalmological examination outside of attack. Appropriate investigations exclude other causes of transient monocular blindness. A recent review suggests that many patients with monocular 'aura' experience retinal infarction of migrainous origin. These patients should be classified as migrainous infarction (1.5.4).

Complications of migraine (1.5)

Chronic migraine (1.5.1), according to the IHS, occurs in those subjects with migraine headaches ≥15 days per month for ≥3 months and **no drug overuse**. Most cases of chronic migraine start as episodic migraine without aura. Therefore, chronicity is regarded as a complication of episodic migraine. If medication overuse is present (acute migraine drugs and/or analgesics >10 days/month), the headaches might represent medication-overuse headache (8.2), a diagnosis which can be assigned with confidence if headaches improve after medication overuse ceases. Otherwise, a diagnosis of *probable chronic migraine with probable medication overuse* should be assigned.

Status migrainosus (1.5.2) refers to an attack of migraine with headache phase lasting more than 72 h despite treatment. Initially the attack resembles an unremarkable attack of migraine. Almost all attacks are accompanied by nausea and vomiting to the point of dehydration. Patient often seeks care in the emergency department. The attack is debilitating. Nondebilitating attacks lasting >72 h are coded 1.6, probable migraine without aura.

Persistent aura without infarction (1.5.3) occurs when aura symptoms persist for more than 2 weeks without radiographic evidence of infarction. It is an unusual form of migraine that is being first included in the IHS classification.

Migrainous infarction (1.5.4) is characterized by one or more migrainous aura symptom not fully reversible within 7 days and/or associated with neuroimaging confirmation of ischemic infarction. A few clues help to distinguish this part of the clinical spectrum of migraine from other causes of stroke: 1 – The neurologic deficit must exactly mimic the migrainous aura of previous attack; 2 – Stroke must occur during the course of a typical migraine attack; 3 – Other cases of stroke must be excluded.

Migraine and seizures are comorbid disorders. Headaches are common in the postictal period, but epilepsy can occur triggered by a migraine (migralepsy). The criteria for *migraine-triggered seizures* (1.5.5) require a seizure fulfilling diagnostic criteria for one type of epileptic attack that occurs during or within 1 h after a migraine aura.

Probable migraine (1.6)

When the International Headache Society (IHS) criteria is applied to patients with migrainous features, between 10% and 45% of them fail to meet the criteria for migraine).[55] If just one migraine criterion is missing, these patients receive the diagnosis of probable migraine (1.6, formerly migrainous headache). A recent study showed that probable migraine was as prevalent as migraine within a health plan.

There are two subtypes of probable migraine: probable migraine without aura (just one criteria for migraine without aura is missing) and probable migraine with aura (one criteria for migraine with aura is missing).

Menstrual migraine

The ICHD-II presents, in the appendix, alternative criteria for the classification of migraine without aura in women, according to the temporal relation with menstruation. *Pure menstrual migraine* (A.1.1.1) is defined by attacks that fulfill criteria for migraine without aura, occurring exclusively from two days prior to the third day (−2 to +3) of menstruation in at least 2 of 3 menstrual cycles, and at no other time. *In menstrually-related migraine* (A.1.1.2), attacks of migraine without aura also occur at least in 2 of 3 menstrual cycles, but also at other times of the cycle. Finally, in *nonmenstrual migraine without aura* (A.1.1.3), attacks meet criteria for migraine without aura without relationship with menstruation.

Suggested reading

1. Abu-Arafeh I, Russel G. Prevalence and clinical features of abdominal migraine compared with those of migraine headache. *Arch Dis Child* 1995; **72**: 413–17.
2. Al-Twaijri WA, Shevell MI. Pediatric migraine equivalents: occurrence and clinical features in practice. *Pediatr Neurol* 2002; **26**: 365–8.
3. Bento MS, Esperanca P. Migraine with prolonged aura. *Headache* 2000; **40**: 52–3.
4. Carrera P, Stenirri S, Ferrari M, *et al.* Familial hemiplegic migraine: a ion channel disorder. *Brain Res Bull* 2001; **56**: 239–41.
5. Couch JR, Diamond S. Status migrainosus. Causative and therapeutic aspects. *Headache* 1983; **23**: 94–101.
6. De Fusco M, Marconi R, Silvestri L, *et al.* Haploinsufficiency of ATP1A2 encoding the Na/K pump a2 subunit associated with familial hemiplegic migraine type 2. *Nat Genet* 2003; advance online publication.
7. Diamond S. Basilar artery migraine. A commonly misdiagnosed disorder. *Postgrad Med* 1987; **81**: 45–6.
8. Drigo P, Carli G, Laverda AM. Benign paroxysmal vertigo of childhood. *Brain Dev* 2001; **23**: 38–41.
9. Ducros A, Denier C, Joutel A, *et al.* The clinical spectrum of familial hemiplegic migraine associated with mutations in a neuronal calcium channel. *N Engl J Med* 2001; **345**: 17–24.
10. Dunn DW, Snyder CH. Benign paroxysmal vertigo of childhood. *Am J Dis Child* 1976; **130**: 1099–1100.
11. Fisher CM. Late-life migraine accompaniments as a cause of unexplained transient ischemic attacks. *Can J Neurol Sci* 1980; **7**: 9–17.
12. Fleisher DR. Cyclic vomiting syndrome and migraine. *J Pediatr* 1999; **134**: 533–5.
13. Haan J, Terwindt GM, Ferrari MD. Genetics of migraine. *Neurol Clin* 1997; **15**: 43–60.
14. Headache Classification Committee of the International Headache Society. Classification and diagnostic criteria for headache disorders, cranial neuralgias and facial pain. *Cephalalgia* 1988; **8** (Suppl 7): 1–96.
15. Headache Classification Committee of the International Headache Society. Classification and diagnostic criteria for headache disorders, cranial neuralgias, and facial pain. Second Edition. *Cephalalgia* 2004; (Suppl 1): 1–160.

16. Hosking G. Special forms: variants of migraine in childhood. In: *Migraine in childhood.* (ed. Hockaday JM). Boston: Butterworths, 1988; 35–53.
17. Klee A, Willanger R. Disturbances of visual perception in migraine. *Acta Neurol Scand* 1966; **42**: 400–14.
18. Kuhn WF, Kuhn SC, Daylida L. Basilar migraine. *Eur J Emerg Med* 1997; **4**: 33–8.
19. Li BU. Cyclic vomiting syndrome: age-old syndrome and new insights. *Semin Pediatr Neurol* 2001; **8**: 13–21.
20. Lippman CV. Certain hallucinations peculiar to migraine. *J Nerv Ment Dis* 1952; **116**: 346.
21. Lipton RB, Ottman R, Ehrenberg BL, *et al.* Comorbidity of migraine: the connection between migraine and epilepsy. *Neurology* 1994; **44**: 28–32.
22. Lipton RB, Pfeffer D, Newman LC, *et al.* Headaches in the elderly. *J Pain Symptom Manage* 1993; **8**: 87–97.
23. Manzoni G, Farina S, Lanfranchi M, *et al.* Classic migraine: clinical findings in 164 patients. *Eur Neurol* 1985; **24**: 163–9.
24. Ophoff RA, Terwindt GM, Vergouwe MN, *et al.* Familial hemiplegic migraine and episodic ataxia type-2 are caused by mutations in the Ca2+ channel gene CACNL1A4. *Cell* 1996; **87**: 543–52.
25. Ophoff RA, Terwindt GM, Vergouwe MN, *et al.* Wolff Award 1997. Involvement of a Ca2+ channel gene in familial hemiplegic migraine and migraine with and without aura. Dutch Migraine Genetics Research Group. *Headache* 1997; **37**: 479–85.
26. Ottman R, Lipton RB. Comorbidity of migraine and epilepsy. *Neurology* 1994; **44**: 2105–10.
27. Panayiotopoulos CP. Basilar migraine: a review. In: *Benign childhood partial seizures and related epileptic syndromes.*(ed Panayiotopoulos CP). London: John Libbey & Company Ltd., 1999; 303–8.
28. Rains JC, Penzien DB, Lipchik GL, *et al.* Diagnosis of migraine: empirical analysis of a large clinical sample of atypical migraine (IHS 1.7) patients and proposed revision of the IHS criteria. *Cephalalgia* 2001; **21**: 584–95.
29. Raskin NH. Treatment of status migrainosus: the American experience. *Headache* 1990; **30** (Suppl 2): 550–3.
30. Rasmussen BK, Jensen R, Olesen J. A population-based analysis of the criteria of the International Headache Society. *Cephalalgia* 1991; **11**: 129–34.
31. Rasmussen BK. Epidemiology of headache. *Cephalalgia* 2001; **21**(7): 774–77.
32. Rothrock JF, Walicke P, Swenson MR, *et al.* Migrainous stroke. *Arch Neurol* 1988; **45**: 63–7.
33. Russel MB, Olesen J. A nosographic analysis of the migraine aura in a general population. *Brain* 1996; **119**: 355–61.
34. Sandrini G, Antonaci F, Pucci E, *et al.* Comparative study with EMG, pressure algometry and manual palpation in tension-type headache and migraine. *Cephalalgia* 1994; **14**: 451–7.
35. Schwartz BS, Stewart WF, Simon D, *et al.* Epidemiology of tension-type headache. *JAMA.* 1998 Feb 4; **279** (5): 381–3.
36. Silberstein SD, Lipton RB. Chronic daily headache, including transformed migraine, chronic tension-type headache, and medication overuse. In: *Wolff's headache and other head pain.* (eds Silberstein SD, Lipton RB, Dalessio DJ). New York: Oxford University Press, 2001: 247–82.
37. Silberstein SD, Lipton RB. Headache epidemiology. Emphasis on migraine. *Neurol Clin* 1996; **14** (2): 421–34.
38. Solomon S, Grosberg BM. Retinal Migraine (abstract). *Headache* 2003; **43**: 510.
39. Staehelin-Jensen T, Olivarius B, Kraft M, *et al.* Familial hemiplegic migraine. A reappraisal and long-term follow-up study. *Cephalalgia* 1981; **1**: 33–9.
40. Thomsen LL, Ostergaard E, Olesen J, *et al.* Evidence for a separate type of migraine with aura: sporadic hemiplegic migraine. *Neurology* 2003; **60**: 595–601.

41. Tietjen GE. The relationship of migraine and stroke. *Neuroepidemiology* 2000; **19**: 13–9.
42. Troost T, Zagami AS. Ophthalmoplegic migraine and retinal migraine. In *The Headaches.* (eds Olesen J, Tfelt-Hansen P, Welch KMA). Philadelphia, Lippincott Willians & Wilkins, 2000: 511–16.
43. Willey RG. The scintillating scotoma without headache. *Ann Ophthalmol* 1979; **11**: 581–5.
44. Withers GD, Silburn SR, Forbes DA. Precipitants and aetiology of cyclic vomiting syndrome. *Acta Paediatr* 1998; **87** (3): 272–7.
45. Ziegler DK, Hanassein RS. Specific headache phenomena: their frequency and coincidence. *Headache* 1990; **30**: 152–60.

10
Migraine with aura and its borderlands

M. K. Eriksen, L. L. Thomsen, and J. Olesen

A detailed knowledge of the aura symptoms is crucial when diagnosing migraine with aura because it is a clinical entity with no diagnostic biological markers. Most descriptions of migraine with aura are from studies of modest size or questionnaire studies.[1–4] Since studies using a validated, semistructured interview done by physicians with experience in headache diagnoses are more likely to increase the understanding of the symptomatology of migraine with aura,[5,6] the aim of the present paper was to review the clinical characteristics of migraine with aura as reported in studies using this approach. For several years, the research groups at the Danish Headache Center have collected empirical data on migraine with non-hemiplegic aura (MA), familial hemiplegic migraine (FHM), and sporadic hemiplegic migraine (SHM) using a similar, valid methodology. The present paper reviews the results from these studies. The paper focuses on the symptom characteristics essential for making a diagnosis of migraine with aura, that is, the common features that characterize the visual, sensory, aphasic and motor aura, and the headache following the aura in MA, FHM, and SHM.

The Danish migraine studies

At the Danish Headache Center patients with familial MA, who represented severe clinic-type MA, FHM, or SHM were recruited from the Danish National Patient Registry comprising patients who had been in contact with Danish Hospitals.[7–10] In addition, files from practicing neurologists were screened, and an advertisement for patients was placed in the major Danish medical journal.[7–10] The studies of MA aimed at identifying migraine families since the patients were used for genetic studies as well. The patients participated in a validated semistructured telephone interview by a trained physician and were diagnosed according to the International Headache Society Classification from 1988 (ICHD-1).[7–11] All patients with hemiplegic migraine had a neurological examination but patients with MA did not. Using this approach, 362 patients with familial MA (from 105 families),[7] 147 patients with FHM (from 44 families),[8,9] and 105 patients with SHM[10] were recruited. Further patients with MA (labeled population-based MA) were recruited for a population-based study among persons drawn from the Danish National Civil Registration System.[1,12] In that study, the patients were diagnosed according to the ICHD-1 by a trained physician using a semistructured interview similar to the interview used in the studies concerning familial MA, FHM, and SHM. Using this approach, 163 patients with population-based MA were recruited of whom nine had hemiplegic aura.[1,12]

Characteristics of migraine with aura

Aura distribution

The distribution of the visual, sensory, aphasic, and motor aura in MA, FHM, and SHM is shown in Fig. 10.1. Almost all patients had a visual aura at least in some attacks, and 39% (142/362) of patients with familial MA[7] and 68% (104/154) of patients with population-based MA[12] had exclusively visual aura. In hemiplegic migraine, 100% (252/252) had at least two aura symptoms in each attack ($p<0.001$ compared with familial MA, Chi-square test) of whom 28% (71/252) had three aura symptoms and 68% (171/252) had four aura symptoms in each attack.[9,10] Basilar-type aura,

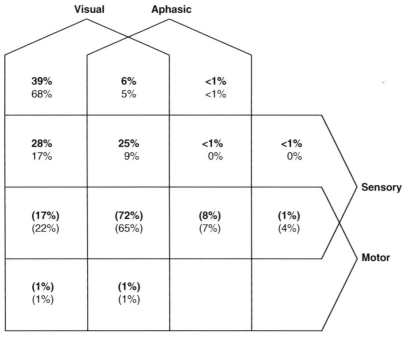

Fig. 10.1 Distribution of aura symptoms: Venn diagram illustrating the distribution of the aura symptoms in familial MA (bold) ($n=362$),[7] population-based MA (not bold) ($n=154$, patients with motor aura excluded),[12] FHM (bold parenthesis) ($n=147$),[9] and SHM (not bold parenthesis) ($n=105$).[10]

which fulfilled the ICHD-1 criteria for basilar-type migraine, was present in 10% (35/362) of patients with familial MA[7] compared with 69% (101/147) of patients with FHM[9] and 72% (76/105) of patients with SHM[10] ($p<0.001$ compared with familial MA, Chi-square test). Basilar-type aura was not recorded in patients with population-based MA[12].

Gradual development of the aura

The migraine aura is characterized by a gradual development. The mean gradual progression time of the aura in MA, FHM, and SHM is shown in Fig. 10.2. The mean progression time of each aura symptom was approximately 20–30 min.[7,9,10,12] However, some patients were not able to describe that their aura developed gradually over more than 5 min. Among patients with any subtype of migraine with aura, only 81–97% ($n=746$) of patients reported a gradually developing visual aura,[7,9,10,12] 85–98% ($n=494$) reported a gradually developing sensory aura[7,9,10,12] and 88–90% ($n=152$) reported a gradually developing motor aura.[9,10] However, if more than one aura symptom was present they occurred in succession in 96% (149/155) of patients with familial MA.[7]

Aura duration

The mean duration of the aura in MA, FHM, and SHM is shown in Fig. 10.3. In MA, the aura duration was 60 min or less in most patients.[7,12] Patients with

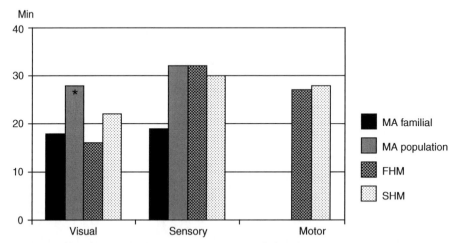

Fig. 10.2 Mean gradual progression time of the aura among patients reporting a gradually developing aura in familial MA ($n=362$),[7] population-based MA ($n=163$).[12] FHM ($n=147$),[9] and SHM ($n=105$).[10] *The mean progression time of the visual aura in population-based MA was reported as 25 min in patients exclusively with visual aura and 33 min in patients with co-occurrence of other aura symptoms.

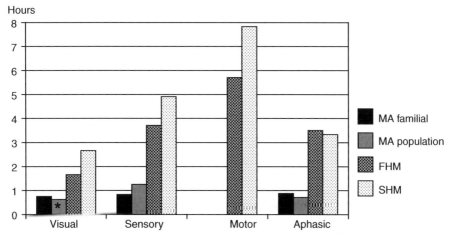

Fig. 10.3 Mean duration of the aura in familial MA (n=362),[7] population-based MA (n=163),[12] FHM (n=147),[9] and SHM (n=105).[10] *The mean duration of the visual aura in population-based MA was reported as 33 min in patients exclusively with visual aura and 44 min in patients with co-occurrence of other aura symptoms.

hemiplegic migraine had a more prolonged aura (duration more than 60 min)[9,10] compared with patients with MA:[7,12] the visual aura was prolonged in 27% of patients with FHM and 27% with SHM (vs. 10% with familial MA and 8% with population-based MA), the sensory aura was prolonged in 54% with FHM and 48% with SHM (vs. 14% with familial MA and 20% with population-based MA), the aphasic aura was prolonged in 36% with FHM and 27% with SHM (vs. 22% with familial MA and 17% with population-based MA), and the motor aura was prolonged in 59% with FHM and 49% with SHM.[7,9,10,12] Though the aura symptoms were prolonged in FHM and SHM the duration of each aura symptom was 24 h or less in 98–100% of the FHM patients[9] and 92–100% of the SHM patients.[10]

Aura location

The migraine aura is known to have a unilateral location. Figure 10.4 illustrates the percentage of patients having a unilateral location of the aura symptoms in MA, FHM, and SHM. The sensory and motor aura was unilateral in most patients.[7,9,10,12] However, only 60–69% (n=746) of all patients described a unilateral visual aura.[7,9,10,12] The distribution of the motor aura varied among patients with hemiplegic migraine. In 59% (n=147) of FHM patients and 50% (n=105) of SHM patients, the motor aura affected the ipsilateral arm *and* leg, that is the motor aura was hemiparetic, while 41% of FHM patients and 50% of SHM patients had a unilateral motor aura affecting only the arm *or* leg, that is the motor aura was nonhemiparetic.[9,10]

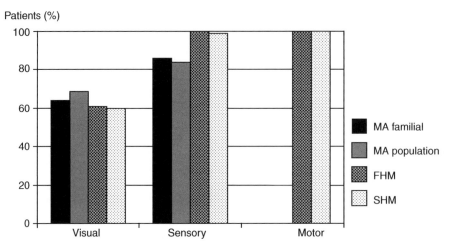

Fig. 10.4 Unilateral location of the aura in familial MA (n=362),[7] population-based MA (n=163),[12] FHM (n=147),[9] and SHM (n=105).[10]

Headache characteristics

The prevalence of a headache related to the aura varied among patients as shown in Fig. 10.5. In familial MA, 64% (234/362) of patients always had a headache[7] compared with 58% (94/163) in population-based MA,[12] 94% (138/147) in FHM,[9] and 93% (98/105) in SHM.[10] Figure 10.6 illustrates how often the headache related to the aura fulfilled the diagnostic subcriteria for migraine without aura (MO) according to the ICHD-1.[13] Most patients fulfilled the pain criteria (moderate/severe intensity, unilateral, pulsating, and aggravation by physical activity) and the criteria for associated symptoms (nausea, vomiting, photophobia, and phonophobia).[1,7,9,10] However, in familial MA, the duration of the headache was less than 4 h in many patients.[7] Therefore, the headache fulfilled every set of sub-criteria for MO in only 57% (189/329) of patients with familial MA[7] compared with 73% in FHM (106/145)[9] and 76% (80/105) in SHM[10] ($p < 0.001$ compared with familial MA, Chi-square test). The proportion of patients fulfilling every set of subcriteria for MO was not reported in patients with population-based MA.[12]

Discussion

Methodological considerations

In the studies reviewed in the present paper, all patients were diagnosed in a validated[6,14] semistructured interview by a physician trained in headache diagnoses to secure the highest possible accuracy and adherence to the formal diagnostic criteria.[1,7–10,12] Furthermore, the physicians that conducted the studies had

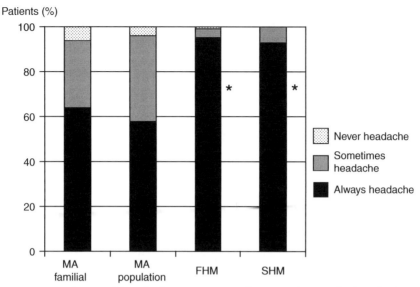

Fig. 10.5 Prevalence of headache in aura attacks. Prevalence of a headache related to the aura in familial MA ($n=362$),[7] population-based MA ($n=163$),[12] FHM ($n=147$),[9] and SHM ($n=105$).[10] *Significantly different from familial MA ($p<0.001$, Chi-square test). In FHM, two patients never had a headache related to the aura.

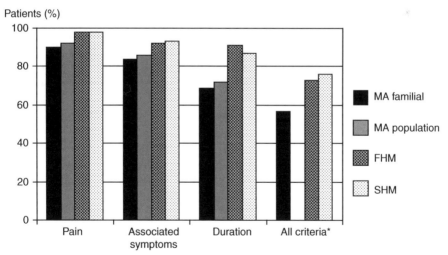

Fig. 10.6 Headache fulfilling subcriteria in migraine without aura. Proportion of patients with a headache related to aura that fulfils the subcriteria of migraine without aura in familial MA ($n=341$),[7] population-based MA ($n=156$),[12] FHM ($n=145$),[9] and SHM ($n=105$).[10] *In MA: except the criterion regarding the number of attacks. In FHM/SHM: including the criterion regarding the number of attacks.

been trained in the same headache center minimizing the interobserver variability.[1,7–10,12] This enabled a more precise comparison of the symptom characteristics between the subtypes of migraine with aura. The patients with migraine with non-hemiplegic aura did not have a physical or neurological examination, since previous studies have shown that this rarely alters the diagnosis of migraine in epidemiological studies.[15]

To summarize, in most MA patients the aura was gradually developing over more than 5 min; it had a duration of 5–60 min; a unilateral location; and was followed by a headache, though it was common to also have attacks of non-hemiplegic aura without headache. Patients with FHM and SHM differed from patients with MA in several aspects: they had a higher number of aura symptoms (at least two symptoms in each attack); longer aura duration (prolonged aura 1–24 h); higher frequency of basilar-type aura; and they almost always had a migraine headache related to the aura.[1,7–10,12]

Suggestions for revised diagnostic criteria for the ICHD-2

Based on empirical findings from the studies reviewed in the present paper[1,7–10,12] the Classification Committee of the International Headache Society revised the diagnostic criteria for MA, FHM, SHM, and basilar-type migraine for the International Classification of Headache Disorders 2nd Edition (ICHD-2).[11] The development of the new ICHD-2 criteria for MA will be described in the following chapter of the present book.[16] The development of the new ICHD-2 criteria for FHM, SHM, and basilar-type migraine was based on the suggestions by Thomsen et al.[9,10] Since hemiplegic migraine differs from non-hemiplegic migraine, Thomsen et al. suggested new separate diagnostic criteria for FHM and SHM, and a better delineation of hemiplegic migraine from basilar-type migraine.[9] According to Thomsen et al., the ICHD-2 criteria for FHM should include patients with some degree of motor weakness or hemiplegia; at least one additional aura symptom besides the motor aura symptom should be present; the criteria should accept a prolonged aura (less than 24 h); the headache related to the aura should fulfil the diagnostic criteria for MO[9]; and the criteria should include second-degree relatives since a reduced penetrance has been reported in FHM.[9] Thomsen et al. suggested that SHM should be diagnosed by separate diagnostic criteria.[9,10] The ICHD-2 criteria for SHM should be identical to the FHM criteria except that no first- or second-degree relative has hemiplegic migraine.[10] According to Thomsen et al., the ICHD-2 criteria for basilar-type migraine should exclude patients with motor weakness—if a motor aura is present, patients should be diagnosed with FHM or SHM.[9,10]

Differential diagnoses

The empirical data presented improve the classification and diagnostic criteria of migraine with aura and, furthermore, help to sharpen the differential diagnoses. The data show that if more than one aura symptom is present, patients almost always have a visual aura besides other aura symptoms. In hemiplegic migraine, patients have at least one additional aura symptom besides their motor aura. In MA, attacks of aura without headache may occur but in hemiplegic migraine, the aura is almost always followed by a migraine headache. The main differential diagnoses of migraine with aura are transient ischemic attacks, stroke, epilepsy (postictal weakness following seizures or Todd phenomenon), functional attacks, and visual disturbances in MO.[17] Diagnostic caution is required when aura-like symptoms are not followed by a headache and if sensory, aphasic, or motor symptoms occur without visual symptoms.[1,7–10,12] In such cases and in cases with other diagnostic uncertainty, appropriate investigations should rule out intracranial pathology.

References

1. Russell MB, Rasmussen BK, Fenger K, et al. Migraine without aura and migraine with aura are distinct clinical entities: a study of four hundred and eighty-four male and female migraineurs from the general population. Cephalalgia 1996; **16** (4): 239–45.
2. Jensen K, Tfelt-Hansen P, Lauritzen M, et al. Classic migraine. A prospective recording of symptoms. Acta Neurol Scand 1986; **73** (4): 359–62.
3. Manzoni GC, Farina S, Lanfranchi M, et al. Classic migraine–clinical findings in 164 patients. Eur Neurol 1985; **24** (3): 163–9.
4. Kallela M, Wessman M, Havanka H, et al. Familial migraine with and without aura: clinical characteristics and co-occurrence. Eur J Neurol 2001; **8** (5): 441–9.
5. Rasmussen BK, Jensen R, Olesen J. Questionnaire versus clinical interview in the diagnosis of headache. Headache 1991; **31** (5): 290–5.
6. Russell MB, Rasmussen BK, Thorvaldsen P, et al. Prevalence and sex-ratio of the subtypes of migraine. Int J Epidemiol 1995; **24** (3): 612–8.
7. Eriksen M, Thomsen L, Olesen J. Clinical characteristics of 362 patients with familial migraine with aura. Cephalalgia 2004; **24**: 564–75.
8. Lykke Thomsen L, Kirchmann Eriksen M, Faerch Romer S, et al. An epidemiological survey of hemiplegic migraine. Cephalalgia 2002; **22** (5): 361–75.
9. Thomsen LL, Eriksen MK, Roemer SF, et al. A population-based study of familial hemiplegic migraine suggests revised diagnostic criteria. Brain 2002; **125** (Pt 6): 1379–91.
10. Thomsen LL, Ostergaard E, Olesen J, et al. Evidence for a separate type of migraine with aura: sporadic hemiplegic migraine. Neurology 2003; **60** (4): 595–601.
11. The International Classification of Headache Disorders 2nd Edition. Cephalalgia 2004; **24** (1): 1–160.
12. Russell MB, Olesen J. A nosographic analysis of the migraine aura in a general population. Brain 1996; **119** (Pt 2): 355–61.
13. Headache Classification Committee of the International Headache Society. Classification and diagnostic criteria for headache disorders, cranial neuralgias and facial pain. Cephalalgia 1988; **8** (7): 1–96.
14. Rasmussen BK, Jensen R, Schroll M, et al. Epidemiology of headache in a general population–a prevalence study. J Clin Epidemiol 1991; **44** (11): 1147–57.
15. Rasmussen BK, Olesen J. Symptomatic and nonsymptomatic headaches in a general population. Neurology 1992; **42** (6): 1225–31.
16. Eriksen M, Thomsen L, Olesen J. Sensitivity and specificity of new diagnostic criteria for migraine with aura. Submitted.
17. The Headaches. Second ed; 2000.

11
Chronic migraine

N. J. Wiendels and M. D. Ferrari

Classification

Chronic daily headache (CDH) is a collective term for primary headaches occurring on more than 14 days per month. The 2nd edition of the International Classification of Headache Disorders (ICHD-II) now includes four types of CDH: chronic migraine (CM), chronic tension-type headache (CTTH), new daily persistent headache (NDPH), and hemicrania continua (HC).[1] CM is classified as a complication of migraine and is described as headache, fulfilling criteria for migraine without aura, occurring on 15 or more days per month for more than three months in the absence of medication overuse. Since most patients start with episodic migraine without aura, chronicity is regarded as a complication of episodic migraine. Clinical experience however, suggests that when the frequency of migraine attacks increases into almost daily headaches, headache characteristics become less prominent and severe, which makes it difficult to discern from CTTH. Many patients experience almost daily tension-type headaches with episodically superimposed migraine attacks (Fig. 11.1). This is why Silberstein and Lipton proposed to add three alternative criteria to support the diagnosis of CM: (1) a prior history of episodic migraine; (2) a period of increasing headache frequency with decreasing severity of migraine features; or (3) superimposed attacks of headaches that meet criteria for migraine without aura except duration.[2] This proposal did not make it to the ICHD-II. According to the new classification, these patients are not to be classified as CM. The requirement that the daily headache meets criteria for

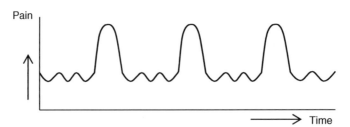

Fig. 11.1 An example of chronic headache with daily headaches of moderate intensity and superimposed migraine attacks.

migraine without aura probably makes CM a rare entity. The difference with status migrainosus, another rare complication of migraine, is not very clear since an interruption due to sleep or medication of the 'unremitting' severe migraine attack can be disregarded for the diagnosis and a maximum number of migraine days is not given. Future studies have to prove existence of pure CM and practical use of this category.

The majority of patients will probably be classified as medication-overuse headache (MOH). The process of transformation of episodic into chronic daily headache is usually accompanied by a gradual increase of the use of analgesics and migraine drugs. Since medication overuse is the most likely cause of chronification, withdrawal of all headache medication and caffeine is the appropriate therapy. When overuse is present, the diagnosis is probable MOH until after withdrawal, plus the antecedent migraine subtype, when there is a history of episodic migraine. Patients do not always provide an accurate and clear history. Sometimes characteristics of the episodic headache type become clear only after withdrawal. A further specified classification of the medication overuse, like triptan-overuse headache or analgesic-overuse headache will not be possible in patients described above. The criteria for triptan-overuse include migraine headache characteristics, thereby excluding tension-type headache characteristics, and vice versa for analgesic-overuse. In practice, the majority of CDH patients with a history of episodic migraine, overusing triptans, have some of both migraine and tension-type headache characteristics.

Epidemiology

The prevalence of CDH in the general population worldwide is around 4%. Studies based on CDH criteria proposed by Silberstein and Lipton were conducted in the general population in Spain, the US, and Taiwan and revealed a prevalence of CDH of 4.7%, 4.1%, and 3.2%, respectively.[3–5] In the Spanish study, 90% of the CDH patients were women (prevalence women 8.7%, men 1%) and the mean age was 50 years (range 18–89). The relative frequencies of CM, CTTH, and NDPH were 51%, 47% and 2%, respectively. HC was not diagnosed. In Taiwan, the prevalence amongst women was 4.3% and men 1.9%, and the mean age was 39 years (range 15–78). The relative frequencies of CM and CTTH in this study were 55% and 44%. In specialized headache centers, 40% of patients have CDH,[6] and up to 14% of patients with episodic migraine may develop CDH within one year.[7] CDH occurs at any age. Mean age of children and adolescents with CDH in a headache clinic is 12 years, with a range of 2–18.[8,9] In Taiwan, 3.9% of elderly suffer from CDH.[10]

Pathophysiology

The exact pathophysiologic mechanisms that lead to CDH are not known. An important theoretical concept is central sensitization. The nucleus caudalis of the trigeminal nerve receives peripheral sensory input from nociceptive and mechanoceptive neurons of meningeal and pericranial structures. Prolonged activation of peripheral nociceptors increases excitability of nociceptive neurons and consecutively central neurons of the nucleus caudalis, expressed as spontaneous pain and induction of pain by non-noxious stimuli (allodynia).[11] Pericranial muscles can suddenly be painful because mechanosensitive neurons project to hyperexcitable, sensitized central neurons. How nociceptors become activated in the first place is not clear. In migraine with aura, a wave of depolarization spreads forward from the occipital cortex followed by neuronal inactivation, a phenomenon called 'cortical spreading depression' (CSD). During CSD the concentration of ions, neurotransmitters, and metabolites increases, which activates nociceptors in pia and dura mater.[12] Vasoactive neuropeptides from trigeminal nerve ends mediate an inflammatory response with vasodilatation and protein extravasation, causing sensitization of trigeminal nociceptive neurons. Dysfunction of central pain modulating systems can induce or prolong central sensitization. Tissue iron levels in the periaquaductal grey matter (PAG) increases with duration (in years) of CDH, which may reflect impaired iron homeostasis associated with neuronal dysfunction or damage.[13] The PAG is part of a descending antinociceptive system, which can facilitate central sensitization when dysfunctioning. Chronic use of painkillers can also influence central pain modulation by decreasing antinociceptive activity.

Treatment

Overuse of headache medication and caffeine is an important risk factor for CDH. Prevalence data on overuse vary depending on setting and definition. In tertiary centers the majority (47–73%) of CDH patients overuse medication, in the general population lower percentages are reported.[6,14] Twenty-five percent of the general population in Spain overused medication and 34% of the population in Taiwan.[3,5] Both studies did not account for caffeine overuse. In The Netherlands 4% suffer from CDH, with 57% overusing medication and 80% overusing medication and/or caffeine. Overuse of caffeine is still an experimental category in the ICHD-II. General practitioners are usually not aware of the frequent use of headache medication because most patients treat themselves with over-the-counter medication and patients are not aware of the paradoxical effect of painkillers causing chronification of their headaches. Some patients take analgesics preventatively or at the slightest signs of headache because of fear of having a migraine attack that day. Relief of pain and associated mood effects after intake of analgesics, sedatives, and/or caffeine reinforce their use (positive reinforcement). Physical adaptation to medication develops; the delayed intake of medication or caffeine results in withdrawal headache (negative reinforcement). Patients often notice that the analgesics do not work as effectively as they used to, so they increase dosage and combine different kinds of medication. Ultimately the patient finds himself in a vicious circle of daily headaches and medication, and/or caffeine use. Many patients wake up with headache and begin their day with intake of analgesics. Their headache worsens with physical or intellectual exertion and is associated with tiredness, nausea, irritation, concentration problems, restlessness, anxiety, and depression.

Physicians should think of MOH at the following frequency of intake:

- Analgesics on ≥3 days a week and/or,
- triptans on ≥2 days a week and/or,
- ergotamine on ≥1 day a week and/or,
- daily use of >5 units of caffeine (coffee, tea, ice-tea, cola, chocolate).

Frequency of intake seems to be important rather than dosage per intake. This means that daily use of 1 tablet of paracetamol is worse than 6 tablets on 1 day a week. Patients often do not regard analgesics as medication, physicians should specifically ask about analgesic use. These criteria for medication overuse are used in the Leiden University Medical Centre (LUMC). Unlike the criteria for MOH in the ICHD II suggest, headache characteristics are not important when overuse is present.

Different methods are possible for withdrawal; abrupt discontinuation, replacement by NSAIDs, with or without immediate start of prophylactic drugs and in- or outpatient treatment.[15] If patients succeed in withdrawal, most patients have a favorable outcome. In the LUMC, we favor abrupt outpatient discontinuation of analgesics, triptans, and ergotamine and caffeine during 3 months without replacement medication. Narcotics, beta-blockers, and benzodiazepines should be tapered to prevent severe withdrawal symptoms. Extensive explanation of physical adaptation to medication, withdrawal symptoms, and motivation of the patient is important. We believe that successful outpatient withdrawal is psychologically better, because patients experience more control over their headaches when they withdraw medication all by themselves and know they can do without, which decreases the risk of relapse. Tapering of acute medication makes withdrawal symptoms less severe, but also lengthens the process, which makes it difficult for the patient to abstain. Prophylactic medication is not effective when overuse is present and should be withdrawn too. After three months, the episodic headache pattern emerges. Choice of further treatment depends on frequency and headache characteristics.

Summary and conclusions

In the ICHD-II, CM is classified as a complication of migraine and is described as migraine headache occurring on 15 or more days per month for more than 3 months in the absence of medication overuse. In clinical practice however, most patients with chronified episodic migraine have less severe and clear headache characteristics, especially when overusing headache medication. A practical approach to the patient with frequent headaches is depicted in Fig. 11.2. When a patient presents with headaches on 3 days a week or more, first determine whether it is a trigeminal autonomic cephalalgia. If not, specifically ask about frequency of acute medication and caffeine use. When overuse is present, start withdrawal,

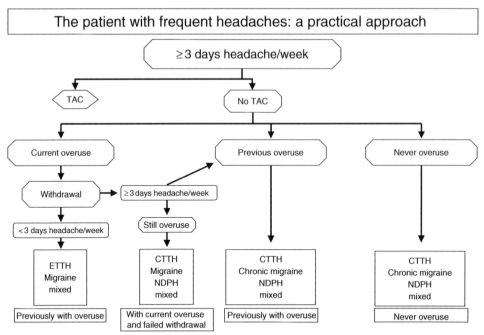

Fig. 11.2 The patient with frequent headaches: a practical approach. TAC – trigeminal autonomic cephalalgia, ETTH – episodic tension-type headache, CTTH – chronic tension-type headache, NDPH – new daily persistent headache, and CM – chronic migraine.

regardless of the headache characteristics. After three months of withdrawal, the former episodic headache usually emerges with clear headache characteristics, which can then be treated accordingly. Use of acute medication should be limited to avoid relapse. Some patients do not improve after withdrawal. When overuse is not, or no longer present, diagnose the chronic headache type according to headache characteristics and treat with the usual prophylactic medication.

References

1. Headache classification subcommittee of the International Headache Society. The International Classification of Headache Disorders. *Cephalalgia* 2004; **24**: 8–160.
2. Silberstein SD, Lipton RB, Sliwinski M. Classification of daily and near-daily headaches: field trial of revised IHS criteria. *Neurology* 1996; **47**: 871–5.
3. Castillo J, Munoz P, Guitera V, *et al*. Epidemiology of Chronic Daily Headache in the General Population. *Headache* 1999; **39**: 190–6.
4. Scher AI, Stewart WF, Liberman J, *et al*. Prevalence of Frequent Headache in a Population Sample. *Headache* 1998; **38**: 497–506.
5. Lu SR, Fuh JL, Chen WT, *et al*. Chronic daily headache in Taipei, Taiwan: prevalence, follow-up and outcome predictors. *Cephalalgia* 2001; **21**: 980–6.
6. Mathew NT. Chronic refractory headache. *Neurology* 1993; **43**: S26–33.

7. Katsarava Z, Schneeweiss S, Kurth T, *et al*. Incidence and predictors for chronicity of headache in patients with episodic migraine. *Neurology* 2004; **62**: 788–90.
8. Abu-Arafeh I. Chronic tension-type headache in children and adolescents. *Cephalalgia* 2001; **21**: 830–6.
9. Hershey AD, Powers SW, Bentti AL, *et al*. Characterization of chronic daily headaches in children in a multidisciplinary headache center. *Neurology* 2001; **56**: 1032–7.
10. Wang SJ, Fuh JL, Lu SR, *et al*. Chronic daily headache in Chinese elderly: prevalence, risk factors, and biannual follow-up. *Neurology* 2000; **54**: 314–9.
11. Burstein R, Cutrer MF, Yarnitsky D. The development of cutaneous allodynia during a migraine attack clinical evidence for the sequential recruitment of spinal and supraspinal nociceptive neurons in migraine. *Brain* 2000; **123**: 1703–9.
12. Bolay H, Reuter U, Dunn AK, *et al*. Intrinsic brain activity triggers trigeminal meningeal afferents in a migraine model. *Nat Med* 2002; **8**: 136–42.
13. Welch KM, Nagesh V, Aurora SK, *et al*. Periaqueductal gray matter dysfunction in migraine: cause or the burden of illness? *Headache* 2001; **41**: 629–37.
14. Solomon S, Lipton RB, Newman LC. Clinical features of chronic daily headache. *Headache* 1992; **32**: 325–9.
15. Zed PJ, Loewen PS, Robinson G. Medication-induced headache: overview and systematic review of therapeutic approaches. *Ann Pharmacother* 1999; **33**: 61–72.

12 Application of diagnostic criteria for migraine without aura*

P. Torelli, E. Beghi, and G. C. Manzoni

Introduction

Thanks to its unquestionable merits, the International Headache Society (IHS) classification published in 1988[1] has been instrumental for a correct scientific and clinical approach to primary and symptomatic headaches.

Fifteen years later, nosographic and clinical knowledge has considerably improved, calling for a revision of the 1988 classification and leading to the publication of the International Classification of Headache Disorders (2nd edition) (ICHD-II) in 2004.[2] Although substantial progress has been made in the last few years, there is still much to be learned in the headache field. To encourage research in this direction, an appendix has been added to the revised classification that describes a number of still-uncoded disorders and proposes an alternative set of diagnostic criteria to be tested as a replacement for the official ones, namely for migraine without aura (MO) (coded to A1.1) and tension-type headache (TTH) (coded to A2.1, A2.2, and A2.3). The aim of this study was to determine whether the criteria described in the Appendix to ICHD-II for MO offer any benefits compared to the ICHD-II official criteria in a group of patients referred to a headache clinic.

Materials and methods

The study population consisted of all patients seen for the first time on a consecutive basis at the University of Parma Headache Center from October 1 to November 30, 2003 ($n=256$). Headache diagnosis was established by two neurologists. The first neurologist

*Appendix to the International Classification of Headache Disorders (2nd Edition): Application of diagnostic criteria for migraine without aura.

Table 12.1 Alternative diagnostic criteria for migraine without aura in the appendix to the international classification of headache disorders (ICHD-II)

A. At least five attacks fulfilling criteria B–D
B. Headache attacks lasting 4–72 h (untreated or unsuccessfully treated)
C. Headache has at least two of the following characteristics:
    1. unilateral location
    2. pulsating quality
    3. moderate or severe pain intensity
    4. aggravation by or causing avoidance of routine physical activity (e.g. walking or climbing stairs)
D. During headache at least two of the following:
    1. nausea
    2. vomiting
    3. photophobia
    4. phonophobia
    5. osmophobia
E. Not attributed to another disorder

(GCM) was a headache specialist who, having reviewed the patients' past medical histories and performed a physical and a neurological examination, based diagnosis on his own experience. Obviously, in his clinical judgement he also considered other clinical aspects that are not listed among the ICHD-II criteria, such as the disease's natural history, its evolution in relation to female reproductive events, family history of headache, associated symptoms, triggering and attenuating factors, and response to drug therapy. The second neurologist (PT) was blind to the diagnosis and established the diagnosis by means of a semi-structured interview based on the ICHD-II criteria and on the criteria proposed in the Appendix to ICHD-II. The Appendix criteria for MO are reported in Table 12.1. For patients with more than one headache subtype, only the more frequent was considered. The MO diagnosis established by the headache specialist was taken as the gold standard against which the ICHD-II Appendix criteria for MO were to be compared. The study was approved by the Ethics Commission of the University of Parma School of Medicine. The patients gave their written consent.

Data analysis was done by SPSS 11.0 for Windows.

Results

The initial sample consisted of 256 subjects (174 women and 82 men; mean age 35.9 years ± 12.3). The headache neurologist diagnosed MO in 119 patients (89 women and 30 men; mean age, 34.8 years ± 10.4) and atypical MO in 23 (18 women and five men; mean age, 33.6 years ± 10.3).

When the ICHD-II criteria were applied to the MO group, 106 patients (89.1%) were codable to 1.1, 12 (10.1%) to 1.6.1, and one (0.8%) to 2.2. When the Appendix criteria were applied to the same group, 103 patients (86.6%) were codable to A1.1, 15 (12.6%) to 1.6.1, and one (0.8%) to 2.4.2. With the new Appendix criteria, four patients (3.4%) codable to 1.1 using the ICHD-II criteria were now coded to 1.6.1, because they reported nausea as the only associated symptom. By contrast, only one patient codable to 1.6.1 using the ICHD-II criteria could now be coded to A1.1, because the reported associated symptoms were osmophobia and nausea. A total of 34 MO patients out of 119 (28.6%) reported osmophobia in addition to the headache, but in 33 (97.1%) osmophobia was associated with at least two of such other symptoms as photophobia, phonophobia, nausea, and vomiting. Using the ICHD-II criteria in the patients diagnosed with atypical MO by the headache specialist, 12 (52.2%) were codable to 1.1, 10 (43.5%) to 1.6.1, and one (4.3%) to 2.2. Using instead the Appendix criteria, 11 (47.8%) were codable to A1.1, 11 (47.8%) to 1.6.1, and one (4.3%) to 2.4.2.

Discussion

Following the publication of the first edition of the IHS classification,[1] several investigations were carried out to validate the diagnostic criteria for MO.[3–7] However, only a few authors have proposed alternative criteria to those of the IHS: Merikangas et al.[3] remarked that the criteria for MO appear to be too unrestrictive for application in the community, particularly among young adults at the peak period of incidence of migraine, and suggested that criterion D (associated symptoms) of the IHS criteria for MO should be modified to require both gastrointestinal symptoms and photophobia and phonophobia. Rains et al.[7] suggested that revisions should include decreasing the minimum headache duration criteria from 4 h to 2 h. The diagnostic criteria for MO introduced in the Appendix to ICHD-II are very similar to those currently in use: the only differences are the addition of osmophobia to the associated symptoms and the requirement that at least two associated symptoms, i.e. photophobia, phonophobia, osmophobia, nausea, and vomiting, be present for a diagnosis of MO. Among the associated symptoms, a few authors[6] have already indicated osmophobia as highly discriminating for MO versus the other primary headaches, even though the high specificity of this parameter is associated with a low sensitivity.

In our study, the application of the ICHD-II diagnostic criteria for MO in a clinical population led to a correct diagnosis in 89.1% of patients with MO. The percentage of patients with MO diagnosed as MO cases using the Appendix criteria was 86.6%. With these criteria, only one patient, previously diagnosed with probable MO (1.6.1) based on the ICHD-II criteria, could actually be included among the true MO cases (A.1.1), while as many as four patients with MO who reported only nausea as an associated symptom were now diagnosed as probable MO cases and had their coding changed from 1.1. to 1.6.1. The differences between the two sets of criteria as to coding of atypical MO were not significant. Our study does have a few limitations: (i) lacking any specific biological markers allowing for discrimination between the various primary headache subtypes, the diagnostic gold standard obviously depends on subjective interpretation of symptoms; (ii) the gold standard was the judgement of only one specialist, not of a group of specialists, which might have helped reduce the subjective variability of diagnosis. In conclusion, the diagnostic criteria for MO in the Appendix to ICHD-II are helpful in diagnosing most of the patients referred to a headache centre, but changes in the D criterion, as proposed in the Appendix, do not appear to offer any benefits over current diagnostic criteria and do not allow for MO diagnosis in those patients reporting only nausea as an associated symptom.

References

1. Headache Classification Committee of the IHS. Classification and diagnostic criteria for headache disorders, cranial neuralgias and facial pain. *Cephalalgia* 1998; **8** (Suppl 7): 1–96.
2. Headache Classification Committee of the IHS. The International Classification of Headache Disorders, 2nd Edition. *Cephalalgia* 2004; **24** (Suppl 1): 1–160.
3. Merikangas KR, Whitaker AE, Angst J. Validation of diagnostic criteria for migraine in the Zurich longitudinal cohort study. *Cephalalgia* 1993; **13** (Suppl 12): 47–53.
4. Rokicki LA, Semenchuk EM, Bruehl S, *et al*. An examination of the validity of the IHS classification system for migraine and tension-type headache in the college student population. *Headache* 1999; **39**: 720–7.
5. Pajaron E, Lainez JM, Monzon MJ, *et al*. The validity of the classification criteria of the International Headache Society for migraine, episodic tension headache and chronic tension headache. *Neurologia* 1999; **14**: 283–8.
6. Merikangas KR, Dartigues JF, Whitaker A, *et al*. Diagnostic criteria for migraine. A validity study. *Neurology* 1994; **44** (6 Suppl 4): S11–6.
7. Rains JC, Penzien DB, Lipchik GL, *et al*. Diagnosis of migraine: empirical analysis of a large clinical sample of atypical migraine (IHS 1.7) patients and proposed revision of the IHS criteria. *Cephalalgia* 2001; **21**: 584–95.

13 Migraine with aura: IHS-subtypes 1988 compared to 2004 in clinical practice

H. Göbel, A. Heinze, K. Heinze-Kuhn,
U. Todt, and C. Kubisch

Introduction

In the second edition of *The International Classification of Headache Disorders*, the subtypes of migraine with aura have been completely revised. For example, a subtype *migraine with prolonged aura*, i.e. with auras lasting more than 60 min is no longer recognized as a separate entity in 2004, whereas the subtypes *typical aura with migraine headache* and *typical aura with non-migraine headache* have been newly created (Tables 13.1 and 13.2). One essential feature determining the subtyping of auras is the time course of the focal neurologic symptoms. Onset and duration of the aura symptoms as well as the temporal relationship to the following headache have to be considered. Obviously, the other important point is the development of the single aura symptom.[1-5] In this study, we investigated the frequencies of the aura subtypes in a large sample of 536 patients using the classifications of both 1988 and 2004. Furthermore, we compared the aura subtypes regarding the duration of both the aura and the headache phase and the frequency of attacks.

Methods

Information on the kind of aura, duration of the aura and the following headache phase, and the frequency of attacks were collected from 536 patients of the Kiel Pain Clinic and the Institute of Human Genetics, University of Bonn, suffering from migraine with aura. The aura subtypes were diagnosed according to the IHS-classifications of both 1988 and 2004. The aura characteristics were recorded in a

MIGRAINE WITH AURA: COMPARISON OF SUBTYPES 1988 AND 2004 **81**

Table 13.1 Classification of migraine aura (1988)

1.2 Migraine with aura

    1.2.1 Migraine with typical aura
    1.2.2 Migraine with prolonged aura
    1.2.3 Familial hemiplegic migraine
    1.2.4 Basilar migraine
    1.2.5 Migraine aura without headache
    1.2.6 Migraine with acute onset aura

1.3 Ophthalmoplegic migraine
1.4 Retinal migraine
1.6 Complications of migraine

    1.6.1 Status migrainosus
    1.6.2 Migrainous infarction

standardized interview based on the diagnostic criteria of both the new and the old classification systems. The interviews were performed by four physicians experienced in the classification of headaches. The features of all individual aura symptoms were recorded if more than one aura symptom was present.

Results

Based on the diagnostic criteria of the first edition of the IHS-classification, 68.5% of the patients suffered from migraine with typical aura, 22.7% of migraine with prolonged aura, 6.2% of aura without headache, 1.8% of hemiplegic migraine,

Table 13.2 Classification of migraine aura (2004)

1.2 Migraine with aura

    1.2.1 Typical aura with migraine headache
    1.2.2 Typical aura with non-migraine headache
    1.2.3 Typical aura without headache
    1.2.4 Familial hemiplegic migraine (FHM)
    1.2.5 Sporadic hemiplegic migraine
    1.2.6 Basilar-type migraine

1.4 Retinal migraine
1.5 Complications of migraine

    1.5.1 Chronic migraine
    1.5.2 Status migrainosus
    1.5.3 Persistent aura without infarction
    1.5.4 Migrainous infarction
    1.5.5 Migraine-triggered seizures

and 0.9% of basilar migraine (Table 13.3). Based on the second edition of the classification, 89.1% of all patients with typical or prolonged auras, according to the 1988 classification, described a related migraine headache, whereas 4.7% had a non-migraine headache (Table 13.4).

When the duration of aura and headache phase (Table 13.5) were compared, *migraine with prolonged aura* (1988) was associated with longer headache phases (501.04 +/– 885.10 min) than *migraine with typical aura* (34.92 +/– 18.70).

Table 13.3 Distribution of different aura subforms using the first edition of the IHS classification (1988)

	Absolute frequency	Relative frequency %
Typical aura	390	68.5
Prolonged aura	129	22.7
Familial hemiplegic aura	10	1.8
Basilar migraine	5	.9
Aura without headache	35	6.2
Total	569	100.0

Table 13.4 Distribution of different headache phenotypes using the second edition of the IHS classification (2004)

	Absolute frequency	Relative frequency %
Aura without headache	35	6.2
Typical aura with migraine headache	507	89.1
Typical aura with non-migraine headache	27	4.7
Total	569	100.0

Table 13.5 Migraine with aura: frequencies of headache duration

	Absolute frequency	Relative frequency %
1–12 h	148	26.0
–24	125	22.0
–48	121	21.3
–72	109	19.2
Longer than 72 h	33	5.8
Total	536	94.2

Conclusions

The new *migraine with aura* subdivision into *typical aura with migraine headache* and *typical aura with non-migraine headache* in the 2004 IHS-classification is supported by the results of this study. About 5% of the patients suffering from migraine with aura report a related headache which does not fulfil the diagnostic criteria of migraine. In these cases, it therefore seems feasible to base the diagnosis of migraine on the fulfilment of the aura criteria only. The pathophysiological relationship between migraine aura and non-migraine headaches is still unknown.

However, there is also meaningful clinical reasons for the former differentiation between *typical* and *prolonged auras* with 23% prolonged auras being the second most common aura subtype. Migraine with aura therefore should be included in the headache classification again.

References

1. Nyholt DR, Gillespie NG, Heath AC, *et al*. Latent class and genetic analysis does not support migraine with aura and migraine without aura as separate entities. *Genet Epidemiol* 2004; **26** (3): 231–44.
2. Eriksen MK, Thomsen LL, Russell MB. Prognosis of migraine with aura. *Cephalalgia* 2004; **24** (1): 18–22.
3. Wober-Bingol C, Wober C, Karwautz A, *et al*. Clinical features of migraine: a cross-sectional study in patients aged three to sixty-nine. *Cephalalgia* 2004; **24** (1): 12–17.
4. Welch KM. Stroke and migraine – the spectrum of cause and effect. *Funct Neurol* 2003; **18** (3): 121–6.
5. The International Classification of Headache Disorders: 2nd edition. *Cephalalgia* 2004; **24** (Suppl 1): 9–160.

14
ICHD-2 applied to 362 patients with migraine with aura according to ICHD-1

M. K. Eriksen, L. L. Thomsen, and J. Olesen

The second edition of the International Classification of Headache Disorders (ICHD-2)[1] subdivides migraine with aura (MA) differently from the first edition of the classification (ICHD-1),[2] and presents new diagnostic criteria for MA (Table 14.1). The ICHD-2 criteria for MA was based on empirical findings and have a high sensitivity and specificity compared with expert diagnosis according to ICHD-1.[3] The frequency and characteristics (apart from those being part of the diagnostic criteria) of the new ICHD-2 subtypes of MA remain to be described. To evaluate how the new classification of MA works in a clinic population and how patients distribute according to the new subtypes, we applied the ICHD-2 criteria for MA to a large sample previously diagnosed with MA according to ICHD-1.[4,5] Furthermore, we describe a number of clinical differences between the ICHD-2 subtypes of MA.

Materials and methods

A computer search of the National Patient Register and a screening of case records from headache clinics and practising neurologists were used for recruiting MA patients from families with at least one sib pair with both siblings affected with MA and patients with hemiplegic migraine for other studies.[4,6] The recruited patients received a letter before they were contacted by telephone.[6] Out of the 1831 recruited patients, 1365 (labelled as probands) took part in a screening telephone interview: 980 probands were diagnosed with MA of which 189 had a family history of a MA sib pair.[4,6] Selected relatives and probands from these families were contacted for an extensive validated semi-structured telephone interview[7] performed by a trained physician.[3–5] Contact was desirable in 736 living relatives of which 643 took

Table 14.1   Subtypes of migraine with aura

International Classification of Headache Disorders second Edition (ICHD-2)	International Headache Society Classification 1988 (ICHD-1)
1.1 Migraine without aura (MO)*	1.1 Migraine without aura
1.2 Migraine with aura (MA)*	1.2 Migraine with aura
1.2.1 Typical aura with migraine headache (MA-MH)*	1.2.1 Migraine with typical aura
1.2.2 Typical aura with non-migraine headache (MA-NMH)*	1.2.2 Migraine with prolonged aura
1.2.3 Typical aura without headache (MA-WOH)*	1.2.3 Familial hemiplegic migraine
1.2.4 Familial hemiplegic migraine (FHM)	1.2.4 Basilar migraine
1.2.5 Sporadic hemiplegic migraine (SHM)	1.2.5 Migraine aura without headache
1.2.6 Basilar-type migraine (MA-B)*	1.2.6 Migraine with acute onset aura
1.6 Probable migraine	1.7 Migrainous disorder not fulfilling above criteria
1.6.1 Probable migraine without aura[†]	
1.6.2 Probable migraine with aura[‡]	

*Non-official abbreviation.
[†]Attacks fulfilling all but one of the criteria for migraine without aura.
[‡]Attacks fulfilling all but one of the criteria for migraine with aura or any of its subtypes.

part in an interview.[3–5] In total, 105 probands and 257 relatives were diagnosed with MA without hemiplegia (probable MA not included), according to ICHD-1 in an extensive interview, and included in the present study.[3–5] Subsequently, the patients were classified according to ICHD-2 for migraine (Table 14.1). The project was approved by the Danish Ethical Committees.

Results

Migraine with aura according to ICHD-1

The age of the 362 MA patients (M : F ratio 1 : 2.7) was 46 ± 16 years (mean ± SD). Most patients had one or more ICHD-1 subtypes of MA: 54% (197/362) had migraine with typical aura, 17% (62/362) had migraine with prolonged aura, 35% (128/362) had migraine aura without headache, 4% (14/362) had migraine with acute onset aura, and 10% (35/362) had basilar migraine (Fig. 14.1). The presence of ataxia was not considered when diagnosing basilar migraine.[5]

Migraine with aura according to ICHD-2

According to ICHD-2, 89% (322/362) of patients had MA and the remainder had probable MA (Fig. 14.2). The MA patients had at least one ICHD-2 subtype

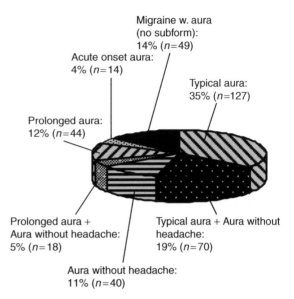

Fig. 14.1 Classification of patients according to the International Headache Society Classification 1988 (ICHD-1) (n=362). All patients were diagnosed with migraine with aura (MA) according to ICHD-1. In addition to the subtypes of MA shown in the diagram, 35 patients had basilar migraine. They were equally distributed among the subgroups of patients. (H: headache).

Migraine w. aura (no subform): 14% (n=49)

Acute onset aura: 4% (n=14)

Typical aura: 35% (n=127)

Prolonged aura: 12% (n=44)

Prolonged aura + Aura without headache: 5% (n=18)

Typical aura + Aura without headache: 19% (n=70)

Aura without headache: 11% (n=40)

of MA: 54% (173/322) had typical aura with migraine headache (MA-MH), 40% (129/322) had typical aura with non-migraine headache (MA-NMH), 37% (120/322) had aura without headache (MA-WOH), and 7% (26/322) had basilar-type migraine (MA-B). In the present study, patients with co-occurring attacks of MA-MH and MA-NMH were only diagnosed with MA-MH although they had both subtypes. Most patients were diagnosed without difficulty. However, six patients had a non-migraine headache beginning before the onset of aura and the headache did not transform into a migraine headache during or after the aura. As a consequence, these patients did not fulfil any of the MA diagnoses and they were diagnosed as probable MA. Another patient had a typical aura followed by a migraine headache with a free interval of 120 min. This patient had to be diagnosed as MA-WOH. In total, 11% of patients did not fulfil the new MA criteria: eight patients had a bilateral prolonged aura, 14 patients had a bilateral acute onset aura, six patients did not fulfil the criterion regarding the associated headache (mentioned above), and 12 patients were unable to remember their aura symptoms in detail. The more recently the patients had had their last MA attack, the better they described their aura ($p=0.022$, Chi-square test).[5]

Co-occurrence of migraine without aura

The co-occurrence of attacks of migraine without aura (MO) was higher in women with MA-MH (patients with MA-B excluded) than in MA-NMH [43% (51/119) vs. 22% (20/91), $p = 0.002$, Chi-square test]. A similar trend was observed in men [30% (9/30) vs. 13% (5/38), $p = 0.13$, Chi-square test]. The co-occurrence of

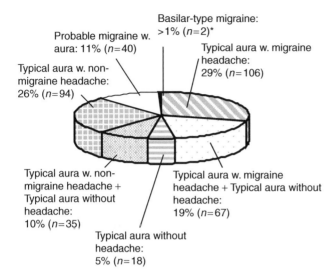

Probable migraine w. aura: 11% (n=40)

Basilar-type migraine: >1% (n=2)*

Typical aura w. non-migraine headache: 26% (n=94)

Typical aura w. migraine headache: 29% (n=106)

Typical aura w. non-migraine headache + Typical aura without headache: 10% (n=35)

Typical aura w. migraine headache + Typical aura without headache: 19% (n=67)

Typical aura without headache: 5% (n=18)

Fig. 14.2 Classification of patients according to the International Classification of Headache Disorders second Edition (ICHD-2) (n = 362). According to ICHD-2 322 patients were diagnosed with migraine with aura (MA) and 40 patients were diagnosed with probable MA. *In addition, 24 patients had basilar-type migraine with co-occurring attacks of typical aura with migraine headache of which eight also had typical aura without headache.

MO attacks in MA-B was identical to the co-occurrence in MA-MH. Three out of 18 patients exclusively with MA-WOH had co-occurrence of MO attacks.

Age at onset, lifetime number of attacks, and attack frequency

The age at onset of MA varied significantly among the ICHD-2 subtypes of MA (Table 14.2). There was a trend towards a higher lifetime number of MA attacks in MA-MH (patients with MA-B excluded) than in MA-NMH: 2–4 attacks in 4 vs. 11 patients, 5–9 attacks in 8 vs. 12 patient, 10–49 attacks in 58 vs. 47 patients, 50–100 attacks in 42 vs. 23 patients, and >100 attacks in 37 vs. 35 patients respectively ($p = 0.054$, Chi-square test on five groups).[5] The lifetime number of attacks in MA-B and MA-WOH was not significantly different from the number of attacks in MA-MH or MA-NMH. The current attack frequency was similar among the ICHD-2 subtypes of MA.

Characteristics of typical aura

The characteristics of the aura symptoms were analysed. Among patients with typical aura according to the ICHD-2, 83% (265/320) of patients fulfilled the criterion of a unilateral aura, 95% (303/320) fulfilled the criterion of a gradual development of the aura, and 85% (271/320) fulfilled the criterion of aura duration.[3,4] Overall, 62% (199/320) of patients with typical aura according to ICHD-2 fulfilled all the criteria just mentioned. Two or more aura symptoms (visual, sensory, or aphasic) occurred in 81% (21/26) of patients with MA-B, 60% (89/149) of patients with MA-MH (patients with MA-B excluded), 70% (90/129) of patients with MA-NMH, and 33% (6/18) of patients with MA-WOH. Patients with MA-B had more aura

Table 14.2 Age at onset between subtypes of migraine with aura according to the International Classification of Headache Disorders, Second Edition (ICHD-2)

	Age at Onset					
	Women (n=238)			Men (n=84)		
Subtype	Mean±SD	(n)	Statistics[†]	Mean±SD	(n)	Statistics[†]
Basilar type migraine	16±7	(19)	p=0.132	22±8	(7)	NS
Typical aura with migraine headache*	20±10	(119)	p=0.044	20±14	(30)	NS
Typical aura with non-migraine headache	23±13	(91)	p=0.024	21±15	(38)	
Typical aura without headache, exclusively	36±18	(9)		31±13	(8)[‡]	p=0.023

*Patients with basilar-type migraine excluded.
[†]Mann–Whitney U test – difference in age at onset between subtypes of migraine with aura. SD – standard deviation. NS – not significant.
[‡]One missing value.

symptoms ($p=0.041$, Chi-square test) and the patients with MA-WOH had less aura symptoms ($p=0.033$, Chi-square test) than patients with MA-MH.

Discussion

Methodological considerations

The patients were diagnosed in a validated[7] semi-structured interview by a trained physician to secure the highest possible accuracy and adherence to the formal diagnostic criteria, and the same physician applied both sets of classification to eliminate inter-observer variability.[3-5] The representativeness of the patients and a comparison to a population-based material have been reported elsewhere.[3-5]

Evaluation of the ICHD-2 criteria for migraine with aura

According to ICHD-2, 89% of our patients (previously diagnosed with MA according to ICHD-1) were diagnosed with MA. Applying ICHD-2 for MA exclusively to patients with current attacks of MA and/or improving the description of the migraine attacks by a diagnostic aura diary would probably improve the sensitivity of the new MA criteria.[8] The ICHD-2 was exhaustive since patients not diagnosed with MA were diagnosed with probable MA (Fig. 14.2). Since only 62% of patients with MA according to ICHD-2 fulfilled each and every sub-criterion for typical aura, our study showed that operational diagnostic criteria are required when diagnosing MA. The ICHD-2 for MA allows variations in symptom characteristics between patients although, the ICHD-2 is less open for subjective interpretations than the ICHD-1.

The ICHD-2 for MA was more effortlessly applied to the patients than ICHD-1. The ICHD-2 outlines exclusively *one* set of criteria for the typical non-hemiplegic *aura* compared to ICHD-1, which outlines *four* different sets of criteria. The ICHD-2 divides MA into various subtypes according to the characteristics of the *headache* related to the aura (Tables 14.1 and 14.2). The new MA criteria acknowledge exclusively a headache beginning during the aura or following the aura within 60 min (Table 14.2). However, in the present study, six patients had a mild headache beginning *before* the onset of aura and consequently they could not be diagnosed with MA according to ICHD-2. These patients certainly suffered from MA since they had a classic visual aura. A prospective recording of the MA attacks of these patients may reveal if the aura begins before the headache. We do not recommend a modification of the MA criteria based on the present finding, since a modification may reduce the specificity of the criteria.

Implications

The classification of MA is intended to delineate homogeneous samples of MA patients. We identified several significant clinical variations between the ICHD-2 subtypes of MA indicating that patients with similar subtype share phenotype and very likely have similar underlying pathology. Thus, our findings suggest that the ICHD-2 subtypes of MA are reasonable and less arbitrary than the ICHD-1 subtypes. MA is a multifactorial, genetically heterogeneous disorder with a complex mode of inheritance but the genes involved have not yet been identified.[9] Previous studies have shown that MA patients predisposed to MA have a more severe phenotype and a lower age at onset.[4,10] Stratifying MA patients by ICHD-2 subtype may be considered in future genetic studies and, furthermore, in experimental studies and drug trials since patients with different MA subtype may show different underlying pathophysiological mechanism and different treatment response. Patients with different ICHD-2 subtype of MA may also require different medical attention. In conclusion, the ICHD-2 for MA is easy to apply, sensitive, and exhaustive. However, it remains to be analysed whether the present MA criteria are the best option or if including other aura characteristics can further improve the validity and reliability of the MA criteria.

References

1. Headache Classification Committee of the International Headache Society. Classification and diagnostic criteria for headache disorders, cranial neuralgias and facial pain. *Cephalalgia* 1988; **8** (7): 1–96.
2. The International Classification of Headache Disorders 2nd Edition. *Cephalalgia* 2004; **24** (1): 1–160.
3. Eriksen M, Thomsen L, Olesen J. Sensitivity and specificity of new diagnostic criteria for migraine with aura. Submitted.
4. Eriksen M, Thomsen L, Olesen J. Clinical characteristics of 362 patients with familial migraine with aura. *Cephalalgia* 2004; **24**: 564–75.
5. Eriksen M, Thomsen L, Olesen J. New international classification of migraine with aura (ICHD-2) applied to 362 migraine patients. *Eur J Neurol* 2004; **11**: 583–91.
6. Lykke Thomsen L, Kirchmann Eriksen M, Faerch Romer S, *et al.* An epidemiological survey of hemiplegic migraine. *Cephalalgia* 2002; **22** (5): 361–75.
7. Russell MB, Rasmussen BK, Thorvaldsen P, *et al.* Prevalence and sex-ratio of the subtypes of migraine. *Int J Epidemiol* 1995; **24** (3): 612–18.
8. Russell MB, Iversen HK, Olesen J. Improved description of the migraine aura by a diagnostic aura diary. *Cephalalgia* 1994; **14** (2): 107–17.
9. Wessman M, Kallela M, Kaunisto MA, *et al.* A susceptibility locus for migraine with aura, on chromosome 4q24. *Am J Hum Genet* 2002; **70** (3): 652–62.
10. Noble-Topham SE, Cader MZ, Dyment DA, *et al.* Genetic loading in familial migraine with aura. *J Neurol Neurosurg Psychiatry* 2003; **74** (8): 1128–30.

15
Validation of new diagnostic criteria (ICHD-2) for migraine with aura

M. K. Eriksen, L. L. Thomsen, and J. Olesen

Migraine with aura (MA) has been diagnosed according to the operational diagnostic criteria of the International Headache Society (ICHD-1) since 1988.[1] The diagnosis of MA relies on the description of symptoms because there are no diagnostic biological markers available. The ICHD-1 for MA was mostly based on expert opinion due to the scarcity of empirical studies. The ICHD-1 for MA was difficult to understand and did not describe the nature of the aura in detail. Therefore, the reliability of the MA diagnosis very likely can be improved. Furthermore, the ICHD-1 for MA comprised a major error as patients could be diagnosed with MA without fulfilling the criterion for presence of any typical aura symptom. For several years, our group has collected data on MA patients for genetic studies. Part of these data were used in a preliminary search for diagnostic criteria for MA with an optimal combination of sensitivity and specificity and the selected criteria were included in ICHD-2.[2,3] In this study, we present the reliability of the new criteria compared with the old one in the sample used for the preliminary search for reliable MA criteria and in an independent sample used for validating the criteria.

Materials and methods

A computer search of the National Patient Register and a screening of case records from headache clinics and practising neurologists were used for recruiting MA patients from families with at least one sib pair with both siblings affected with MA and patients with hemiplegic migraine for other studies.[4,5] The recruited patients received a letter before they were contacted by telephone.[4] Out of the 1831 recruited patients, 1365 (labelled as probands) took part in a screening telephone interview: 980 probands were diagnosed with MA of which 189 had a family history of a MA sib pair.[4,6] Selected relatives and probands from these families were contacted for an extensive validated semi-structured telephone interview[7] performed by a trained physician.[2,6] Contact was desirable in 736 living relatives of which 643 took part in an interview.[2,6] In total, 105 probands and 257 relatives were diagnosed with MA without hemiplegia according to the ICHD-1 in an extensive interview and included in the present study.[2,6] During the recruitment procedure, we furthermore recruited 112 patients with other reversible visual disturbances.[2] Their visual disturbances were not judged to be migraine aura and did not fulfil the ICHD-1 for MA.

The 474 participants were separated into two sub-samples: A training sample of 200 patients (141 randomly selected MA patients plus 59 patients with non-migraine visual disturbances) and a validation sample of 274 patients (the remainder participants). The training sample was used for testing several sets of selected criteria for MA comprising different combinations of three aura characteristics selected a priori in general agreement by the International Headache Classification Committee.[2] The diagnoses made according to the selected criteria were compared to the ICHD-1 diagnoses to select the criteria with the highest sensitivity and specificity for inclusion in the ICHD-2. The accepted criteria were validated on the validation sample. Due to time pressure, the diagnoses made according to the selected diagnostic criteria in the training sample were based exclusively on the *visual symptoms*, whereas the diagnoses made according to the accepted criteria in the validation sample were based on *all aura symptoms*. The project was approved by the Danish Ethical Committees.

Results

Patient characteristics

The age of the 362 MA patients (M : F ratio 1:2.7) was 46 ± 16 years (mean ± SD). Among the MA patients, 61% (220/362) had a combination of aura symptoms and 39% (142/362) had visual aura exclusively (Table 15.1). When more than one aura symptom was observed, they occurred in succession in 96% (149/155) and simultaneously in 4% (6/155) of the MA patients (65 missing values). The age of the 112 patients with non-migraine visual disturbances (M : F ratio 1:2.5) was 41 ± 14 years. The non-migraine visual disturbances were often characterized by flickering light lasting less than 5 min or by general blurring of vision lasting more than 60 min, but they did not fall into well-defined categories (Table 15.1). The headache related to the non-migraine visual disturbances fulfilled the ICHD-1 for migraine without aura (MO) in 37% (41/112) of patients, migrainous disorder without aura in 4% (4/112), and episodic tension-type headache in 16% (18/112) – however, 40% (45/112) had an unspecified headache and 3% (4/112) had no headache.

Testing of selected sets of diagnostic criteria for MA

Five sets of selected criteria for MA were tested on the training sample. The diagnoses made according to the selected sets of criteria were compared to the ICHD-1

Table 15.1 Characteristics of migraine with aura (MA) and other reversible visual disturbances (no MA)

| | MA (n=362) | | | | | | No MA (n=112) | |
| | Visual aura (n=358) | | Sensory aura (n=196) | | Aphasic aura (n=116) | | Visual disturbances (n=112) | |
Symptoms	%*	n	%*	n	%*	n	%*	n
Progression								
Acute onset	19	65	25	47	–	–	87	89
Developing ≥5 min	72	250	62	117	–	–	7	7
Patient cannot say	9	30	12	23	–	–	6	6
Duration†								
<1 min	–	–	–	–	–	–	15	17
1–4 min	<1	1	–	–	–	–	24	27
5–60 min	90	319	86	163	78	81	15	16
>60 min	10	36	14	26	22	23	46	51
Location								
Unilateral	64	225	86	165	–	–	27	29

*Only subjects with valid values included for statistical analysis.
†Recorded as numerical data.

diagnoses (Table 15.2). The set of criteria presented at the top of Table 15.2 was suggested by the Classification Committee but due to the low sensitivity, this set of criteria was rejected. The set of criteria presented at the bottom of Table 15.2 had a high sensitivity (84%) and specificity (97%), and was accepted by the Classification Committee for inclusion in the ICHD-2 for MA.

Validation of accepted diagnostic criteria for MA

The accepted set of criteria for MA was validated on the validation sample: the diagnosis according to the accepted criteria had a sensitivity of 90% and a specificity of 96% when compared to the ICHD-1 diagnosis (Table 15.3). The likelihood ratio of a positive result of the criteria was 23(0.90/[1 – 0.96]) and the likelihood ratio of a negative result was 0.10([1 – 0.90]/0.96).[2]

Discussion

Study design and representativeness

We developed the new diagnostic criteria of MA for the ICHD-2 from one material and tested it on another to avoid random errors and false positive results. Patients were

Table 15.2 Testing of selected sets of diagnostic criteria for migraine with aura (training sample, n = 200)

Set of criteria	Sensitivity (n = 141*)			Specificity (n = 59†)		
	n	%	95% CI	n	%	95% CI
Aura fulfils all of the following three characteristics: 1. Homonymous visual symptoms. 2. The visual symptom develops gradually over ≥5 min 3. The visual symptom lasts ≥5 min and ≤60 min	65	**46**	38–54	59	**100**	98–100
Aura fulfils all of the following three characteristics: 1. Homonymous or *bilateral* visual symptoms. 2. The visual symptom develops gradually over ≥5 mins 3. The visual symptom lasts ≥5 min and ≤60 min	100	**71**	63–78	59	**100**	98–100
Aura fulfils the following characteristic: 1. Homonymous visual symptoms and at least one of the following two characteristics: a. The visual symptom develops gradually over ≥5 min b. The visual symptom lasts ≥5 min and ≤60 min	88	**62**	54–70	56	**95**	89–100
Aura fulfils the following characteristic: 1. Homonymous or *bilateral* visual symptoms and at least one of the following two characteristics: a. The visual symptom develops gradually over ≥5 min b. The visual symptom lasts ≥5 min and ≤60 min	139	**99**	97–100	45	**76**	65–87
Aura fulfils at least two of the following three characteristics: 1. Homonymous visual symptoms. 2. The visual symptom develops gradually over ≥5 min 3. The visual symptom lasts ≥5 min and ≤60 min	118	**84**	79–89	57	**97**	95–99

*Patients with migraine with aura according to the ICHD-1. The sensitivity is the proportion of patients fulfilling the selected set of diagnostic criteria.
†Patients with non-migraine visual disturbances. The specificity is the proportion of patients not fulfilling the selected set of diagnostic criteria.

Table 15.3 Validation of accepted diagnostic criteria for migraine with aura (validation sample, n = 274)

Set of criteria	Sensitivity (n = 221*)			Specificity (n = 53†)		
	n	%	95% CI	n	%	95% CI
Aura fulfils at least two of the following three characteristics: 1. Homonymous visual symptoms and/or unilateral sensory symptoms. 2. At least one aura symptom develops gradually over ≥5 min or different symptoms occur in succession over ≥5 min 3. Each symptom lasts ≥5 min and ≤60 min	199	**90**	86-94	51	**96**	91-100

*Patients with migraine with aura according to ICHD-1. The sensitivity is the proportion of patients fulfilling the selected set of diagnostic criteria.
†Patients with non-migraine visual disturbances. The specificity is the proportion of patients not fulfilling the selected set of diagnostic criteria.

selected from specialist practices and diagnosed in a validated physician-conducted interview. The proportion of patients with unilateral aura and the duration of the aura is identical to those in a population-based study.[6,8] Yet, a gradual develop-ment of the aura is reported less often in the present study (visual aura: 81% vs. 97%, sensory aura: 75% vs. 98%) and a combination of aura symptoms more often (60% vs. 31%) than in the population-based study.[6,8] Some of the variations might increase and some might decrease the sensitivity of the ICHD-2 for MA when applied to population samples.[2] The non-migraine visual disturbances resemble the transient visual disturbances reported in MO. The positive visual dis-turbances in MO may be explained by a suggested lower cortical threshold for visual stimulation and presence of cortical hypersensitivity.[9]

Assessment of reliability and validity

The reliability of the ICHD-2 for MA is believed to be improved compared to ICHD-1 as the criteria are further operationalized and a description of the typical aura is included.[3] The MA diagnosis now relies less on a clinical judgement. Overall, ICHD-1 has been shown to have good reliability but the studies included few MA patients.[10] Future studies will show if the ICHD-2 for MA live up to the expectedly increased reliability. The validity of the ICHD-2 for MA is believed to be fair because it is based on a large material in which the MA diagnoses were supported by a long history of MA, a history of previous MA diagnosis and treatment, and a strong family predisposition to MA.[6] Furthermore, the criteria were developed in agreement by experts and in agreement with empirical findings of aura characteris-tics.[8] Eventually, the validity of the ICHD-2 for MA may be tested against the genetic constitution of MA, the response to novel selective drugs such as tonabersat that may prevent cortical spreading depression, or the characteristic cerebral blood flow change during MA attacks.

Implications

The ICHD-2 for MA accepts only three kinds of aura: visual, sensory, and aphasic aura.[3] However, it must be remembered that additional symptoms do not affect the diagnosis. Thus, the new criteria will enable an analysis of how often other symp-toms may co-occur. Analysing further aura characteristics using regression models may reveal if including other characteristics can further improve the criteria. Since a headache related to aura is a variable feature in MA,[6,8] the presence and the char-acteristics of the headache is used only for sub-diagnosing MA patients in the ICHD-2.[3] However, diagnostic caution is required when aura is not followed by headache and if sensory and aphasic symptoms occur without visual aura.[6] Whenever there is diagnostic uncertainty, appropriate investigations should rule out intracranial pathology even if the patient fulfils the MA criteria. In conclusion, the ICHD-2 for MA has a high sensitivity and specificity when compared to ICHD-1 diagnoses. The new criteria are more operational and probably delineate a more homogeneous sample of MA patients than ICHD-1. By narrowing the definition of the trait, one will include only individuals likely to have a similar aetiology leading to the disease phenotype. The ICHD-2 for MA has significant implications for case finding in future research and in clinical diagnosis.

References

1. Headache Classification Committee of the International Headache Society. Classification and diagnostic criteria for headache disorders, cranial neuralgias and facial pain. *Cephalalgia* 1988; **8** (7): 1–96.
2. Eriksen M, Thomsen L, Olesen J. Sensitivity and specificity of new diagnostic criteria for migraine with aura. Submitted.
3. The International Classification of Headache Disorders 2nd Edition. *Cephalalgia* 2004; **24** (1): 1–160.
4. Lykke Thomsen L, Kirchmann Eriksen M, Faerch Romer S, *et al.* An epidemiological survey of hemiplegic migraine. *Cephalalgia* 2002; **22** (5): 361–75.
5. Thomsen LL, Eriksen MK, Roemer SF, *et al.* A population-based study of familial hemiplegic migraine suggests revised diagnostic criteria. *Brain* 2002; **125** (Pt 6): 1379–91.
6. Eriksen M, Thomsen L, Olesen J. Clinical characteristics of 362 patients with familial migraine with aura. *Cephalalgia* 2004; **24**: 564–75.
7. Russell MB, Rasmussen BK, Thorvaldsen P, *et al.* Prevalence and sex-ratio of the subtypes of migraine. *Int J Epidemiol* 1995; **24** (3): 612–18.
8. Russell MB, Olesen J. A nosographic analysis of the migraine aura in a general population. *Brain* 1996; **119** (Pt 2): 355–61.
9. Mulleners WM, Chronicle EP, Palmer JE, *et al.* Suppression of perception in migraine: evidence for reduced inhibition in the visual cortex. *Neurology* 2001; **56** (2): 178–83.
10. Granella F, D'Alessandro R, Manzoni GC, *et al.* International Headache Society classification: interobserver reliability in the diagnosis of primary headaches. *Cephalalgia* 1994; **14** (1): 16–20.

Session

III

The primary headaches: Part II

16 Tension-type headache: what is new in the second edition of the International Classification of Headache Disorders?

L. Bendtsen and R. Jensen

Introduction

The classification of tension-type headache is not simple. Tension-type headache is the most common of primary headaches with a lifetime prevalence of 30%–78% thus known to almost everybody, but it is also the most featureless of headaches, which obviously makes classification difficult. It is also the headache type with the highest socioeconomic impact of all primary headaches and yet one of the least studied headaches, which hampers progress in classification.

In the second edition of The International Classification of Headache Disorders,[1] several important changes have been made including the subdivision of episodic tension-type headache into infrequent and frequent forms, the segregation of a new entity called new daily-persistent headache, and, important with regard to chronic tension-type headache, the criteria for medication-overuse headache have been strengthened and specified in more detail. The basic criteria for headache characteristics and accompanying symptoms, however, are largely unchanged.

Subdivision on the basis of headache frequency

In the first edition of the headache classification,[2] tension-type headache was divided arbitrarily into an episodic and a chronic form on the basis of whether headache frequency was below or equal/above 15 days per month. The disability of tension-type headache is closely related to frequency. Thus, having tension-type headache of mild intensity for a few hours a month is only a minor problem, not a disease; while tension-type headache of moderate intensity lasting from when the patient wakes up till he or she goes to bed each and every day is a heavy burden. Moreover, since the number of patients with daily or almost daily tension-type headache is far greater than the analogous situation in other primary headache disorders, chronic tension-type headache is a major problem not only for the individual sufferer but also for the society. Equally important, the episodic and the chronic forms have proved to differ in pathophysiological aspects.[3,4] Thus, although tension-type headache was arbitrarily divided on the basis of frequency in the first edition of the headache classification, this division has proved to be highly meaningful. The episodic form has been further divided in the new edition, into infrequent and frequent episodic tension-type headache (Table 16.1). The infrequent form occurs less than once per month and has therefore very little impact on the individual and the society. Persons with this very infrequent type of headache are usually regarded as healthy individuals, although not completely headache-free. The frequent episodic form occurs between one and fifteen days per month and may cause significant disability as well as a risk of analgesic overuse and chronification of headache.

The discrepancies in prevalence of tension-type headache in former epidemiological studies are mainly due to this sub-grouping of episodic tension-type headache, as some studies have included subjects with very few headache episodes per year and have found a very high last year prevalence of up to 74%,[5] whereas others may have included only those subjects that suffered from more frequent episodes and found prevalence rates at about 38%.[6,7] When the new subdivision is applied to a recent epidemiological material, 43% of a general population have infrequent episodic tension-type headache and 37% suffer from frequent episodic tension-type headache (Lyngberg et al., submitted). These new data indicate that the subdivision of episodic tension-type headache in the revised classification will lead to more consistent results between epidemiological studies. In addition, the subdivision will probably stimulate pathophysiological research in frequent tension-type headache. In particular, it is of major importance to identify mechanisms and risk factors for transformation of frequent episodic to chronic tension-type headache.

Subdivision on the basis of pericranial tenderness

In the first edition of the headache classification, tension-type headache was divided into forms associated and not associated with a muscular factor on the basis of one of the three measurements, (a) pericranial tenderness to manual palpation,

Table 16.1   Diagnostic criteria for episodic tension-type headache.
The International Classification of Headache Disorders, 2nd edition

---

2.1. Infrequent episodic tension-type headache

    A. At least 10 episodes occurring on <1 day per month on average
        (<12 days per year) and fulfilling criteria B–D
    B. Headache lasting from 30 minutes to 7 days
    C. Headache has at least two of the following characteristics:

        1. bilateral location
        2. pressing/tightening (non-pulsating) quality
        3. mild or moderate intensity
        4. not aggravated by routine physical activity such as walking or
           climbing stairs

    D. Both of the following.

        1. no nausea or vomiting (anorexia may occur)
        2. no more than one of photophobia or phonophobia

    E. Not attributed to another disorder[1]

Note:
    1. History and physical and neurological examination do not suggest any
        of the disorders listed in groups 5–12, or history and/or physical and/or
        neurological examinations do suggest such disorders but it is ruled out by
        appropriate investigations, or such disorder is present but headache does
        not occur for the first time in close temporal relation to the disorder.

2.2. Frequent episodic tension-type headache

    A. At least 10 episodes occurring on ≥1 but <15 days per month for
        at least 3 months (≥12 and <180 days per year) and fulfilling criteria B–D
    B. Same as 2.1
    C. Same as 2.1
    D. Same as 2.1
    E. Same as 2.1

(b) electromyographic (EMG) activity, and (c) pressure pain thresholds. Since then, it has been demonstrated that manual palpation, but not EMG or pressure algometry, can be used to discriminate between subjects with and without a muscular factor.[8] In the revised classification, subdivision into forms associated or not associated with a muscular factor is therefore based on the presence or absence of myofascial tenderness to manual palpation. On the third digit level, subjects are subdivided into both episodic and chronic tension-type headaches with (1) designating increased pericranial tenderness on manual palpation and (2) designating no increased tenderness.

    A palpometer that allows the control of palpation pressure has been developed. By means of this device, it has been demonstrated that although there is great variability in the pressure exerted between physicians, the pressure exerted by the individual physician is stable from week to week.[4] Thus, in daily clinical practice, tenderness can be measured by manual palpation without the need of an apparatus as long as the observer is the same. Pericranial tenderness is the most significant abnormal finding in tension-type headache and tenderness is related to the intensity and frequency of headache[3] as well as to the efficacy of prophylactic treatments.[9] Therefore, the subdivision is relevant both in daily clinical practice and in research, but whether tenderness is a cause or an effect of headache is not yet clear.

New daily persistent headache

Chronic tension-type headache usually evolves over time (several years) from episodic tension-type headache.[10] This is most likely due to the development of central sensitization caused by prolonged nociceptive input from pericranial myofascial tissues.[3,4] It is therefore conceivable that tension-type like headache that is daily and unremitting from start is a separate disorder. This is supported by clinical observations.[11] The revised classification has therefore included a new entity called 4.8 *New daily-persistent headache*. This entity has headache characteristics and accompanying symptoms identical to chronic tension-type headache, but instead of having evolved from episodic tension-type headache, it has become daily and unremitting from within 3 days of onset. It is important that this development is unambiguously remembered by the patient. If not, the headache should be classified as 2.3 *Chronic tension-type headache* (Table 16.2, Note 1). The segregation of *New daily-persistent headache* from *chronic tension-type headache* will hopefully stimulate studies of whether the two entities differ clinically, pathophysiologically, and with respect to treatment as *New daily-persistent headache* usually is fairly refractory to any kind of treatment.

Medication overuse

The utmost importance of considering medication overuse when treating chronic headaches has been known for many years, but before 1988 only limited research had been done in this area. Since the publication of the first edition of the classification, several important studies have investigated this problem.[12,13] As a consequence, the diagnostic criteria for 8.2 *Medication-overuse headache* have been strengthened and specified in more detail. An important note regarding medication-overuse headache has been added to the diagnostic criteria for chronic tension-type headache (Table 16.2, Note 3), which emphasizes that medication intake has to be considered before the diagnosis of chronic tension-type headache is given.

If the patient has an intake of medications that exceeds the limits specified in 8.2 *Medication-overuse headache*, the default rule is to code for 2.4.3 *Probable chronic tension-type headache* plus 8.2.7 *Probable medication-overuse headache*. Two months after overuse has stopped, a final diagnosis can be applied, i.e. 2.3 *Chronic tension-type headache* if the headache is still chronic or 8.2 *Medication-overuse headache* if headache has resolved or reverted to its previous pattern.

Table 16.2 Diagnostic criteria for chronic tension-type headache.
The International Classification of Headache Disorders, 2nd edition

2.3. Chronic tension-type headache

   A. Headache occurring on ≥15 days per month on average for >3 months
(≥180 days per year)[1] and fulfilling criteria B–D
   B. Headache lasts hours or may be continuous
   C. Headache has at least two of the following characteristics:

     1. bilateral location
     2. pressing/tightening (non-pulsating) quality
     3. mild or moderate intensity
     4. not aggravated by routine physical activity such as walking or
climbing stairs

   D. Both of the following:

     1. no more than one of photophobia, phonophobia, or mild nausea
     2. neither moderate or severe nausea nor vomiting

   E. Not attributed to another disorder[2,3]

Notes:

1. 2.3 *Chronic tension-type headache* evolves over time from episodic
tension-type headache; when these criteria A–E are fulfilled by headache that,
unambiguously, is daily and unremitting within 3 days of its first onset, code as
4.8 *New daily-persistent headache*. When the manner of onset is not remembered
or is otherwise uncertain, code as 2.3 *Chronic tension-type headache*.
2. Same as note 1 for episodic tension-type headache.
3. When medication overuse is present and fulfils criterion B for any of the
subforms of 8.2 *Medication-overuse headache*; it is uncertain whether this
criterion E is fulfilled until 2 months after medication has been withdrawn
without improvement.

Tension-type headache versus migraine without aura

It can be difficult to differentiate between episodic tension-type headache and mild
migraine without aura, in particular in patients who suffer from both entities and
treat their migraine attacks very early as recently recommended.[14] In the committee,
it was suggested to tighten the criteria for tension-type headache so that three out of
four pain characteristics should be fulfilled and no accompanying symptoms should
be allowed in order to better separate the two conditions. However, this would
lower the sensitivity of the criteria. The subcommittee estimated that approximately 12% of headaches would be classified as 2.4 *Probable tension-type headache*
or 1.6 *Probable migraine* if at least three out of four pain characteristics should be
fulfilled. The population-based epidemiological study by Rasmussen *et al.*[15] showed
that 10% of patients with episodic tension-type headaches had phonophobia and
7% photophobia. The problem with lack of sensitivity is more prominent in

chronic tension-type headache, where 42% of headaches could not be classified if no accompanying symptoms were allowed, 25% due to nausea, 12% due to photophobia, and 4% due to phonophobia.[15] These findings were confirmed in a recent clinical study based on four-week headache diaries, where 46% of chronic tension-type headaches were associated with nausea (25%) or photophobia or phonophobia (21%) (unpublished data from the authors). The subcommittee concluded that the strict criteria would result in unacceptable loss of specificity and therefore chose to include the more strict alternative criteria as an appendix to the new edition of the classification. The alternative diagnostic criteria requires that at least three pain characteristics are fulfilled (instead of two) and that no accompanying symptoms are present. Previously, it has also been suggested that the accompanying symptoms should be graded to increase specificity,[15] but this would probably complicate daily clinical work too much. The inclusion of the appendix to the second edition of the classification will hopefully stimulate research on these aspects.

Chronic tension-type headache versus other chronic primary headaches

The classification of frequent headaches is the part of the first classification that has been most discussed and much effort has been spent with various attempts to improve the diagnostic criteria of frequent headaches. In 1994, Silberstein suggested the term 'chronic daily headache' to designate headaches lasting 4 h or more and occurring 15 days or more per month.[16] Chronic daily headache includes chronic migraine, chronic tension-type headache, new daily-persistent headache, and hemicrania continua. Chronic daily headache has not been included in the revised classification, but the suggested three novel entities mentioned above have. The inclusion of 1.5.1 *Chronic migraine* constitutes a problem, because headaches can theoretically fulfil both the criteria for this entity and for 2.3 *Chronic tension-type headache* if two, and only two, of the four pain characteristics are present and if headaches at the same time are associated with nausea and no other accompanying symptoms. To minimize this problem and better differentiate between chronic tension-type headache and chronic migraine, the criteria for the degree of nausea allowed in chronic tension-type headache have been strengthened in the revised classification, so that only mild nausea, not moderate and severe nausea, is allowed (see 2.3.D in Table 16.2). This means that headaches fulfil criteria for both chronic tension-type headache and chronic migraine only if two, and only two, of the four pain characteristics are present and if headaches at the same time are associated with *mild* nausea and no other accompanying symptoms. When this rare situation happens, one must make the best choice between the two possible diagnoses from other available clinical evidence.

We find that the term chronic daily headache should only be used as an unspecific, clinical working description and never as a final diagnosis due to lack of specificity.[17]

Most patients in specialized headache clinics suffer from several different primary and secondary headaches at the same time[11] and deserve a careful characterization before a rational therapy can be initiated.

Conclusions

The basic diagnostic criteria for tension-type headache have been kept largely unchanged in the revised classification, which is of paramount importance for the acceptance and continued use of the classification among colleagues less familiar with headaches. However, important changes have been made on the second and third digit levels allowing more detailed classification with regard to, e.g. headache frequency, evolution of headache over time, and medication overuse. Hopefully, these improvements in the classification will lead to better clinical characterization of patients with tension-type headache and stimulate research in pathophysiological mechanisms and treatment of this very prevalent disorder.

References

1. The International Classification of Headache Disorders: 2nd edition. *Cephalalgia* 2004; **24** (Suppl 1): 9–160.
2. Headache Classification Committee of the International Headache Society. Classification and diagnostic criteria for headache disorders, cranial neuralgias and facial pain. *Cephalalgia* 1988; **8** (Suppl 7): 1–96.
3. Jensen R. Pathophysiological mechanisms of tension-type headache: a review of epidemiological and experimental studies. *Cephalalgia* 1999; **19**: 602–21.
4. Bendtsen L. Central sensitization in tension-type headache – possible pathophysiological mechanisms. *Cephalalgia* 2000; **20**: 486–508.
5. Rasmussen BK, Jensen R, Schroll M, *et al*. Epidemiology of headache in a general population – a prevalence study. *J Clin Epidemiol* 1991; **44**: 1147–57.
6. Göbel H, Petersen-Braun M, Soyka D. The epidemiology of headache in Germany: a nationwide survey of a representative sample on the basis of the headache classification of the International Headache Society. *Cephalalgia* 1994; **14**: 97–106.
7. Schwartz BS, Stewart WF, Simon D, *et al*. Epidemiology of tension-type headache. *JAMA* 1998; **4**: 381–3.
8. Jensen R, Rasmussen BK. Muscular disorders in tension-type headache. *Cephalalgia* 1996; **16**: 97–103.
9. Bendtsen L, Jensen R. Amitriptyline reduces myofascial tenderness in patients with chronic tension-type headache. *Cephalalgia* 2000; **20**: 603–10.
10. Langemark M, Olesen J, Poulsen DL, *et al*. Clinical characterization of patients with chronic tension headache. *Headache* 1988; **28**: 590–6.
11. Bigal ME, Sheftell FD, Rapoport AM, *et al*. Chronic daily headache in a tertiary care population: correlation between the International Headache Society diagnostic criteria and proposed revisions of criteria for chronic daily headache. *Cephalalgia* 2002; **22**: 432–8.
12. Limmroth V, Katsarava Z, Fritsche G, *et al*. Features of medication overuse headache following overuse of different acute headache drugs. *Neurology* 2002; **59**: 1011–14.

13. Katsarava Z, Limmroth V, Finke M, *et al*. Rates and predictors for relapse in medication overuse headache: a 1-year prospective study. *Neurology* 2003; **60**: 1682–3.
14. Burstein R, Collins B, Jakubowski M. Defeating migraine pain with triptans: a race against the development of cutaneous allodynia. *Ann Neurol* 2004; **55**: 19–26.
15. Rasmussen BK, Jensen R, Olesen J. A population-based analysis of the diagnostic criteria of the International Headache Society. *Cephalalgia* 1991; **11**: 129–34.
16. Silberstein SD, Lipton RB, Solomon S, *et al*. Classification of daily and near-daily headaches: proposed revisions to the IHS criteria. *Headache* 1994; **34**: 1–7.
17. Jensen R, Bendtsen L. Is chronic daily headache a useful diagnosis? *J Headache Pain* In press, 2004.

17
Trigeminal autonomic cephalalgias

P. J. Goadsby

Introduction

The Trigeminal Autonomic Cephalalgias (TACs) is a grouping of headache syndromes recognized in the second edition of the International Headache Society classification.[1] The term was coined to reflect some part of the pathophysiology of these conditions that is a common thread, viz., excessive cranial parasympathetic autonomic reflex activation to nociceptive input in the ophthalmic division of the trigeminal nerve.[2] The TACs are classified in Section III of the second edition of the classification,[1] and include cluster headache,[3] paroxysmal hemicrania, and short-lasting unilateral neuralgiform headache attacks with conjunctival injection and tearing (SUNCT).[4] In an early draft, hemicrania continua was included but this was finally classified in Section IV. I will briefly review the underlying physiology of the trigeminal autonomic reflex that underpins these conditions, set out their classification, and point out the limitations and some directions for future research.

Pathophysiology of TACs

Any pathophysiological construct for TACs must account for the two major clinical features characteristic of the various conditions that comprise this group: trigeminal distribution pain and ipsilateral cranial autonomic features.[2] The pain-producing innervation of the cranium projects through branches of the trigeminal and upper cervical nerves[5,6] to the trigeminocervical complex[7] from whence nociceptive pathways project to higher centers.[8]

Experimental studies

Stimulation of the trigeminal ganglion in the cat produces cranial vasodilation[9] and neuropeptide release, notably calcitonin gene-related peptide (CGRP) and substance P.[10] The dilation is mediated by antidromic activation of the trigeminal nerve, 20% of the effect, and orthodromic activation through the cranial parasympathetic outflow via the facial (VIIth) cranial nerve, the other 80%. The afferent arm of the trigeminal-parasympathetic reflex traverses the trigeminal root,[9] synapses in the trigeminal nucleus, and then projects to neurons of the superior salivatory nucleus in the pons.[11] There is a glutamatergic excitatory receptor[12] and projection via the facial nerve[13] without synapse in the geniculate ganglion. The greater superficial petrosal nerve supplies classical autonomic pre-ganglionic fibers to the sphenopalatine (pterygopalatine in humans) and otic ganglia.[14] The sphenopalatine synapse is a hexamethonium-sensitive nicotinic ganglion.[14] The VIIth cranial nerve effect is associated with release of vasoactive intestinal polypeptide (VIP)[15] and blocked by VIP antibodies.[16] In terms of brain blood flow, it is frequency dependent[17,18] and cerebral metabolism independent.[19] There is VIP in the sphenopalatine ganglion,[20] as well as nitric oxide synthase, which is also involved in the vasodilator mechanism.[21]

Human studies

This basic science work implies an integral role for the ipsilateral trigeminal nociceptive pathways in TACs, and predicts in some patients cranial parasympathetic autonomic activation. The ipsilateral autonomic features seen clinically are consistent with cranial parasympathetic activation (lacrimation, rhinorrhea, nasal congestion, and eyelid edema) and sympathetic hypofunction (ptosis and miosis). The latter is likely to be a neurapraxic effect of carotid swelling[22,23] with cranial parasympathetic activation. Some degree of cranial autonomic symptomatology is, therefore, a normal physiologic response to cranial nociceptive input.[24–26] Indeed other primary headaches, notably migraine,[27] or patients with facial pain such as trigeminal neuralgia,[28] would be expected to have cranial autonomic activation, as they do. The distinction between the TACs and other headache syndromes is the degree of cranial autonomic activation, not its presence alone.[29]

Permitting trigeminal-parasympathetic activation

What is the basis for the cranial autonomic symptoms being so prominent in the TACs? Is it due to a central disinhibition of the trigeminal-autonomic reflex?[29] Evidence from functional imaging studies: positron emission tomography studies in cluster headache[30,31] and a functional MRI study in SUNCT syndrome,[32] has demonstrated ipsilateral posterior hypothalamic activation. Posterior hypothalamic activation seems specific to these syndromes and is not seen in episodic[33,34] or chronic[35] migraine, or in experimental ophthalmic trigeminal distribution head pain.[36] There are direct hypothalamic-trigeminal connections[37] and the hypothalamus is known to have a modulatory role on the nociceptive and autonomic pathways. Hence, cluster headache and SUNCT syndrome are probably due to an abnormality in the region of the hypothalamus with subsequent trigeminovascular and cranial autonomic activation. Imaging data with paroxysmal hemicrania is keenly awaited.

Differential diagnosis of TACs

The TACs need to be differentiated from secondary TAC-producing lesions, from other primary headaches, and from each other. The differentiation from secondary causes is not that problematic if one images patients but can be extremely difficult if one does not. An MRI of the brain with attention to the pituitary fossa and cavernous sinus will detect most secondary causes. It is easy to make an argument given the rarity of paroxysmal hemicrania and SUNCT that MRI would be a reasonable part of the initial review of such patients. It is more complex for cluster headache. There are no clear studies, our impression from a cohort that now exceeds 400 (the National Hospital for Neurology and Neurosurgery, Queen Square, London) is that MRI would detect no more than 1 in 100 cases of lesions in episodic cluster headache, so we cannot recommend it. For chronic cluster headache, an MRI seems reasonable given that very difficult nature of the long-term management and developments in neuromodulation as a treatment.

For other primary headaches, migraine is the single biggest problem for cluster headache differential diagnosis. Migraine can *cluster* and despite the best intentions of the IHS classification committee, short attacks do occur. Moreover, while cranial autonomic symptoms do not occur they are well-reported,[27] and the neuropeptide changes are the same[38] as in cluster headache.[39] The occurrence of attacks together does not seem to have the seasonal preponderance that is so typical of cluster headache, and this can be a useful differential diagnostic feature. This author regards the term *cluster migraine* as unhelpful and is yet to see a convincing case of a distinct biological entity usefully described by this name. The criterion for the effect of movement was added to cluster headache to sharpen the difference with migraine. The Committee hoped this would draw attention to the fact that most cluster headache patients feel restless or agitated,[40] while most migraine patients are quiescent, as IHS-I recognized.[41] In clinical practice, this symptom and the periodicity are extremely helpful in differential diagnosis. The other feature of cluster headache, and this is a feature of TACs when compared to migraine, is that patients with TACs often complain of unilateral, homolateral photophobia, where migraineurs complain of bilateral photophobia. Bilateral photophobia in TAC patients could be speculated to occur in about 25% purely by the chance of them having some migrainous biology.

The TACs themselves (Table 17.1) can often be differentiated by their attack length. This is certainly true when comparing cluster headache to SUNCT/SUNA. The IHS criteria for TACs does betray an uncomfortable naivety with regard to the timing by setting up the ranges. The A, C, D, E/F criteria are rather similar for each TAC (Tables 17.2–17.4). It seems neat in some way to have SUNCT be up to 4 min long, paroxysmal hemicrania from 2 to 30 min, and cluster headache from 15 min onwards. The overlap seems minimal. It almost goes without saying that this must be wrong in absolute terms but does provide a very useful way to identify cases of sufficient similarity to make meaningful biological studies. If these

Table 17.1 Clinical features of trigeminal autonomic cephalalgias (TACs)

	Cluster headache	Paroxysmal hemicrania	SUNCT syndrome
Sex F:M	1:4	2:1	1:2
Pain			
Type	Stabbing, boring	Throbbing, boring, stabbing	Burning, stabbing, sharp
Severity	Excruciating	Excruciating	Moderate to severe
Site	Orbit, temple	Orbit, temple	Periorbital
Attack frequency	1/alternate day –8 daily	1–40/day	1/day–30/h
Duration of attack	15–180 min	2–30 min	5–240 s
Autonomic features	Yes	Yes	Yes (prominent conjunctival injection *and* lacrimation)
Migrainous features*	Yes	Yes	No**
Alcohol trigger	Yes	Occasional	No
Indomethacin effect	–	++	–

*Nausea, photophobia (often ipsilateral to the pain) or phonophobia.
**May have photophobia ipsilateral to the pain.

Table 17.2 Cluster headache

3.1 Diagnostic criteria:
  A. At least five attacks fulfilling B-D.
  B. Severe or very severe unilateral orbital, supraorbital, and/or temporal pain lasting 15–180 min if untreated.
  C. Headache is accompanied by at least one of the following:
    1. ipsilateral conjunctival injection and/or lacrimation
    2. ipsilateral nasal congestion and/or rhinorrhoea
    3. forehead and facial sweating
    4. ipsilateral eyelid oedema
    5. ipsilateral forehead and facial sweating
    5. ipsilateral miosis and/or ptosis
    6. a sense of restlessness or agitation
  D. Attacks have a frequency from 1 every other day to 8 per day.
  E. Not attributed to another disorder.

3.1.1 *Episodic cluster headache*
  Description: Occurs in periods lasting 7 days to 1 year separated by pain-free periods lasting one month or more
  Diagnostic criteria:
  A. All fulfilling criteria A–E of 3.1.
  B. At least 2 cluster periods lasting from 7 to 365 days and separated by pain-free remissions of ≥1 month.

3.1.2 *Chronic cluster headache*
  Description: Attacks occur for >1 year without remission or with remissions lasting <1 month.
  Diagnostic criteria:
  A. All alphabetical headings of 3.1.
  B. Attacks recur over >1 year without remission periods or with remission periods <1 month

conditions behave as other human conditions we will see a distribution with tails that provide overlap; however, if we use the well-defined cases for our studies we should be able to understand the overlaps and subtleties better.

Challenges for the TACs

The classification and biology of the TACs has come a long way in a short time. The syndromes are well-established, and although rare compared to migraine they are sufficiently common, with cluster headache affecting about 0.2% of the population,[42] to demand neurological and headache specialist's attention. There are some particular issues of classification that are not currently clear.

Table 17.3 Paroxysmal hemicrania

3.2 Diagnostic criteria:
   A. At least 20 attacks fulfilling B–D.
   B. Severe unilateral orbital, supraorbital, or temporal pain lasting 2–30 min.
   C. Headache is accompanied by at least one of the following:
      1. ipsilateral conjunctival injection and/or lacrimation
      2. ipsilateral nasal congestion and/or rhinorrhoea
      3. forehead and facial sweating
      4. ipsilateral eyelid oedema
      5. ipsilateral forehead and facial sweating
      5. ipsilateral miosis and/or ptosis
   D. Attacks have a frequency above 5 per day for more than half the time, although periods with lower frequency may occur
   E. Attacks are prevented completely by therapeutic dose of indomethacin
   F. Not attributed to another disorder

3.2.1 *Episodic paroxysmal headache*
      Description: Occurs in periods lasting 7 days to 1 year separated by pain–free periods lasting 1 month or more.
3.2.2 *Chronic paroxysmal headache*
      Description: Attacks occur for >1 year without remission or with remissions lasting <1 month.

Cluster headache

A patient with a first attack of cluster headache is now simply classified as cluster headache (3.1). This takes the top-down view, i.e. diagnose what you can and fill in the detail as it is available. Such cases are unsuitable for almost any study except natural history studies, where they are ideally the starting point. A similar problem is how to refer to patients who have one type of TAC, typically an episodic form, and then evolve to the chronic form. The old classification differentiated

Table 17.4 Short-lasting Unilateral Neuralgiform headache attacks with Conjunctival injection and Tearing (SUNCT)

3.3 Diagnostic criteria:
   A. At least 20 attacks fulfilling criteria B–E
   B. Attacks of unilateral, orbital, supraorbital, or temporal stabbing or pulsating pain last 5–240 s
   C. Pain is accompanied by ipsilateral conjunctival injection and lacrimation
   D. Attacks occur with a frequency from 3 to 200 per day
   E. Not attributed to another disorder

Table 17.5 Treatment effects on TACs

	Cluster headache	Paroxysmal hemicrania	SUNCT syndrome
Indomethacin effect	–	++	–
Abortive treatment	◆ Sumatriptan s/c or NS ◆ Oxygen	Nil	Nil
Preventive treatment	◆ Verapamil ◆ Methysergide ◆ Lithium ◆ Prednisone	◆ Indomethacin	◆ Lamotrigine ◆ Topiramate ◆ Gabapentin

primary from secondary chronic cluster headache depending on whether there was a period of episodic headache first. This argument would apply equally to chronic paroxysmal hemicrania. There seems little evidence that the clinical characteristics or therapeutic behavior of primary or secondary chronic cluster headache are different. Moreover, the main clinical imperative when the timing changes would be review, perhaps with investigation, but this is a generic principle in the management of headache that does, of itself, not justify the two terms. For the moment, the distinction has been dropped. It will be interesting to see if studies can reinstate it.

Paroxysmal hemicrania (PH)

The diagnosis of PH by the IHS criteria requires a response to indomethacin. This is very difficult. It is not clear what the basis for the indomethacin effect is, although it is perfectly clear that the effect is clinically very meaningful (Table 17.5). Patients with PH who are treated with indomethacin have an almost unbelievably spectacular resolution. We have recently explored this response in comparison to placebo in a single-blind randomized fashion (Cittadini and Goadsby, unpublished data). A typical hemicrania continua patient is shown in Fig. 17.1 as an example. The response is rapid, clear, and lasts many hours. However, there are patients with short-lasting headache attacks, lasting 20–30 min who fit all the other criteria and yet are unresponsive to indomethacin.[43] For the moment, these patients are classified with cluster headache and time will reveal whether this is correct. Indeed, brain imaging may be helpful in general biological terms if it differentiates PH from cluster headache, although the greatest gains will come from understanding how indomethacin works. Our impression is that indomethacin may be no better than placebo in cluster headache, taking 1 h as a lower limit of attacks to test to avoid overlap with longer lasting PH that may be indomethacin-insensitive, if that exists.

In regard to insensitivity, we have certainly seen a requirement for a single dose, given first thing in the morning, of 300 mg indomethacin to produce a complete response. It is entirely possible that there are dosing requirements that are unrecognized. There is certainly a timing requirement and again we have seen patients turn off but only after 10 days at the dose of 275 mg daily.

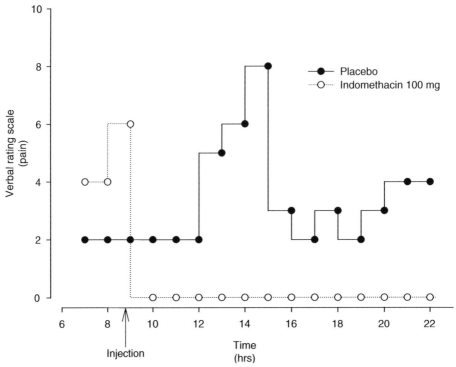

Fig. 17.1 A placebo-controlled indomethacin test, where a patient has single blinded an injection of either saline or indomethacin (100 mg at the same fixed time of the day (↑) and records their pain on a verbal rating scale for the following 24 h while they are awake. The case is an example of hemicrania continua, although the principle may be applied to any of the indomethacin-sensitive headaches. Placebo produces no clear response while indomethacin markedly and for many hours suppresses the headache syndrome.

SUNCT

For SUNCT, the most immediate challenge must be to define the phenotype properly. We certainly have seen patients who fulfil criteria for SUNA (Table 17.6) but not SUNCT (Table 17.4). Typically the eye is not red, but we have also seen, for example external auditory canal swelling and peri-aural flushing as the sole cranial autonomic symptom (Cohen *et al.*, unpublished data), as has been reported for PH.[44] It seems possible, given the relative proportion of patients with cluster headache who have lacrimation and conjunctival injection as compared to other cranial autonomic symptoms,[40] that these symptoms are for some reason biologically more likely. This is supported by the same relative changes being seen in experimentally induced head pain.[45] Thus research criteria for a more encompassing syndrome are proposed (Table 17.5).

Table 17.6   Short-lasting Unilateral Neuralgiform headache attacks with cranial Autonomic symptoms (SUNA)

A 3.3 Diagnostic criteria:

   A. At least 20 attacks fulfilling criteria B–E
   B. Attacks of unilateral orbital, supraorbital, or temporal stabbing pain lasting from 2 s to 10 min
   C. Pain is accompanied by one of:

   1. conjunctival injection and/or tearing
   2. nasal congestion and or rhinorrhoea
   3. eyelid oedema

   D. Attacks occur with a frequency of ≥1 per day for more than half the time
   E. Not attributed to another disorder

A 3.3.1 *Episodic SUNA*
   Description: SUNA attacks occurring for 7 days to 1 year with pain–free intervals longer than 1 month

A 3.3.2 *Chronic SUNA*
   Description: At least two attack periods lasting for 7 days to 1 year separated by remission periods of <1 month (untreated).

Conclusions

The TACs represent a great success story in headache. From a classification point of view, the syndromes share much biology so their agglomeration in Section III draws attention to them and to the trigemino-parasympathetic reflex. It is highly desirable that headache classification moves to a more biological and pathophysiological basis and the TACs are a step in that direction. The TACs also represent excellent clinical opportunities to take a careful history and offer effective therapy to otherwise highly disabled and suffering patients. Last, further investigations of the TACs are bound to illuminate physiological processes whose understanding will be useful to the range of primary headache syndromes.

References

1. Headache Classification Committee of The International Headache Society. The International Classification of Headache Disorders (second edition). *Cephalalgia* 2004; **24** (Suppl 1): 1–160.
2. Goadsby PJ, Lipton RB. A review of paroxysmal hemicranias, SUNCT syndrome and other short-lasting headaches with autonomic features, including new cases. *Brain* 1997; **120**: 193–209.
3. Goadsby PJ. Pathophysiology of cluster headache: a trigeminal autonomic cephalalgia. *Lancet Neurology* 2002; **1**: 37–43.

4. Matharu MS, Boes CJ, Goadsby PJ. Management of trigeminal autonomic cephalalgias and hemicrania continua. *Drugs* 2003; **63**: 1637–77.
5. McNaughton FL, Feindel WH. Innervation of intracranial structures: a reappraisal. In: *Physiological aspects of clinical neurology* (ed., Rose FC). Oxford: Blackwell Scientific Publications, 1977: 279–93.
6. Feindel W, Penfield W, McNaughton F. The tentorial nerves and localization of intracranial pain in man. *Neurology* 1960; **10**: 555–63.
7. Goadsby PJ, Hoskin KL. The distribution of trigeminovascular afferents in the nonhuman primate brain *Macaca nemestrina*: a c-fos immunocytochemical study. *J Anat* 1997; **190**: 367–75.
8. May A, Goadsby PJ. The trigeminovascular system in humans: pathophysiological implications for primary headache syndromes of the neural influences on the cerebral circulation. *J Cereb Blood Flow Metabol* 1999; **19**: 115–27.
9. Lambert GA, Bogduk N, Goadsby PJ, *et al.* Decreased carotid arterial resistance in cats in response to trigeminal stimulation. *J Neurosurg* 1984; **61**: 307–15.
10. Goadsby PJ, Edvinsson L, Ekman R. Release of vasoactive peptides in the extracerebral circulation of man and the cat during activation of the trigeminovascular system. *Ann Neurol* 1988; **23**: 193–6.
11. Spencer SE, Sawyer WB, Wada H, *et al.* CNS projections to the pterygopalatine parasympathetic preganglionic neurons in the rat: a retrograde transneuronal viral cell body labeling study. *Brain Res* 1990; **534**: 149–69.
12. Nakai M, Tamaki K, Ogata J, *et al.* Parasympathetic cerebrovascular center of the facial nerve. *Circ Res* 1993; **72**: 470–5.
13. Goadsby PJ, Lambert GA, Lance JW. Effects of locus coeruleus stimulation on carotid vascular resistance in the cat. *Brain Res* 1983; **278**: 175–83.
14. Goadsby PJ, Lambert GA, Lance JW. The peripheral pathway for extracranial vasodilatation in the cat. *J Auto Nerv Syst* 1984; **10**: 145–55.
15. Goadsby PJ, Shelley S. High frequency stimulation of the facial nerve results in local cortical release of vasoactive intestinal polypeptide in the anesthetised cat. *Neurosci Lett* 1990; **112**: 282–9.
16. Goadsby PJ, Macdonald GJ. Extracranial vasodilatation mediated by VIP (Vasoactive Intestinal Polypeptide). *Brain Res* 1985; **329**: 285–8.
17. Goadsby PJ. Characteristics of facial nerve elicited cerebral vasodilatation determined with laser Doppler flowmetry. *Am J Physiol* 1991; **260**: R255–62.
18. Seylaz J, Hara H, Pinard E, *et al.* Effect of stimulation of the sphenopalatine ganglion on cortical blood flow in the rat. *J Cereb Blood Flow Metabol* 1988; **8**: 875–8.
19. Goadsby PJ. Effect of stimulation of the facial nerve on regional cerebral blood flow and glucose utilization in cats. *Am J Physiol* 1989; **257**: R517–21.
20. Uddman R, Tajti J, Moller S, *et al.* Neuronal messengers and peptide receptors in the human sphenopalatine and otic ganglia. *Brain Res* 1999; **826**: 193–9.
21. Goadsby PJ, Uddman R, Edvinsson L. Cerebral vasodilatation in the cat involves nitric oxide from parasympathetic nerves. *Brain Res* 1996; **707**: 110–18.
22. Ekbom K, Greitz T. Carotid angiography in cluster headache. *Acta Radiologica* 1970; **10**: 177–86.
23. May A, Buchel C, Bahra A, *et al.* Intra-cranial vessels in trigeminal transmitted pain: a PET Study. *Neuroimage* 1999; **9**: 453–60.
24. Drummond PD, Lance JW. Pathological sweating and flushing accompanying the trigeminal lacrimation reflex in patients with cluster headache and in patients with a confirmed site of cervical sympathetic deficit. Evidence for parasympathetic cross-innervation. *Brain* 1992; **115**: 1429–45.
25. Drummond PD. Autonomic disturbance in cluster headache. *Brain* 1988; **111**: 1199–209.
26. May A, Buchel C, Turner R, *et al.* MR-angiography in facial and other pain: neurovascular mechanisms of trigeminal sensation. *J Cereb Blood Flow Metabol* 2001; **21**: 1171–6.

27. Barbanti P, Fabbrini G, Pesare M, *et al.* Unilateral cranial autonomic symptoms in migraine. *Cephalalgia* 2002; **22**: 256–9.
28. Benoliel R, Sharav Y. Trigeminal neuralgia with lacrimation or SUNCT syndrome? *Cephalalgia* 1998; **18**: 85–90.
29. Goadsby PJ, Matharu MS, Boes CJ. SUNCT syndrome or trigeminal neuralgia with lacrimation. *Cephalalgia* 2001; **21**: 82–3.
30. May A, Bahra A, Buchel C, *et al.* Hypothalamic activation in cluster headache attacks. *Lancet* 1998; **352**: 275–8.
31. May A, Bahra A, Buchel C, *et al.* PET and MRA findings in cluster headache and MRA in experimental pain. *Neurology* 2000; **55**: 1328–35.
32. May A, Bahra A, Buchel C, *et al.* Functional MRI in spontaneous attacks of SUNCT: short-lasting neuralgiform headache with conjunctival injection and tearing. *Ann Neurol* 1999; **46**: 791–3.
33. Weiller C, May A, Limmroth V, *et al.* Brain stem activation in spontaneous human migraine attacks. *Nat Med* 1995; **1**: 658–60.
34. Bahra A, Matharu MS, Buchel C, *et al.* Brainstem activation specific to migraine headache. *Lancet* 2001; **357**: 1016–17.
35. Matharu MS, Bartsch T, Ward N, *et al.* Central neuromodulation in chronic migraine patients with suboccipital stimulators: a PET study. *Brain* 2004; **127**: 220–30.
36. May A, Kaube H, Buechel C, *et al.* Experimental cranial pain elicited by capsaicin: a PET-study. *Pain* 1998; **74**: 61–6.
37. Malick A, Burstein R. Cells of origin of the trigeminohypothalamic tract in the rat. *J Comp Neurol* 1998; **400**: 125–44.
38. Goadsby PJ, Edvinsson L, Ekman R. Vasoactive peptide release in the extracerebral circulation of humans during migraine headache. *Ann Neurol* 1990; **28**: 183–7.
39. Goadsby PJ, Edvinsson L. Human *in vivo* evidence for trigeminovascular activation in cluster headache. *Brain* 1994; **117**: 427–34.
40. Bahra A, May A, Goadsby PJ. Cluster headache: a prospective clinical study in 230 patients with diagnostic implications. *Neurology* 2002; **58**: 354–61.
41. Headache Classification Committee of The International Headache Society. Classification and diagnostic criteria for headache disorders, cranial neuralgias and facial pain. *Cephalalgia* 1988; **8** (Suppl 7): 1–96.
42. Sjaastad O, Bakketeig LS. Cluster headache prevalence. Vaga study of headache epidemiology. *Cephalalgia* 2003; **23**: 528–33.
43. Boes CJ, Dodick DW. Refining the clinical spectrum of chronic paroxysmal hemicrania: a review of 74 patients. Headache 2002; **42**: 699–708.
44. Boes CJ, Swanson JW, Dodick DW. Chronic paroxysmal hemicrania presenting as otalgia with a sensation of external acoustic meatus obstruction: two cases and a pathophysiologic hypothesis. *Headache* 1998; **38**: 787–91.
45. Frese A, Evers S, May A. Autonomic activation in experimental trigeminal pain. *Cephalalgia* 2003; **23**: 67–8.

18 Other primary headaches: old concepts and new views

G. Nappi, G. Sandrini, N. Ghiotto,
A. P. Cecchini, C. Tassorelli, and G. Sances

Since the appearance, in 1988, of the International Headache Society's Classification and Diagnostic Criteria for Headache Disorders, Cranial Neuralgias and Facial Pain,[1] numerous papers have been published, aiming to validate the proposed criteria or to identify new nosographic entities.

In the recently published second edition of the classification (International Classification of Headache Disorders, ICHD-II),[2] Chapter IV, previously named 'Primary Miscellaneous Headaches', emerges as one of the chapters to have undergone the most profound revision, as indicated by its title, which has now been changed to *Other Primary Headaches*.

It has become increasingly clear, over recent years, that many of the forms included in this chapter raise major problems as regards their differential diagnosis from other conditions. Therefore, the ICHD-II subcommittee has made a considerable effort to emphasize and address this particular aspect.

With the exception of anecdotal reports and the demonstration of indomethacin efficacy in specific forms, very little is known about the effective therapeutical strategies for these headaches. Similarly, the pathophysiological mechanisms underlying most of them is largely unknown or controversial.

ICHD-II: a new Chapter IV

Because of their low prevalence, and the potential heterogeneity of their patho-genetic mechanisms, the headaches listed in Chapter IV have, to date, received much less attention than the other three groups of primary headaches (i.e. migraine, tension-type headache, and cluster headache + trigeminal-autonomic cephalalgias).

However, the increase in the number of reports appearing in the literature in recent years has made it clear that these 'miscellaneous' headaches are an important consideration in neurological practice because some of them may mimic, especially at their onset, serious forms of symptomatic headache due to organic disease of underlying structures. This new chapter has been enriched by the addition of newly identified entities, whose clinical features have been adequately documented in the literature. These new entities are: *primary thunderclap headache, hypnic headache, hemicrania continua,* and *new daily-persistent headache,* and they have been added to: *primary stabbing headache, primary cough headache, primary exertional headache,* and *primary headache associated with sexual activity.*

On the other hand, other forms originally included in the 'Miscellaneous Primary Headaches' chapter of the first classification, such as the 'external compression headache' or the 'cold-stimulus headache', have, in view of their specific pathogenetic mechanism, been moved to Chapter XIII of ICHD-II (*Cranial Neuralgias and Central Causes of Facial Pain*).

The main changes made to Chapter IV of the classification are shown in Table 18.1.

The pathogenetic mechanisms underlying the headaches listed in Chapter IV, as mentioned above, are largely unknown and existing hypotheses are based mainly on indirect suggestions, e.g. pain characteristics or the response to treatments (Table 18.2).

In this latter regard, it must be noted that the total lack of controlled studies in the literature is another characteristic feature of the *Other Primary Headaches*. A positive response to indomethacin has been reported in some of them and has been elevated to the role of diagnostic criterion in the case of *hemicrania continua.*

Table 18.1   Chapter IV: comparison of the first and second International Headache Society (IHS) classifications

HIS Classification 1988	IHS Classification 2004
◆ Idiopathic stabbing headache	◆ Primary stabbing headache
◆ External compression headache	◆ ⇒ Chapter 13
◆ Cold stimulus headache	◆ ⇒ Chapter 13
◆ Benign cough headache	◆ Primary cough headache
◆ Benign exertional headache	◆ Primary exertional headache
◆ Headache associated with sexual activity	◆ Primary headache associated with sexual activity
	◆ New entities:
	Hypnic headache
	Primary thunderclap headache
	Hemicrania continua
	New daily-persistent headache (NDPH)

Table 18.2 Other primary headaches: suggested pathogenetic mechanisms

		Vascular	Tensional	Neuronal
4.1	Primary stabbing headache			+
4.2	Primary cough headache	+		
4.3	Primary exertional headache	+		
4.4.1	Preorgasmic headache		+	
4.4.2	Orgasmic headache	+		
4.5	Hypnic headache	+		+
4.6	Primary thunderclap headache	+		
4.7	Hemicrania continua	+		+
4.8	New daily-persistent headache		+	

Primary stabbing headache

This form of idiopathic headache is characterized by sudden pain, which manifests itself as a single stab or as a series of stabs. These stabs are brief (lasting from less than a second to 3 s), and generally felt in the distribution of the first division of the trigeminal nerve. Stabs occur repetitively in the course of the day, and periods of *status* last up to several days and are separated by remission phases. Primary stabbing headache is a benign condition in most cases, but caution is warranted when stabs are strictly located in a specific area and do not 'migrate' (even though this is a warning based on anecdotal reports rather than on solid scientific studies).

Primary stabbing headache is more commonly experienced by people suffering from migraine or cluster headache. A positive response to indomethacin has been reported, but controlled studies are lacking.

Notwithstanding the total absence of human and animal evidence, it has been suggested that stabs may be ascribed to an abnormal discharge in the peripheral trigeminal terminals, probably secondary to a condition of 'central activation'.[3]

Recent investigations have suggested that *primary stabbing headache* is more prevalent than previously supposed[4] and have helped to define more clearly its clinical features and, consequently, its diagnostic criteria[5] (i.e. temporal criteria relating to attacks and total absence of accompanying symptoms and/or signs).

Primary cough headache

This headache is defined by the abrupt onset of pain (*onset*, not worsening of pain, the latter being a non-specific phenomenon) following coughing, straining, or Valsalva manoeuvre; the duration is usually short.

ICHD-II draws attention to the possibility that, in 40% of cases, cough headache is secondary to other conditions, especially disorders of the posterior fossa. Arnold-Chiari malformation accounts for the great majority of symptomatic cases, although carotid or vertebro-basilar diseases and cerebral aneurysms have also been found to be involved. An accurate clinical examination and a thorough diagnostic workup is always necessary to exclude secondary causes.

In accordance with the general suggestions regarding response to treatments, it is noteworthy that in the case of primary cough headache, a good response to indomethacin is not a sufficient diagnostic criterion to exclude secondary forms.[6]

Recent reports suggest that this headache may be related to increased intracranial pressure[7] or to an alteration of intraocular haemodynamics.[8]

Primary exertional headache

The pain is typically triggered by physical exercise, especially when this is intense and performed in a hot environment or at high altitude. Its quality is pulsating, while bilateral location of the pain is no longer considered a diagnostic criterion. *Primary exertional headache* may last from 5 min to 48 h (maximal duration was 24 h in the first edition of the classification) and may be prevented by exercise avoidance. This latter feature, being tautological, is no longer accepted as a diagnostic criterion in ICHD-II. Subarachnoid haemorrhage and arterial dissection must be ruled out when the onset is abrupt. Occurrence of the pain during or after physical exertion is a mandatory criterion.

As in the case of cough headache, a fairly high percentage of exertional headaches are secondary, therefore thorough clinical and instrumental evaluation is always recommended.

It has been suggested that a common, similar mechanism, probably vascular, may underlie the pain in *primary cough headache, primary exertional headache,* and *primary headache associated with sexual activity*. This hypothesis is supported by the similarity of the trigger mechanisms in these conditions, as well as by the frequent co-existence of these forms of primary headache in the same individual.[9]

A positive response to ergotamine or indomethacin treatment has been reported in isolated cases of *primary exertional headache*.

Primary headache associated with sexual activity

This form of headache, previously termed 'coital headache' or 'sex headache', is characterized by onset during sexual intercourse. Typically, it begins as sexual excitement increases and becomes intense at orgasm, and has been reported to last from 1 min to 3 h. It is not clear whether the distinction that has been made between 'dull' and 'explosive' types really corresponds to significant clinical or pathogenetic differences. The 'dull' type used to be considered associated with a 'tensional' mechanism, and the 'explosive' type with vascular mechanisms. In a recent investigation, Frese *et al.*[10] did not highlight differences between the two types.

As with other headaches listed in Chapter IV, *primary headache associated with sexual activity* is frequently observed in migraine patients (50% of cases).

For comments on the differential diagnosis of this headache and its supposed pathogenetic mechanisms, please refer to the paragraph on *primary exertional headache*. Very recently, Evers *et al.*[11] suggested that this type of headache may be ascribed to metabolic-related cerebral haemodynamic changes.

The 'postural' headache type associated with sexual activity has been removed from this chapter because it is now considered secondary to cerebrospinal fluid (CSF) leakage and should therefore be coded as *Headache attributed to spontaneous (or idiopathic) low CSF pressure*.

Hypnic headache

Hypnic headache is a rare and benign condition originally described by Raskin in 1988. This peculiar form of headache, which is strictly related to sleep, was recently added to the *Other Primary Headaches* group because, since the publication of Goadsby and Lipton's proposed criteria in 1997,[12] which were based on the eight cases that had been described in the literature at that time, several new reports have appeared (see ref. 13 for a review), contributing to a better definition of its clinical picture.

Hypnic headache is a late-onset headache that awakens the patient from sleep (nocturnal or diurnal), and whose main characteristics, according to the seminal description by Raskin, are: short duration, bilateral and diffuse pain, and absence of autonomic symptoms.

The diagnostic criteria adopted by the ICHD-II do not take into account the main characteristics of pain – location, duration, and intensity – but focus instead on its occurrence during sleep, its persistence for at least 15 min after awakening the patient, the absence of associated – local or general – autonomic symptoms, the frequency of attacks, and the age at onset. This is probably because the almost 70 cases described in the literature show a considerable variation of the pain features. Pain intensity, for instance, has been reported as severe in 34.6% of cases, moderate in 37.7%, and mild in 13.1%. Bilaterality of pain is reported in 66.3% of cases and cranial-facial autonomic symptoms are reported in 6.6% of literature patients. An attack duration shorter than 180 min has been reported in 83.7%, but reports of longer durations (up to 540 min) also exist in the literature.

In the typical case, with onset after 50 years, it is important to rule out, through appropriate and thorough clinical and instrumental examinations, the existence of intracranial disorders. In particular, a polysomnographic evaluation is recommended in order to exclude a sleep apnea condition, as well as other minor alterations in the pattern of nocturnal respiration.

Hypnic headache must be differentiated from primary headaches, which may occur preferably or frequently during sleep (i.e. cluster headache and migraine). In this case, the strict occurrence of hypnic headache during sleep, together with the absence of cranial–facial autonomic symptoms and the scarcity of associated general autonomic symptoms is usually diagnostic. Secondary causes of headaches occurring during nocturnal sleep include arterial hypertension, substance withdrawal, increased intracranial pressure, and sleep apnea.

As regards the pathogenesis of hypnic headache, the strict and sometimes cyclical occurrence of attacks during the sleep phase has suggested that this headache is an REM-related phenomenon, in which attacks are associated with REM-related inhibition of the activity of the locus coeruleus and of the dorsal raphe, and with brain serotonin reduction.[14] A strict, though non-exclusive relationship between hypnic headache and REM phase is further suggested by polysomnographic recordings, which show that nearly 69% of attacks occur during an REM phase, although very recently these data were not confirmed by our group.[15]

The observation that most patients suffering from *hypnic headache* report the occurrence of attacks at the same time of night (alarm clock headache) has prompted the hypothesis that this peculiar type of headache may be regarded as a chronobiological disorder. This suggestion is supported by reports describing the effectiveness of lithium salt, a drug with a proven role in the treatment of definite chronobiological disturbances, such as cluster headache and bipolar disorder.[16]

An intriguing hypothesis recently advanced by the Pavia group suggests that *hypnic headache* may be a phenotypical variation of migraine over time.[13] This hypothesis is based on several factors: the partial overlapping of clinical features, the tendency of migraine to disappear in elderly people, the typical onset of hypnic headache after the age of 50, and the observation that 20% of patients suffering from *hypnic headache* have a history of migraine. According to this line of reasoning, one may hypothesize that changes in external factors (menopause, retirement, etc.) may act upon a predisposed terrain and cause the appearance of different clinical characteristics over time ('phenotypical heterochronia').

From the therapeutic point of view, several drugs have been reported to be effective in *hypnic headache*, including lithium salt, caffeine, flunarizine, verapamil, indomethacin, and gabapentin.[13] More recently, a case report has described the effectiveness of acetazolamide.[17]

Primary thunderclap headache

This is one of the chapter's 'new entries'. The term 'thunderclap' underlines the violence of the pain, together with the swiftness of its presentation. This form is indeed characterized by the sudden and swift onset (<30 s) of violent headache, lasting for between 1 h and 10 days. Pain may recur within 7 days of the onset, but generally there is no tendency for attacks to recur regularly during the weeks or months following its appearance.

The primary form of thunderclap headache closely mimics secondary forms, e.g. headache attributed to subarachnoid haemorrhage, therefore appropriate instrumental investigation is absolutely mandatory to rule out possible organic causes (these are listed in detail in the comments section of ICHD-II).

The close similarity between secondary and primary thunderclap headaches has led to the hypothesis that the primary forms are the result of the inadequacy of instrumental diagnostics to identify the organic cause. Further studies are needed to clarify this issue.

Hemicrania continua

Hemicrania continua (HC) is a rare headache disorder first described in 1984 by Sjaastad and Spierings,[18] and better defined in subsequent years.[19–21] It is characterized by continuous, moderate to severe unilateral pain with absolute response to indomethacin. The partial overlapping of its clinical features with those of other forms of primary headache, trigeminal autonomic cephalalgias (TACs), in particular, has generated debate over its correct nosological framing.

The ICHD-II subcommittee eventually decided to insert HC as a new headache entity in Chapter IV, and not among the trigeminal-autonomic cephalalgias (TACs), because, unlike TACs – which are typically intermittent and short-lasting headaches – HC is characterized by continuous pain that varies in intensity from mild to moderate, with exacerbations that are superimposed on the continuous basal pain. These exacerbations occur spontaneously, in the absence of clear trigger factors, and may last from 20 min to several days, occurring also at night in one-third of cases. In addition, while pain location in TACs follows the anatomical distribution of the trigeminal nerve (I division), the pain in HC often extends to extra-trigeminal areas (occipital region, neck). Ipsilateral cranial autonomic features may be present during exacerbations in HC, but are usually less prominent than in cluster headache (CH) or chronic paroxysmal hemicrania (CPH).

The ICHD-II criteria take into account the unilaterality, persistence, and intensity of the pain and its exacerbations, as well as the response to indomethacin and the presence of at least one cranial autonomic sign, while the location of pain and other general accompanying symptoms are disregarded.

Although no definitely secondary forms of HC have been observed to date, there are reports of HC associated with other pathologies: head injury, HIV infection, mesenchymal tumour in the sphenoid bone, and C7 root irritation. In addition to these conditions, the differential diagnosis of HC should also take into account all the other primary headaches with a chronic temporal pattern, especially those characterized by long-lasting unilateral headache: unilateral chronic migraine (with/without medication overuse), new daily-persistent headache, and cervicogenic headache. The short duration of TACs usually makes it easy to distinguish between them and HC; however, a chronic paroxysmal hemicrania occurring in association with an interictal dull ache may sometimes be confusing. The clinical changes induced by parenteral administration of indomethacin, the so-called 'indotest',[22] may be helpful in order to distinguish HC from other unilateral primary chronic daily headaches. However, since there are reports of HC with unresponsiveness to indomethacin and of HC with partial or complete response to other NSAIDs and to COX-2 inhibitors, this issue will remain controversial until the underlying pathophysiology of HC and the mode of action of indomethacin are better understood.

Very little is known about HC pathophysiology. A recent report of four cases of HC associated with typical visual aura[23] has suggested that HC may be a migraine variant. Some authors have suggested that it may have the same underlying mechanisms as paroxysmal hemicrania, on the basis of the clinical similarities between the two conditions: unilaterality of pain, prevalence in women, and complete response to indomethacin.[24]

Treatment of HC is usually based on the use of indomethacin, at a dose varying from 50 to 300 mg/day, although many patients discontinue the treatment because of side effects. Alternative therapeutic options are: ibuprofen, piroxicam beta-cyclodextrin, and rofecoxib. We recently described a case with a partial response to sphenopalatin blockade (Nappi *et al.*, this book).

New daily-persistent headache

New daily-persisted headache (NDPH) has a clinical picture that is very similar to that of chronic tension-type headache.[25] The only difference between the two forms lies in the 'unremitting from onset or from <3 days from onset' characteristic that is a specific diagnostic criterion for NDPH. This new entity is associated with some controversial issues, two of which are clearly indicated in the comments section. NDPH is often secondary (e.g. post-traumatic)[26] and, in this case, must be coded according to the causative factor. It is unknown what proportion of secondary NDPHs remains undetected because of misdiagnosis (e.g. post-infectious forms).

Patients with medication overuse should be submitted to the established protocol for differentiating probable forms from definite ones.

The existence of two subtypes of NDPH ('self-limiting' and 'refractory') has been proposed but additional studies are required to establish their clinical characteristics.

Conclusions

Headaches listed in Chapter IV of ICHD-II are probably more common than previously thought. Correct nosographic framing of these forms is necessary because most of them show clinical pictures very similar to those of secondary forms and it is crucial to be able to differentiate primary forms from secondary ones. Most of these forms are first observed in emergency departments because of the suddenness of their onset.

Pharmacological treatment of these headaches differs in part from that undertaken in most common primary headache forms (migraine, tension-type headache, and cluster headache), but additional, controlled studies are needed to test the effectiveness of options suggested in case reports. Further studies are also needed in order to clarify their pathogenetic mechanisms, about which little is currently known.

References*

1. Headache Classification Committee of the International Headache Society. Classification and diagnostic criteria for headache disorders, cranial neuralgias and facial pain. *Cephalalgia* 1988; **8** (Suppl 7): 1–96.
2. Olesen J, Bousser M-G, Diener H, *et al.* for the International Headache Society. The International Classification of Headache Disorders. 2nd Edition. *Cephalalgia* 2004; **24** (Suppl 1): 1–160.
3. Lance JW, Goasdby PJ. Miscellaneous headaches unassociated with a structural lesion. In: *The Headaches—Second Edition* (eds Olesen J, Tfelt-Hansen P, and Welch KMA). Philadelphia: Lippincott Williams & Wilkins, 2000; pp 751–62.
4. Sjaastad O, Pettersen H, Bakketeig LS. Extracephalic jabs/idiopathic stabs. Vågå study of headache epidemiology. *Cephalalgia* 2003; **23**: 50–4.
5. Pareja JA, Ruiz J, de Isla C, *et al.* Idiopathic stabbing headache (jabs and jolts syndrome). *Cephalalgia* 1996; **16**: 93–6.
6. Buzzi MG, Formisano R, Colonnese C, *et al.* Chiari-associated exertional, cough, and sneeze headache responsive to medical therapy. *Headache* 2003; **43**: 404–6.
7. Boes CJ, Matharu MS, Goasby PJ. Benign cough headache. *Cephalalgia* 2002; **22**: 772–9.
8. Gupta VK. Is benign cough headache caused by intraocular haemodynamic aberration? *Medical Hypotheses* 2004; **62**: 45–8.
9. Pascual J, Iglesia F, Oterino A, *et al.* Cough, exertional, and sexual headaches: an analysis of 72 benign and symptomatic cases. *Neurology* 1996; **46**: 1520–4.
10. Frese A, Eikermann A, Frese K, *et al.* Headache associated with sexual activity. Demography, clinical features, and comorbidity. *Headache* 2003; **61**: 796–800.
11. Evers S, Schmidt O, Frese A, *et al.* The cerebral hemodynamics of headache associated with sexual activity. *Pain* 2003; **102**: 73–8.
12. Goadsby PJ, Lipton RB. A review of paroxysmal hemicranias, SUNCT syndrome and other short-lasting headaches with autonomic feature, including new cases. *Brain* 1997; **120**: 193–209.
13. Ghiotto N, Sances G, Di Lorenzo G, *et al.* Report of eight new cases of hypnic headache and mini-review of the literature. *Funct Neurol* 2002; **17**: 211–19.
14. Dodick DW, Eross EJ, Parish JM. Clinical, anatomical, and physiologic relationship between sleep and headache. *Headache* 2002; **43**: 282–92.
15. Manni R, Sances G, Terzaghi M, *et al.* Hypnic headache PSG evidence of both REM- and NREM-related attacks. *Neurology* 2004; **62**: 1411–13.
16. Costa A, Nappi G. Cluster headache as a disorder of inner temporal organization. In:*Cluster Headache Syndrome in General Practice*, 2000 (eds Sjaastad O and Nappi G). London: Smith-Gordon, 2003; pp 25–34.
17. Sibon I, Ghorayeb I, Henry P. Successful treatment of hypnic headache syndrome with acetazolamide. *Neurology* 2003; **61**: 1157–8.
18. Sjaastad O, Spierings EL. Hemicrania continua: another headache absolutely responsive to indomethacin. *Cephalalgia* 1984; **4**: 65–70.
19. Newman LC, Lipton RB, Solomon S. Hemicrania continua: ten new cases and a review of the literature. *Neurology* 1994; **44**: 2111–14.
20. Pareja JA, Palomo T, Gorriti MA, *et al.* Hemicrania continua. The first Spanish case: a case report. *Cephalalgia* 1990; **10**: 143–5.
21. Newman LC, Lipton RB, Solomon S. Hemicrania continua: ten new cases and a review of the literature. *Neurology* 1994; **44**: 2111–14.
22. Antonaci F, Pareja JA, Caminero AB, *et al.* Chronic paroxysmal hemicrania and hemicrania continua. Parenteral indomethacin: the "Indotest". *Headache* 1998; **8**: 235–6.

*Key references can be found in reference n. 2.

23. Peres MFP, Siow HC, Rozen TD. Hemicrania continua with aura. *Cephalalgia* 2002; **22**: 246–8.

24. Pareja JA, Vincent M, Antonaci F, *et al*. Hemicrania continua: diagnostic criteria and nosologic status. *Cephalalgia* 2001; **21**: 874–7.

25. Li D, Rozen TD. The clinical characteristics of new daily-persistent headache. *Cephalalgia* 2002; **22**: 66–9.

26. Goadsby PJ, Boes C. New daily-persistent headache. *J Neurol Neurosurg Psychiatry* 2002; **72** (Suppl II): ii6–ii9.

19
A case of hemicrania continua overlapping with other forms of strictly unilateral headaches associated with autonomic symptoms

G. Nappi, C. Tassorelli, G. Sances,
A. P. Cecchini, E. Guaschino, and G. Sandrini

At two decades from its first description[1] Hemicrania Continua (HC) remains an enigma in the field of primary headaches in terms of etiology and pathogenesis.[2] In the recently released second edition of the International Classification of Headache Disorders (ICHD-II),[3] HC has been aggregated to the fourth group 'Other Primary Headaches', not without a vivacious and prolonged discussion among the members of the Classification Subcommittee. Here we report an intriguing case of unilateral daily headache that meets ICHD-II criteria for HC, but at the same time that raises interesting issues as regards the proper place of this headache among the primary forms.

Case report

Clinical picture

A Caucasian male, aged 49, started to experience five years before – during a period of intense stress associated with frequent intercontinental trips – sporadic episodes of mild pain located in the occipital and temporal regions (more frequently on the right side, but sometimes bilateral) and described as a pressure associated with stiffness. Paroxysms of sudden, severe pulsating/stabbing pain located in the right orbital, supraorbital, and temporal regions were superimposed onto the baseline painful condition, and were associated with nausea and autonomic signs (conjunctival injection, lacrimation, nasal congestion, and mild ptosis), all of which were ipsilateral to the pain side.

The initial frequency of the disturbance was of one attack per month. Subsequently, the frequency rapidly increased and became daily within a couple of years. Possible precipitating factors were recognized only at the beginning in alcohol intake, quick neck movement, and long car trips behind the wheel were recognized as possible precipitating factors.

At the time of the observation at our Center, the pain had become strictly unilateral (always on the right side), continuous with exacerbations that usually occurred once a day, starting approximately 30 min after the patient had got up from his bed. Exacerbations lasted several hours (up to six) if untreated, but rapidly responded to ergotamine. Twice a week, mostly on weekends, the patient reported a second daily paroxysm, which occurred in the late afternoon or in the evening. The peak intensity of pain during the paroxysms was reached in 5 min. Occasionally – 2 to 3 episodes per year – the pain experienced during the paroxysms reached an excruciating intensity, being in that case associated with intense anger and restlessness.

Pharmacological history

The initial effectiveness of ergotamine faded in a few months. Subsequently, the patient tried other acute therapies: sumatriptan (ineffective orally; rapidly and completely effective subcutaneously), oral indomethacin (ineffective) or ketorolac (rapidly effective only for a short period of time), and oxygen inhalation (ineffective). Prophylactic treatments such as verapamil and gabapentin partially and temporarily improved the clinical condition, while lithium, propranolol, pizotifen, and paroxetine were completely ineffective. Steroids proved of limited efficacy, as the attacks promptly reappeared upon discontinuation.

Diagnostic workup

Neuroimaging of the brain, cerebral circulation, and cranial bones showed:

(i) a slightly ectasic cavernous/supraclinoid internal carotid artery associated with slight elongation and tortuosity. These findings were bilateral, but more marked on the right side.
(ii) a slight deviation of the nasal septum* with mucosal thickening of the right maxillary sinus.

---

*The patient previously underwent a septal reconstruction with endoscopic ethmoidectomy that failed to induce any clinically -relevant changes.

The INDOTEST, performed at our Department – according to the methodology of the Trondheim group[4] – five years after the onset, induced a prompt remission of the pain.

No affective/personality disorder emerged from the evaluation of the psychopathological profile, in particular no 'addictive' personality trait could be detected.

Diagnosis

The patient was diagnosed as suffering from Hemicrania Continua, according to the criteria of the second edition of International Classification of Headache Disorders (ICHD-II), though a clinical overlapping with other unilateral headaches was observed (Table 19.1).

Treatments

The patient was put on indomethacin treatment (25 mg three times a day), which induced the disappearance of the exacerbations and associated autonomic signs. Unfortunately, indomethacin had to be discontinued after a few weeks because of gastric intolerance. Celecoxib was proposed as a substitute of indomethacin, but it proved useless.

The injection of the muscles located in the cervical and frontal and temporal regions with botulin toxin (40 U) induced only a partial and temporary improvement.

Six months ago, the patient underwent the right sphenopalatine ganglion block, which caused a partial and so far stable benefit in terms of reduced frequency of paroxysmal attacks (<1/day) and restored the response to ergotamine (complete pain response to 0.5 mg in 20 min).

Discussion

The most robust characteristics of HC are represented by the strict unilaterality and the absolute response to indomethacin. Our patient showed both these characteristics, as well as all the others included in the diagnostic criteria of ICHD-II (see Table 19.1). It seems noteworthy that a partial overlap was also observed with the trigeminal autonomic cephalalgias (TACs): chronic cluster headache, chronic paroxysmal hemicrania, and SUNCT.

The concomitant internal carotid artery abnormalities can be considered paraphysiological and do not seem to represent a causative factor. However, the slight asymmetry observed between and within paroxysms probably represents a local predisposing condition, which may be responsible for pain lateralization and cranial autonomic dysfunction.

HC has been linked in the past to migraine: Evers et al. reported a patient with familial hemiplegic migraine plus HC and many migraine-associated symptoms

Table 19.1 Fulfillment of the ICHD-II diagnostic criteria for Hemicrania Continua and for other types of strictly unilateral headaches associated with autonomic symptoms. Note that for comparative purposes, diagnostic criteria were broken down to the various clinical characteristics considered in the sets of criteria for the different types of headaches

Diagnostic criteria	Our patient	Hemicrania continua	Chronic cluster headache	Chronic paroxysmal hemicrania	SUNCT*
(1) Pain quality	(1) Continuous mild-moderate pain described as pressure associated stiffness (baseline pain) (2) Sharp exacerbations of severe pulsating/stabbing pain (1–2/day)	Continuous pain of moderate intensity with exacerbations of severe intensity	Attacks of severe or very severe pain (separated by pain-free periods)	Attacks of severe pain (separated by pain-free periods)	Attacks of stabbing or pulsating pain (separated by pain-free periods)
(2) Temporal pattern	No pain-free periods Daily for >3 years	Daily for >3 months	Daily or almost daily for >1 year, with remission periods lasting <1month	Daily or almost daily for >1 year, with remission periods lasting <1 month	–
(3) Frequency of exacerbations/attacks	1–2 per day	–	From 1 every other day to 8 per day	>5 per day for more than half of the time	3–200 per day

Continued

Table 19.1 Fulfillment of the ICHD-II diagnostic criteria for Hemicrania Continua and for other types of strictly unilateral headaches associated with autonomic symptoms. Note that for comparative purposes, diagnostic criteria were broken down to the various clinical characteristics considered in the sets of criteria for the different types of headaches—Cont'd

Diagnostic criteria	Our patient	Hemicrania continua	Chronic cluster headache	Chronic paroxysmal hemicrania	SUNCT*
(4) Duration of exacerbations/attacks	30–180 min	–	15–180 min	2–30 min	5–240 s
(5) Location	Occipital and temporal region for baseline pain; Orbital, supraorbital, and temporal for exacerbations	–	Orbital, supraorbital, and/or temporal	Orbital, supraorbital, or temporal	Orbital, supraorbital, or temporal
(6) Side (7) Ipsilateral autonomic symptoms	Strictly unilateral Conjunctival injection, lacrimation, eyelid ptosis, nasal congestion	Strictly unilateral At least one of: ◆ conjunctival injection and/or lacrimation ◆ nasal congestion and/or rhinorrhea ◆ ptosis and/or miosis	Strictly unilateral At least one of: ◆ conjunctival injection and/or lacrimation ◆ nasal congestion and/or rhinorrhea ◆ eyelid edema ◆ forehead and facial sweating ◆ miosis and/or ptosis ◆ a sense of restlessness or agitation	Strictly unilateral At least one of: ◆ conjunctival injection and/or lacrimation ◆ nasal congestion and/or rhinorrhea ◆ eyelid edema ◆ forehead and facial sweating ◆ miosis and/or ptosis	Strictly unilateral Conjunctival injection and lacrimation

(8) Response to therapeutic doses of indomethacin	Complete	Complete	–	Complete	–

CONCORDANCE				
	Complete	Pain intensity, duration, and location of exacerbations/attacks Unilaterality Autonomic signs	Pain intensity of exacerbations/attacks Unilaterality Autonomic signs Response to indomethacin	Pain quality of exacerbations/attacks Unilaterality Autonomic signs

*Short-lasting Unilateral Neuralgiform headache with conjunctival injection and tearing.

(including visual auras) have been reported during HC exacerbations.[5–8] In our patient, the strict unilaterality of pain, the presence of exacerbations – with pain located in 'trigeminal' areas – associated with oculocephalic autonomic symptoms, the response to indomethacin rather suggest a clinical and pathophysiological proximity with the TACs group (cluster headache and paroxysmal hemicrania, *in primis*).[9] The closeness of HC to TACs is further suggested, in this patient, by the quick and complete response of exacerbations to subcutaneous sumatriptan, coupled with the inefficacy of the oral route, by the improvement observed following the sphenopalatine ganglion block[10] as well as by the restless behavior observed in particularly intense paroxysms.

If we try and analyse unilateral headaches by plotting pain duration with relevance of oculocephalic autonomic symptomatology (Fig. 19.1), TACs would fit in the sector corresponding to short-lasting headaches with medium-to-marked oculocephalic autonomic symptomatology, migraine would fit in the area corresponding to long-lasting headache with slight-to-none oculocephalic autonomic involvement. In order to fit in the plot, HC would probably need to be split into two attack subtypes: (i) continuous baseline pain, which would fall in the sector corresponding to long-lasting headache with slight-to-none autonomic symptomatology sector and (ii) exacerbations, which would fit in the area corresponding to medium-to-short-lasting attacks associated with slight-to-moderate autonomic symptomatology.

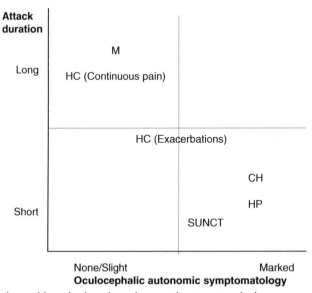

Fig. 19.1 Unilateral headache plotted according to attack duration and cranial autonomic symptomatology. M = migraine; HC – hemicrania continua; CH – cluster headache; PH – paroxysmal hemicrania; SUNCT – short-lasting unilateral neuralgiform headache with conjunctival injection and tearing.

In conclusion, this case report suggests that HC may be closer to TACs than to the groups of headaches included in Chapter IV of ICHD-II. In addition, it also prompts the need for a better characterization of exacerbations in terms of pain characteristics, frequency, duration, and response to treatments. It seems likely that this additional information might allow a better nosographic framing of HC.

Acknowledgments

We thank Prof. N. T. Mathew for sharing with us his long-time expertise in the field of Trigeminal Autonomic Cephalalgias and for his contribution to the evaluation of patients.

We are also grateful to Prof. O. Sjaastad and Dr. F. Antonaci for their precious input as regards the INDO test.

References

1. Sjaastad O, Spierings ELH. 'Hemicrania continua'. Another headache absolutely responsive to indomethacin. *Cephalalgia* 1984; **4**: 65–70.
2. Pareja JA, Vincent M, Antonaci F, *et al.* Hemicrania continua: diagnostic criteria and nosologic status. *Cephalalgia* 2001; **21**: 874–7.
3. Headache Classification Committee of the International Headache Society. The International Classification of Headache Disorders, 2nd Edition. *Cephalalgia* 2004; **24** (Suppl 1): 1–160.
4. Antonaci F, Costa A, Ghirmai S, *et al.* Parenteral indomethacin (the INDOTEST) in cluster headache. *Cephalalgia* 2003; **23**: 193–6.
5. Evers S, Bahara A, Goadsby PJ. Coincidence of familial hemiplegic migraine and hemicrania continua? A case report. *Cephalalgia* 1999; **19**:533–55.
6. Bordini C, Antonaci F, Stovner LJ, *et al.* 'Hemicrania continua': a clinical review. *Headache* 1991; **31**: 20–6.
7. Newman LC, Lipton RB, Solomon S. Hemicrania continua: ten new cases and a review of the literature. *Neurology* 1994; **44**: 2111–14.
8. Espada F, Escalza I, Morales-Asin F, *et al.* Hemicrania continua: nine new cases. *Cephalalgia* 1999; **19**: 442.
9. Sjaastad O, Nappi G, eds. Cluster headache syndrome in general practice. London: Smith-Gordon, 2000.
10. Sanders M, Zuurmond WW. Efficacy of sphenopalatine ganglion blockade in 66 patients suffering from cluster headache: a 12- to 70-month follow-up evaluation. *J Neurosurg* 1997; **87**: 876–80.

20
Appendix to the International Classification of Headache Disorders (2nd edition): application of diagnostic criteria for tension-type headache

P. Torelli, E. Beghi, and G. C. Manzoni

Introduction

The new revised edition of the International Classification of Headache Disorders (2nd Edition (ICHD-II),[1] published 15 years after the first edition,[2] also includes an interesting Appendix. In addition to being the first step to remove a few disorders included as diagnostic entities from the classification in the 1st Edition (sufficient evidence for this has still not been published) the Appendix contains criteria for entities that have not been sufficiently validated by research studies proposes an alternative set of criteria to those in the main body of the classification, namely for migraine without aura (MO) (coded to A1.1) and for tension-type headache (TTH) (coded to A2.1, A2.2, A2.3). The aim of this study was to determine whether the criteria for TTH described in the Appendix to ICHD-II offer any benefits compared to the ICHD-II official criteria in a group of patients referred to a headache clinic.

Materials and methods

The study population consisted of all patients seen for the first time on a consecutive basis at the University of Parma Headache Centre from October 1 to November 30 2003 ($n=256$). Headache diagnosis was established by two neurologists. The first neurologist (GCM) was a headache specialist who, having reviewed the patients' past medical histories and performed a physical and a neurological examination, based diagnosis on his own experience. Obviously, in his clinical judgement he also considered other clinical aspects that are not listed among the ICHD-II criteria, such as the disease's natural history, its evolution in relation to female reproductive events, family history of headache, associated symptoms, triggering and attenuating factors, and response to drug therapy. The second neurologist (PT) was blind to the diagnosis and established the diagnosis by means of a semi-structured interview based on the ICHD-II criteria and on the criteria proposed in the Appendix to ICHD-II. The Appendix criteria for TTH are reported in Table 20.1. We define patients affected by chronic TTH fulfilling all but one criteria as 'probable chronic TTH' (code 2.4.3) even if this definition is not included in ICHD-II. For patients with more than one headache subtype, only the more frequent one was considered. The TTH diagnosis established by the headache specialist was taken as the golden standard against which the ICHD-II Appendix criteria for TTH were to be compared. The study was approved by the Ethics Commission of the University of Parma School of Medicine. The patients gave their written consent.

Data analysis was done by SPSS 11.0 for Windows.

Results

The initial sample consisted of 256 subjects (174 women and 82 men; mean age 35.9 years ± 12.3). Fifty patients had TTH (25 women and 25 men; mean age,

Table 20.1 Alternative diagnostic criteria for tension-type headache in the Appendix to the International Classification of Headache Disorders (ICHD-II)

A. Episodes, or headache, fulfilling criterion A for [whichever of 2.1 *Infrequent episodic tension-type headache*, 2.2 *Frequent episodic tension-type headache*, or 2.3 *Chronic tension-type headache*] and criteria B–D below
B. Headache lasting from 30 min to 7 days
C. At least three of the following pain characteristics:
   1. bilateral location
   2. pressing/tightening (non-pulsating) quality
   3. mild or moderate intensity
   4. not aggravated by routine physical activity such as walking or climbing stairs
D. No nausea (anorexia may occur), vomiting, photophobia, or phonophobia
E. Not attributed to another disorder

35.2 years ± 14.8), including 27 with frequent episodic TTH and 23 with chronic TTH. Twelve patients had atypical TTH (five women and seven men; mean age, 36.4 years ± 17.0), including nine with the frequent episodic form and three with the chronic form.

When the ICHD-II criteria were applied to the TTH group, 23 patients (46.0%) were codable to 2.2, 23 (46.0%) to 2.3, and four (8.0%) to 2.4.2. When the Appendix criteria were applied to the same group, 11 patients (22.0%) were codable to A2.2, 15 (30.0%) to A2.3, 16 (32.0%) to 2.4.2, and 8 (16.0%) to 2.4.3. In 20 patients, TTH diagnosis was certain with the ICHD-II criteria (coding to 2.2 and 2.3) and probable with the ICHD-II Appendix criteria (coding to 2.4.2 or 2.4.3). Five patients (25.0%) had their coding changed due to the nature of pain (the patients did not report at least three of the following characteristics: bilateral location, pressing/tightening quality, mild to moderate intensity, not worsened by routine physical activity), three (15.0%) to the clinical features and the presence of associated symptoms, and 12 (60.0%) to the presence of associated symptoms (five patients out of 12, or 41.7%, reported photophobia; 5/12, or 41.7%, phonophobia; and 2/12, or 16.6%, mild nausea). Using the IHCD-II criteria in the patients diagnosed with atypical TTH by the headache specialist, seven (58.3%) were codable to 2.2, two (16.7%) to 2.3, two (16.7%) to 2.4.2, and one (8.3%) to 2.4.3. Using instead the IHCD-II Appendix criteria, two (16.7%) were codable to A2.2, one (8.3%) to A2.3, and nine (75.0%) to 2.4 (fulfilling criteria for 2.4.2 and 2.4.3). Of the six patients diagnosed with certain TTH using the ICHD-II criteria (coding to 2.2 or 2.3) and with probable TTH using the Appendix criteria (coding to 2.4.2 or 2.4.3), five had their coding changed because they did not fulfill criterion C and only one of them fulfilled criterion D.

Discussion

Following publication of the 1st Edition of the IHS classification,[2] the studies aimed at testing the validity of diagnostic criteria for TTH have been few in number.[3–5] Although some authors have reported a poor sensitivity of criteria for TTH, in particular for the chronic form,[5] no changes have been proposed so far to the parameters currently in use. In the Appendix to ICHD-II, editors thought it helpful to introduce a set of criteria representing a core TTH syndrome. In our study, the application of the ICHD-II criteria led to a correct diagnosis in 92.0% of TTH cases, including 100% (23 patients out of 23) with chronic TTH and 85.2% (23/27) with frequent episodic TTH, but only in 25.0% of patients diagnosed with atypical TTH by the headache specialist. By contrast, the application of the Appendix criteria led to a diagnosis of certain TTH in only 52.0% patients with TTH, including 40.7% (11 patients out of 27) of those with frequent episodic TTH and 65.2% (15 patients out of 23) of those with chronic TTH, and to a diagnosis of probable TTH, either episodic or chronic, in 75.0% of those with atypical TTH based on the gold standard.

Our study does have a few limitations: (1) lacking any specific biological markers allowing for discrimination between the various primary headache subtypes, the diagnostic gold standard obviously depends on subjective interpretation of symptoms; (2) the gold standard was the judgement of only one specialist, not of a group of specialists, which might have helped reduce the subjective variability of diagnosis.

As was also implied in the commentary to the Appendix, the results of our study indicate that the alternative diagnostic criteria proposed as a replacement to the current ones are more restrictive. As such, they might be preferred in those investigative fields that require the selection of more homogenous and consistent samples. Given that, when the Appendix criteria are applied, in most cases, the coding change from a certain to a probable diagnosis of TTH is due to the presence of an associated symptom (i.e. photophobia, phonophobia, and nausea), the D criterion should perhaps be reconsidered.

References

1. Headache Classification Committee of the IHS. The International Classification of Headache Disorders, 2nd Edition. *Cephalalgia* 2004; **24** (Suppl 1): 1–160.
2. Headache Classification Committee of the IHS. Classification and diagnostic criteria for headache disorders, cranial neuralgias and facial pain. *Cephalalgia* 1988; **8** (Suppl 7): 1–96.
3. Cano Garcia FJ, Rodriguez Franco L. The validity of the International Headache Society criteria and the modifications put forward in 2002 in the diagnosis of migraine and tension type headaches. *Rev Neurol* 2003; **36**: 710–14.
4. Rokicki LA, Semenchuk EM, Bruehl S, *et al*. An examination of the validity of the IHS classification system for migraine and tension-type headache in the college student population. *Headache* 1999; **39**: 720–7.
5. Pajaron E, Lainez JM, Monzon MJ, *et al*. The validity of the classification criteria of the International Headache Society for migraine, episodic tension headache and chronic tension headache. *Neurologia* 1999; **14**: 283–8.

21 Phenotype of chronic tension-type headache

H. Göbel, A. Heinze, and K. Heinze-Kuhn

Introduction

International epidemiological studies have demonstrated that between 40% and 90% of the population suffer from episodic tension-type headache. About 3% of the population describe a chronic tension-type headache with headaches on more than 15 days a month. Tension-type headache is by far the most common headache type and one of the most common of all disorders. This headache type may lead to grave consequences for the patients' life and is responsible for significant costs. In a Danish study, the average number of days off-work was estimated 270 working days per 1000 employees per year for migraine. The corresponding figure for tension-type headache was significantly higher with 920 working days per 1000 employees per year of work.[1]

In contrast to the episodic subtype, chronic tension-type headache is an especially disabling headache type. The main clinical characteristics as defined in the IHS classification can be found in most patients. However, there are additional features commonly described by patients.[2,3] We analysed the headache phenotype of patients referred to a specialized headache center with the diagnosis of chronic tension-type headache.

Methods

One hundred and five patients referred because of chronic tension-type headache were analysed using a standardized interview and questionnaire. Furthermore, patients were asked to keep a prospective headache diary. All patients were diagnosed according to the *International Classification of Headache Disorders*. Only patients fulfilling the diagnostic criteria for chronic tension-type headache completely were included in the study.

Table 21.1   Pain localization and intensity

Headache characteristics		Frequency distribution %		
Pain localization	Localized 28.6	Diffuse 33.7	Moving 37.7	
Pain radiation	Neck and shoulder 32.1	Temples and forehead 60.4	Neck only 7.6	
Pain intensity	Weak 1.0	Moderate 12.4	Severe 46.4	Very severe 40.2
Pain-free days	Yes 14.3	No 85.7		

Results

Of the patients 56.2% were female and 43.8% male. 94.3% fulfilled the IHS criteria for chronic tension-type headache completely. 31.4% of the patients described a diffuse pain localization, in contrast to 68.6% who were able to specify the painful region (Table 21.1). In 64.8% of the patients, the pain was always localized in the same area. 46.7% of the patients described a pain radiating from the neck to the forehead and temples. The pain was characterized as pressing or tightening by 72.4% of the patients (Table 21.2). 86.6% rated the pain intensity as severe or very severe. Common accompanying symptoms (Table 21.3) were sensitivity to touch (23.8%), sweating (32.4%), conjunctival injection (20%), photophobia (34.3%), phonophobia (41.9%), dizziness (31.4%), tiredness (43.8%), and vertigo (47.6%). Only 9.5% of the patients stated no accompanying symptoms.

Table 21.2   Pain characteristics

Features	% of patients
Cutting	6.9
Pulsating	26.5
Dull	55.0
Stabbing	11.4
Throbbing	25.5
Cramp-like	19.6
Stinging	33.3
Sharp	4.9
Pressing	40.2
Aching	23.5
Probing	24.5
Lancinating	9.8
Burning	16.7

Table 21.3 Frequency of accompanying symptoms

Accompanying symptoms	% patients
Pallor	14.7
Swelling	10.8
Allodynia	24.5
Sweating	33.3
Paresthesia	10.8
Sensory disturbance	16.7
Lacrimation	9.8
Conjunctival injection	20.6
Double vision	5.9
Blurred vision	25.5
Photophobia	35.3
Phonophobia	43.1
Nasal obstruction	7.8
Muscle weakness	16.7
Tiredness	45.1
Vertigo	49.0
Nausea	13.3
None	9.8

Conclusions

The IHS criteria for chronic tension-type headache certainly are sensitive, yet they only give an incomplete picture of the phenotype met in clinical practice.[4–6] This includes both pain characteristics and accompanying symptoms.

For diagnosing purposes, the diagnostic IHS criteria are sufficient, allowing for an easy and uncomplicated diagnosing process. However, for the complete clinical phenotype of chronic tension-type headache rather more features are of importance.

Accompanying symptoms may become important when they influence the choice of treatment. Before deciding on the treatment, the entire phenotype of chronic tension-type headache ought to be described and not only by means of the IHS criteria.

References

1. Rasmussen BK, Olesen J. Epidemiology of migraine and tension-type headache. *Curr Opin Neurol* 1994; **7** (3): 264–71.
2. The International Classification of Headache Disorders: 2nd edition. *Cephalalgia* 2004; **24** (Suppl 1): 9–160.
3. Levin M. Chronic daily headache and the revised international headache society classification. *Curr Pain Headache Rep* 2004; **8** (1): 59–65.

4. Mongini F, Deregibus A, Raviola F, *et al.* Confirmation of the distinction between chronic migraine and chronic tension-type headache by the McGill Pain Questionnaire. *Headache* 2003; **43** (8): 867–77.
5. Conti A, Freitas M, Conti P, *et al.* Relationship between signs and symptoms of temporo-mandibular disorders and orthodontic treatment: a cross-sectional study. *Angle Orthod* 2003; **73** (4): 411–7.
6. Cassidy EM, Tomkins E, Hardiman O, *et al.* Factors associated with burden of primary headache in a specialty clinic. *Headache* 2003; **43** (6): 638–44.

22
Discussion summary, the primary headaches: Part II

S. Silberstein

Session III: the primary headaches – part II

Lars Bendtsen highlighted the changes in the new IHS Classification of Headache (ICHD-2).[1] Tension-type headache (TTH) is now subdivided based on frequency and tenderness. New to the classification is the subdivision of episodic TTH into infrequent (<1 day/month) and frequent (>1 and <15 days/month) varieties. The committee felt that the infrequent subtype has very little impact on the individual and did not deserve much attention from the medical profession. However, frequent sufferers often have considerable disability that sometimes warrants expensive drugs and prophylactic medication. Chronic TTH, a subtype of TTH continued from the previous classification, is usually associated with disability and high personal and socioeconomic costs.

Population-based studies from Denmark have shown that approximately 35% of the population have infrequent TTH and 35% have frequent TTH. This may account for the difference in estimates of episodic TTH in different studies. (Denmark's high prevalence may be because the studies have taken infrequent TTH into account.) Stricter criteria for CTTH are now in the Appendix of ICHD-2. They do not allow for any nausea, vomiting, photophobia, or phonophobia. Torelli and Manzoni presented a poster comparing the two different versions of the TTH criteria. The appendix criteria increase the specificity but decrease the sensitivity of the diagnosis. Some argued that the increased sensitivity was due to including cases more similar to chronic migraine.

Peter Goadsby reviewed the pathogenesis and classification of the trigeminal autonomic cephalalgias (TACs), a new entity in the classification that encompasses cluster headache, paroxysmal hemicrania, and short-lasting unilateral neuralgiform headache attacks with conjunctival injection and tearing (SUNCT). Episodic cluster headache now requires a one-month (as opposed to a two-week) break to differentiate it from chronic cluster headache. In addition, a new accompanying symptom has been added: associated with a sense of restlessness or agitation. It was felt that despite the fact that the addition would not increase the sensitivity of the diagnostic criteria, it was so characteristic of cluster headache that it should be included. Paroxysmal hemicrania now has an episodic subtype (EPH) in addition to the chronic variety (CPH). Attacks occur in periods lasting 7 days–1 year separated by pain-free periods lasting ≥1 month.

The diagnosis of SUNCT is new to the classification. This syndrome is characterized by short-lasting attacks of unilateral pain that are much briefer than those seen in any other TAC and very often accompanied by prominent lacrimation and redness of the ipsilateral eye. To make a diagnosis, pain must be accompanied by ipsilateral conjunctival injection and lacrimation. However, some patients have only one of these symptoms. SUNCT may be a subform of short-lasting unilateral neuralgiform headache attacks with cranial autonomic symptoms (SUNA), described in the appendix, and cases missing one of the criteria for SUNCT can be classified here.

Giorgio Sandrini reviewed the other primary headaches, which are clinically heterogeneous. This group includes four new clinical entities: primary thunderclap headache, hypnic headache, hemicrania continua (HC), and new daily-persistent headache (NDPH). The heading 'primary headache associated with sexual activity' encompasses benign sex headache, coital cephalalgia, benign vascular sexual headache, and sexual headache. Sexual headache type 3, postural headache beginning after orgasm, is now classified as headache attributed to spontaneous (or idiopathic) low CSF pressure.

Hypnic headache (hypnic headache syndrome, 'alarm clock' headache) consists of attacks of dull headache that always awaken the patient from sleep. Primary thunderclap headache (benign thunderclap headache) is a high-intensity headache of abrupt onset that mimicks the headache that accompanies ruptured cerebral aneurysm. HC is a persistent, strictly unilateral headache that is responsive to indomethacin. NDPH is daily and unremitting from very soon after onset (within 3 days at most).

NDPH, as defined by ICHD-2, has the characteristics of sudden-onset CTTH. Many have argued, and Li and Rozen[2] have reported, that NDPH often has migraine or chronic migraine features. The suggestion was made to either delete the headache characteristics of NDPH or have both TTH and migraine subtypes.

Migraine with autonomic symptoms (typically associated with migraine without aura) occurs more commonly than recognized. It may be difficult to separate very frequent migraine from HC. The only way to differentiate the disorders may be by their response to indomethacin.

Some argued that requiring a complete response to indomethacin as part of the criteria to HC, EPH, and CPH may be too strict. What if there is a 95% reduction in headaches? It was agreed that there is no easy answer. Many felt that clinical judgment should prevail, but stricter criteria are needed for research.

A discussion took place regarding differentiating long-lasting (~5 min) SUNCT from CPH, cluster headache, and trigeminal neuralgia (TN). SUNCT, like TN, often has cutaneous trigger zones; unlike TN it does not have refractory periods after attacks. SUNCT has associated autonomic features, but TN does not. CPH is defined, and differentiated, by indomethacin responsiveness. CPH with interictal pain and allodynia can mimic HC. Both are indomethacin responsive and the differential can be a diagnostic but not therapeutic problem.

References

1. Headache Classification Committee. The International Classification Of Headache Disorders, 2nd Edition. *Cephalalgia* 2004; **24**: 1–160.
2. Li D, Rozen Td. The clinical characteristics of new daily persistent headache. *Cephalalgia* 2002; **22**: 66–9.

Session
IV

The secondary headaches: Part I

23 Headache attributed to infection

F. Sakai

Introduction

Headache is a common accompaniment of systemic viral infection such as influenza. In intracranial infection, headache is usually the first and the most frequently encountered symptom. Unfortunately, there are no good prospective studies of the headache associated with intracranial infection and precise diagnostic criteria for those subtypes of headache cannot be developed in all cases.

The objectives of the present communication are to summarize what are new in the second edition of the classification and to consider mechanisms for secondary headache.

Old and new classification

In the previous classification, ICHD-I (1988), headache was associated with infection and were classified in different chapters. In the new classification, infection-related headaches were put together to form one group of headache classification for infection. Headache attributed to infection is the new classification (Table 23.1) including intracranial infection, systemic infection, HIV and AIDS, and chronic post-infection headache. Inclusion of chronic post-infection headache to the new classification is a new addition to the ICHD-II.

Headache attributed to intracranial infection includes headache attributed to bacterial meningitis, lymphocyte meningitis, encephalitis, brain abscess, and subdural emphysema.

Diagnostic criteria

When a new headache occurs for the first time in close temporal relation to an infection, it is coded as a secondary headache attributed to infection. A diagnosis of headache attributed to an infection usually becomes definite only when the headache resolves or greatly improves after effective treatment or spontaneous remission of the infection.

Table 23.1 Headache attributed to infection

9.1 Headache attributed to intracranial infection
9.1.1 Headache attributed to bacterial meningitis
9.1.2 Headache attributed to lymphocytic meningitis
9.1.3 Headache attributed to encephalitis
9.1.4 Headache attributed to brain abscess
9.1.5 Headache attributed to subdural emphysema
9.2 Headache attributed to systemic infection
9.2.1 Headache attributed to systemic bacterial infection
9.2.2 Headache attributed to systemic viral infection
9.2.3 Headache attributed to other systemic infections
9.3 Headache attributed to HIV/AIDS
9.4 Chronic post-infection headache
9.4.1 Chronic post-bacterial meningitis headache

Pathophysiology of headache

Pathophysiology of headache for intracranial infection includes irritation and compression of the meningeal or arterial structures, dilatation and congestion of intracranial vessels, increased intracranial pressure, and reaction to toxic products of the infecting agents.

Mechanism for headache

Mechanism for headache attributed to bacterial meningitis is important to consider primary headaches. Bacterial products (toxins), mediators of inflammation, play a role by inducing primary pain sensitization and causing pain. Central sensitization and hyperalgesia seem to be present and are likely to be mediated by glutamate and/or substance p. Therefore, the hypothesis that headache is due to bacterial meningitis may be augmented as a model to study the mechanism of primary headaches by several investigators.[1,2]

Figure 23.1 illustrates the non-contrast CT and contrast CT of a patient with tuberculosis meningitis. Contrast CT scans show marked plasma extravasations, or contrast media extravasations in the meninges and probably the perivascular spaces. Similar observation is reported during migraine headache, although to a much lesser extent detected by contrast-enhanced MRI.[3]

The mechanism for headache attributed to systemic infection has not been well studied. In addition to the effect of fever, direct effects by the microorganisms are considered to influence brainstem nuclei to release substances to cause headache or endotoxins to activate inducible NOS. The exact nature of these mechanisms remains to be investigated.

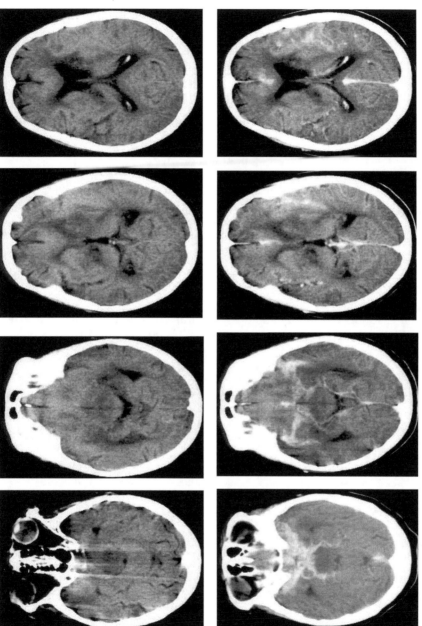

Fig. 23.1 Non-contrast and Contrast CT scans of a 63-year-old woman with tuberculosis meningitis.

The mechanism for headache attributed to HIV/AIDS is divided into three categories: (1) dull lateral headache (may be a part of the symptomatology of HIV infection), (2) aseptic meningitis during HIV infection (but not exclusively in the AIDS stage), and (3) secondary meningitis or encephalitis associated with opportunistic infections or neoplasms (AIDS).

Chronic post-infection headache is a new entity introduced in the new classification. According to Bohr et al,[4] 32% of survivors of bacterial meningitis suffer from persistent headache. This new diagnostic criterion was added in order to encourage the study, because sensitized or damaged brain may persist to ache for a long time.

Conclusion

Headaches attributed to infection are put together into one chapter of classification. Headache disorders attributed to extracranial infections of the head (such as ear, eye, and sinus infections) are coded as subtypes of 11; Headache or facial pain attributed to disorder of the cranium, neck, eyes, nose, sinuses, teeth, mouth, or other facial or cranial structures.

Chronic post-infection headache is a new concept in this chapter. When the causative infection is effectively treated or remits spontaneously but the headache persists after 3 months, the diagnosis changes to chronic post-infection headache. Chronic post-bacterial meningitis headache is so far the only such headache which has good evidence. Other headaches, such as chronic non-bacterial infection headache, are described only in the appendix as research is needed to establish better criteria for causation.

References

1. Weber JR, Angstwurm K, Bove GM, et al. The trigeminal nerve and augmentation of regional cerebral blood flow during experimental bacterial meningitis. J Cereb Blood Flow Metab 1996 Nov; 16 (6): 1319–24.
2. Hoffman O, Keilwerth N, Bille MB, et al. Triptans reduce the inflammatory response in bacterial meningitis. J Cereb Blood Flow Metab 2002 Aug; 22 (8): 988–96.
3. Smith M, Cros D, Sheen V. Hyperperfusion with vasogenic leakage by fMRI in migraine with prolonged aura. Neurology 2002; 58: 1308–10.
4. Bohr V, Hansen B, Kjersen H, et al. Sequelae from bacterial meningitis and their relation to the clinical condition during acute illness, based on 667 questionnaire returns. J Infect 1983; 7: 102–10.

24
Headache attributed to cranial or cervical vascular disorder*

M. G. Bousser

Vascular disorders affecting the head are among the most frequent causes of secondary headaches because, firstly, vascular disorders that directly or indirectly involve the brain are extremely frequent, and secondly, headache is a frequent feature of many of them.

Varieties of headache-attributed cranial or cervical disorders can be schematically grouped according to three main clinical situations:

- the first one is an acute headache overshadowed by other neurological signs such as in the case of stroke, focal deficits, or disorders of consciousness. The diagnosis of headache and its causal link with the underlying vascular disorder is usually easy and we will therefore be brief about this variety of headache.
- The second situation is far more difficult because headache is the first and – at least for some time – the only symptom of the vascular disorder: this is frequent in subarachnoid hemorrhage (SAH) and giant cell arteritis, reversible (or benign) central nervous system angiopathy; but it can also occur in a number of other conditions such as cerebellar hemorrhages, unruptured vascular malformations, cervical or intracranial arterial dissections, and cerebral venous thrombosis (CVT). In such cases, the misdiagnosis of the underlying vascular conditions can lead to disastrous consequences. The diagnosis may be particularly difficult when the vascular disease occurs in a patient who already suffers a primary headache disorder, particularly migraine. A clue that should immediately point to an underlying cause, mostly vascular, is that the patient is experiencing a new headache, so far unknown to him and recognized as different from this previous headache. The pattern of headache is variable: it is usually acute and severe, sometimes of the thunderclap type, which immediately points to SAH but can occur in numerous – mostly vascular – other conditions. Occasionally, the onset of headache is progressive over days or even weeks as in giant cell arteritis or in CVT with isolated intracranial hypertension.

---

*HIS classification of headache disorders. 2nd edition, Chapter 6.

◆ The third situation is completely different: it relates to symptomatic migraine – mostly migraine with aura – which may occur on a chronic basis in a number of cerebral arterial disorders.

We will briefly review the main changes that took place between the first and second editions of the HIS classification, and the main varieties of headache occurring in head and neck vascular disorder emphasizing those headaches which may be the first sign of the vascular disorder.

Changes in Chapter 6 between the 1988 and 2004 classifications

As in all other secondary headaches, the title of this chapter has been modified in replacing 'associated with' by 'attributed to', in order to strengthen the causal link that exists between headache and the underlying vascular disorder. The other important change in the title is that the new chapter is restricted to 'cranial or cervical vascular disorders' instead of 'vascular disorders'.

The various sections present in the two classifications are indicated to (Table 24.1). The main changes are the suppression of arterial hypertension, now in Chapter 10, the suppression of traumatic intracranial hemorrhages which are now in Chapter 5, and the addition of a new group of 'other intracranial vascular disorders', which is a 'pot pourri' of various cerebrovascular diseases and which will most likely be modified in the third edition of the classification.

As regards diagnostic criteria, their presentation is different from that of 1988 and they have included whenever possible:

A. Headache with one (or more) of the stated characteristics (if any are known) and fulfilling criteria C and D.

Table 24.1 Headache and vascular disorders in the first and second editions of the International Classification of Headache Disorders

1988: Headache associated with vascular disorders	2004: Headache attributed to cranial or cervical vascular disorders
1. Acute ischemic CVD	1. Ischemic stroke of TIA
2. Intracranial hematoma	2. Non-traumatic intracranial hemorrhage (ICH, SAH)
3. Subarachnoid hemorrhage	3. Unruptured vascular malformation
4. Unruptured vascular malformation	4. Arteritis
5. Arteritis	5. Carotid or vertebral artery pain
6. Carotid or vertebral artery pain	6. Cerebral venous thrombosis
7. Cerebral venous thrombosis	7. Other intracranial vascular disorders
8. Arterial hypertension	
9. Other vascular disorders	

B. Major diagnostic criteria of the vascular disorder.
C. The temporal relationship of the association with, and/or other evidence of causation by, the vascular disorder.
D. Improvement or disappearance of headache within a defined period after its onset, or after the vascular disorder has remitted, or after its acute phase.

It should however be noted that criterion D is sometimes missing because there were not enough published data to give any reasonable time limit for improvement or disappearance of the headache.

Headache attributed to ischemic stroke or transient ischemic attack (TIA)

Ischemic stroke

The criteria are straightforward: any acute headache developing simultaneously with, or in very close temporal relation to, an ischemic stroke. The headache of ischemic stroke is accompanied by focal neurological signs and/or alterations in consciousness usually allowing easy differentiation from the primary headaches. It is usually of moderate intensity and has no specific characteristics.

Headache accompanies ischemic stroke in 17–34% of cases; it is more frequent in basilar- than in carotid-territory strokes. It is of little practical value in establishing stroke etiology except that headache is very rarely associated with lacunar infarcts but extremely common in arterial dissection.

Transient ischemic attack (TIA)

Headache attributed to TIA occurs simultaneously with the onset of the focal deficit, which characterizes the TIA. Headache is more frequent in basilar TIA than in carotid, and it is usually mild. It is very rare in lacunar TIAs. Although headache has been reported in up to 65% of patients with TIA, it is very rarely a prominent symptom and it is hardly ever a reason for seeking medical advice. The focal deficit is the crucial symptom. If a TIA (or an ischemic stroke) is associated with headaches, it points to a common underlying cause such as arterial dissection, arteritis, or reversible CNS angiopathy.

The differential diagnosis between TIA with headache and an attack of migraine with aura may be particularly difficult. The mode of onset is crucial: the focal deficit is typically sudden in a TIA and more frequently progressive in a migrainous aura. Furthermore, positive phenomena (e.g. scintillating scotoma) are far more common in migrainous aura than in TIA, whereas negative phenomena are more usual in TIA.

The 24-h duration is the classical one of TIA but there is a strong case for reducing it to 1 h, given the MR diffusion data which show that after 1 h there is already changes suggestive of a small infarct.[1]

Headache attributed to non-traumatic intracranial hemorrhage

Intracerebral hemorrhage

Headache almost always develops simultaneously with intracerebral bleeding. It is more common (23–68%) and more severe than in ischemic stroke. It is usually overshadowed by focal deficits or coma, but it can be the prominent early feature of cerebellar hemorrhage, which may require emergency surgical decompression. It can also be the only sign of a temporal lobe hemorrhage in the non-dominant hemisphere. The plain CT that should be performed for any acute unexplained headache will easily show these hemorrhages.

Subarachnoid hemorrhage (SAH)

This is the major variety of headache due to an intracranial vascular disorder. It is both frequent and severe, and it requires an urgent treatment. Subarachnoid hemorrhage is by far the most common cause of intense and incapacitating headache of abrupt onset (thunderclap headache) and remains a serious condition (50% of patients die following SAH, often before arriving at hospital, and 50% of survivors are left disabled).

Excluding trauma, 80% of cases result from ruptured saccular aneurysms.

The headache of SAH is often unilateral at onset but it rapidly becomes diffuse and it is accompanied by nausea, vomiting, disorders of consciousness, and nuchal rigidity and less frequently by fever and cardiac dysrhythmia. However, it may be less severe and without associated signs. The abrupt onset is the key feature. Any patient with headache of abrupt onset or thunderclap headache should be evaluated for SAH. Diagnosis is confirmed by CT scan without contrast or MRI (flair sequences) which have a sensitivity of over 90% in the first 24 h. If neuroimaging is negative, equivocal, or technically inadequate, a lumbar puncture should be performed. However, lumbar puncture itself may be negative either if it is done too early or if the SAH is localized, present only in a few sulci on MR flair. SAH is a diagnostic and therapeutic emergency, which has benefited from the development of endovascular treatment which is now proven to have a better benefit/risk ratio than surgery.[2]

Headache attributed to unruptured vascular malformations

This is one of the most difficult topics of Chapter 6 because it is almost impossible to prove a causal relationship between an unruptured malformation and a headache when headache is the only symptom. The criteria C, similar for the four varieties of vascular malformations, is thus never met in the absence of other concomitant neurological signs. In clinical practice, the most frequent situation is that of a patient with migraine or tension-type headache, who undergoes neuroimaging investigations leading to the discovery of an aneurysm, which is most likely to be an incidental finding, but will create an extreme anxiety for the patient. Given the frequency of these primary headaches and the 1% prevalence of aneurysms, there is indeed a high probability that the two coexist without causal relationship. For the four varieties of vascular malformation, it is considered in the classification that any new headache with neuroimaging evidence for a vascular malformation could be attributable to it. This is particularly important for aneurysm, given the recent study questioning the benefit of surgery for asymptomatic aneurysm.[3]

Saccular aneurysm

Headache is reported by approximately 34% of patients with unruptured cerebral aneurysm. It usually has no specific features. However, thunderclap headache occurs *prior to* confirmed aneurysmal SAH in about 50% of patients. Although thunderclap headache may occur in the absence of vascular malformations, such malformations should be looked for by appropriate non-invasive investigations (MRA or CT angiography) and, in doubtful cases, by conventional angiography. A classic variety of 'warning pain' (signaling impending rupture or progressive enlargement) is an acute third nerve palsy with retro-orbital pain and a dilated pupil, indicating an aneurysm of the posterior communicating cerebral artery or end of carotid artery. Thus both thunderclap headache and a painful third nerve palsy with mydriasis should be investigated on an emergency basis, even in the absence of SAH.

There are reports of migraine with visual aura in patients with a posterior cerebral artery aneurysm but whether the aneurysm is the cause of the migraine or just a triggering factor remains unknown.

Arteriovenous malformation (AVM)

The prevalence of AVM is 0.1% so that the likelihood of an indicental association with primary headache is far less frequent than that for aneurysms. Furthermore, by contrast to aneurysms, which are mainly located on the circle of Willis below the brain, most AVMs are located, at least partly, within the brain so that isolated headache is very rare. Cases have been reported highlighting the association of AVM with a variety of headaches such as cluster headache, chronic paroxysmal hemicrania (CPH), and short-lasting unilateral neuralgiform headache with conjunctival injection and tearing (SUNCT), but these cases had atypical features. There is no good evidence of a relationship between AVM and these primary headaches when they are typical.

Migraine with aura has been reported in up to 58% of women with AVM. A strong argument in favor of a causal relationship is the overwhelming correlation between the side of the headache or of the aura and the side of the AVM. There is thus a strong suggestion that AVM can cause attacks of migraine with aura (symptomatic migraine). Yet in large AVM series, migraine as a presenting symptom is rare, much less common than hemorrhage, epilepsy, or focal deficits.

Dural arteriovenous fistula

Studies devoted to headache with dural arteriovenous fistula are lacking. A painful pulsatile tinnitus can be a presenting symptom, as well as headache with other signs of intracranial hypertension due to decrease in venous outflow and sometimes to sinus thrombosis. Carotido-cavernous fistulae may present as painful ophthalmoplegia.

Cavernous angioma

Cavernous angiomas are increasingly recognized on MRI, but, unless they bleed, they are not visualized on CT scan or at angiography. They can be sporadic or familial (autosomal-dominant), single or multiple, and two responsible genes have been identified in affected families.[4] There are so far no systematic studies devoted to headache associated with cavernous angiomas. Headache is commonly reported as a consequence of cerebral hemorrhage or of seizures, but it is unlikely that headache could be a manifestation of uncomplicated cavernous angiomas. A few cases of SUNCT, atypical facial or headpain, and migraine have been reported but once again the causal link remains obscure.[5]

Encephalotrigeminal (or leptomeningeal) angiomatosis (Sturge Weber syndrome)

This syndrome is defined as a facial angioma associated with an ipsilateral meningeal angioma. Neurologic manifestations include seizures, mental retardation, and focal deficits, such as hemiplegia, aphasia, and hemianopia, which may have a fluctuating course. Headache does not seem more frequent than in the general population but there are a few well-documented cases of symptomatic migraine, with prolonged auras, possibly related to chronic oligemia.

Headache attributed to arteritis

This section is divided into three subsections: (1) giant cell arteritis, (2) primary central nervous system (CNS) angiitis, (3) secondary CNS angiitis. The characteristics of headache in CNS angiitis being similar in primary and secondary varieties, will be discussed together.

Giant cell arteritis (GCA)

Of all arteritides and collagen vascular diseases, giant cell arteritis is the disease most conspicuously associated with headache, which is due to inflammation of head arteries, mostly branches of the external carotid artery. It is one of the very few vascular disorders for which criterion D is based on facts and has a crucial value 'Headache resolves or greatly improves within 3 days of high-dose steroid treatment'. By contrast, the requirement to have either 'a swollen tender scalp artery with elevation ESR and or CRP' or a 'temporal artery biopsy demonstrating GCA' seems too restrictive, since the palpation of temporal arteries may be normal. In a subject over 60 years who has a high ESR or CRP and a recent persisting headache which disappears after 3 days of steroid treatment, the diagnosis of GCA can reasonably be accepted even if the biopsy is negative. Indeed the variability in the characteristics of headache and other associated symptoms of GCA (polymyalgia rheumatica, jaw claudication) are such that any recent persisting headache in a patient over 60 years of age should suggest GCA and lead to appropriate investigations; similarly, recent repeated attacks of amaurosis fugax associated with headache are very suggestive of GCA and should prompt urgent investigations.

The major risk is of blindness due to anterior ischemic optic neuropathy, which can be prevented by immediate steroid treatment; the time interval between visual loss in one eye and in the other is usually less than 1 week and there are also risks of cerebral ischemic events and of dementia. Duplex scanning of the temporal arteries may visualize the thickened arterial wall (as a halo on axial sections) and may help to select the site for biopsy.

On histological examination, the temporal artery may appear uninvolved in some areas (skip lesions) pointing to the necessity of serial sectioning.

Primary or secondary CNS angiitis

Central nervous system angiitis is an infrequent disorder in which headache is the most frequent sign and sometimes the presenting symptom. However, it has no specific features and is therefore of little positive diagnostic value until other signs appear such as focal deficits, seizures, altered cognition, or disorders of consciousness which will then overshadow the headache. By contrast, the absence of headache associated with a normal CSF has a high negative value. The pathogenesis of the headache is multifactorial: inflammation, stroke (ischemic or hemorrhagic), raised intracranial pressure and/or SAH.

There are two main diagnostic situations: the most frequent one is that of a patient known to have a systemic vasculitis and who complains of a new recent headache: even in the absence of other symptoms, CNS angiitis is likely if CSF is abnormal and MRA shows diffuse vasoconstriction. The treatment of the underlying vasculitis will be modified accordingly. In the second – and very difficult situation – primary CNS angiitis is suspected because there are no signs – at an extensive workup – of an underlying disease. The classification accepts (criterion C) that the diagnosis be suspected on the basis of 'angiographic signs' (or proven by biopsy). Since diffuse vasoconstriction at angiography is not specific, an histological proof is crucial because primary CNS angiitis is a severe condition requiring a major treatment with high-dose steroids and immunosuppressants.

Carotid or vertebral artery pain

This section has been noticeably modified:

◆ suppression of idiopathic carotidynia which is now in the appendix because it was not found to be a validated entity[6] despite a few recent case reports using this eponym.[7]
◆ adjunction to post-endarterectomy headache [6.5.2] or headache related to other vascular procedures; angioplasty [6.5.3], intracranial endovascular procedures [6.5.4], and angiography [6.5.5.]. The classification mentions only carotid angioplasty but headache is also frequent with vertebral angioplasty.

There is no diagnostic difficulty as regards headache occurring during, or rapidly after, arterial surgery or endovascular procedures. The only difficult and sometimes life-threatening condition is the hyperperfusion syndrome, which can occur after carotid surgery or angioplasty. Headache, usually unilateral, severe, and pulsatile, occurs around the third day post procedure. It often precedes a rise in blood pressure and the onset of seizures or neurological deficits around the seventh day. Urgent treatment is required since these symptoms can herald an often lethal cerebral hemorrhage.

Arterial dissection

Cervical and intracranial artery dissections are increasingly recognized as causes of ischemic stroke, particularly in the young, accounting for up to 20% of ischemic stroke in this population. They are also increasingly recognized as causes of acute headache or neck pain. Indeed, headache with or without neck pain can be the only manifestation of cervical artery dissection. It is by far the most frequent symptom (55–100% of cases) and it is also the most frequent inaugural symptom (33–86% of cases).

Headache, facial pain, and neck pain are usually unilateral (ipsilateral to the dissected artery), severe, and persistent (for a mean of 4 days). However, it has no specific pattern and it can sometimes be very misleading, mimicking other headaches such as migraine, cluster headache, primary thunderclap headache and SAH (particularly since intracranial vertebral artery dissection can itself present with SAH). Associated signs are frequent: signs of cerebral or retinal ischemia and local signs. A painful Honer's syndrome or a painful tinnitus of sudden onset are highly suggestive of carotid dissection. Similarly, episodes of transient monocular blindness with homolateral facial or head pain should in the young or middle-aged subjects point to carotid dissection (and not to retinal migraine).

In carotid dissection, headache is frequently associated with other 'local' signs, whereas in vertebral artery dissection, headache and neck pain may be isolated, mimicking torticolis, or cervicogenic headache, thus eventually leading to cervical manipulations with sometimes dramatic consequences such as brain stem infarct.[8]

Headache in dissection usually precedes the onset of ischemic signs and therefore requires early diagnosis and treatment. Diagnosis is based on Duplex scanning, MRI, MRA and/or helical CT and, in doubtful cases, conventional angiography. Several of these investigations are commonly needed since any of them can be normal. There have been no randomized trials of treatment but there is a consensus in favor of heparin followed by warfarin for 3–6 months according to the quality of the arterial recovery. Angioplasty with stenting has recently been advocated but needs evaluation.

There are interesting but so far mysterious relationships between migraine and dissection. In two case control studies with dissections as cases and either subjects or patients with ischemic stroke not due to dissection normal as controls, migraine was found twice as frequent in dissections as in controls ($p < 0.005$).[9]

Headache attributed to cerebral venous thrombosis (6.6)

The diagnostic criteria are straightforward: any new headache developing in close temporal relation to CVT. However, in practice, CVT remains a diagnostic challenge, particularly when headache is the only symptom.

Headache is by far the most frequent symptom of CVT (present in 80–90% of cases) and it is also the most frequent inaugural symptom. It has no specific characteristics. Most often it is diffuse, progressive, severe, and associated with other signs of intracranial hypertension. It can also be unilateral and sudden, and sometimes very misleading, mimicking migraine, primary thunderclap headache, CSF hypotension, or SAH (of which it can be a cause). Headache can be the only manifestation of CVT but, in over 90% of cases, it is associated with focal signs (neurological deficits or seizures) and/or signs of intracranial hypertension, subacute encephalopathy, or cavernous sinus syndrome.

Given the absence of specific characteristics, any recent persisting headache should raise suspicion, particularly in the presence of an underlying prothrombotic condition. Diagnosis is based on neuroimaging (MRI/MRA or CT scan/CT angiography) in doubtful cases. Heparin treatment should be started as early as possible.

Headache attributed to other intracranial vascular disorders

This section is a mixture of four conditions which have little in common: the first two are chronic diseases in which there is an unusually high frequency of migraine with aura, i.e. symptomatic migraine with aura. Diagnostic criterion D can obviously not be applied in these chronic conditions for which there is, at present, no cure. The last two are acute conditions often manifesting as thunderclap headache.

Cerebral Autosomal Dominant Arteriopathy with Subcortical Infarcts and Leukoencephalopathy (CADASIL)

CADASIL is a recently identified autosomal dominant (with some sporadic cases) small artery disease of the brain, characterized clinically by recurrent small deep infarcts, subcortical dementia, mood disturbances, and migraine with aura.

Migraine with aura is present in one-third of cases and, in such cases, it is usually the first symptom of the disease, appearing at a mean age of 30, some 15 years before ischemic strokes and 20–30 years before death. Attacks are typical of 1.2 *Migraine with aura* except for an unusual frequency of prolonged aura.[10]

MRI is always abnormal with striking white matter changes on T2W1. The disease involves the smooth muscle cells in the media of small arteries and it is due to mutations of Notch 3 gene. The diagnosis is based on genetic testing or on a skin biopsy with Notch 3 antibodies immunostaining.

Mitochondrial Encephalopathy, Lactic Acidosis, and Stroke-like episodes (MELAS)

It is debatable whether mitochondrial disorders should have been included in Chapter 6 because they are not primarily vascular disorders. Nevertheless, there are vascular changes in MELAS, and migraine with aura is more frequent in this condition than in the general population. This has led to the hypothesis that mitochondrial mutations could play a role in migraine with aura but the 3243 mutation was not detected in two groups of subjects with migraine with aura. Other mutations may play a role since migraine attacks also occur in other mitochondrial disorders.

Benign (or reversible) angiopathy of the central nervous system

This is a poorly understood clinico-radiological syndrome characterized by headache with or without other neurological signs and a reversible vasoconstriction of cerebral arteries.[11] It has been reported under different names. It was been associated with pregnancy (post-partum angiopathy), migraine 'sex headache', sympathomimetic drugs, pheochromocytoma, serotonergic drugs, and triptans. The term 'reversible' is preferable to that of 'benign' since cases have been reported with epilepsy, ischemic or hemorrhagic stroke, and even death. However 'benign' forms are probably underdiagnosed because MR angiography may not visualize the 'string and beads' appearance on distal arteries and conventional angiography is nowadays rarely performed in a patient with isolated headache.

Headache is the leading symptom, present in all cases, and often the only one; the most characteristic pattern is that of a flurry of thunderclap headache lasting from a few minutes to a few hours and recurring over a period of 2–6 weeks. A single episode is also possible as well as a more progressive headache. Whatever the mode of onset, it is usually diffuse and severe. Nimodipine treatment has been suggested, but remains debated in this condition, which is sometimes given a short course of steroids because of the diagnostic difficulty with primary CNS angiitis.

Pituitary apoplexy

This rare clinical syndrome is an acute, sometimes benign, sometimes life-threatening condition, characterized by spontaneous hemorrhagic infarction of the pituitary gland. It is one of the causes of thunderclap headache.

Magnetic resonance imaging is more sensitive than CT scan for detecting intrasellar pathology. This illustrates once again that a workup for acute or thunderclap headache restricted to CT scan and CSF study is not sufficient in a number of cases.

Conclusions

Most headaches related to vascular disorders have an acute onset. They are of variable severity but quite often they are both sudden and severe. In a number of vascular disorders, headache is the main – and occasionally the only – initial symptom. These warning headaches are crucial to recognize in order to correctly diagnose the underlying vascular disorders and start appropriate treatment as early as possible, thus potentially preventing devastating neurological consequences. The clue to early diagnosis is to perform the appropriate neuroimaging investigations, often followed by lumbar puncture and vascular investigations.

Many topics need further research:

- unruptured vascular malformations: what type of headache should point to them? What is their relationship with migraine?
- arterial dissections: what is the yield of various investigations when a patient presents with isolated headache or neck pain? What is the risk of cerebral infarction in dissections with headache and local signs as presenting symptoms?
- cerebral venous thrombosis: what pattern of headache should point to CVT? What is the best treatment for headache in CVT? Can d-dimers be a useful tool for the diagnosis of CVT (or to rule it out)?
- reversible CNS angiopathy: what pattern of headache should point to it? What is the best treatment? In which cases should angiography be performed?
- identification of other chronic vascular conditions associated with migraine with aura. Some have already been reported and should be included in the next edition: hereditary cerebral and retinal vascular diseases,[12] and hereditary infantile hemiparesis, retinal arterial tortuosity, and leukoencephalopathy.[13] These conditions, as well as CADASIL and MELAS, are good models to study the pathophysiology of migraine with aura.

Acknowledgments

I wish to thank most warmly, all the members of the working group on Headache attributed to cranial or cervical vascular disorders, JP Castel, A Ducros, J Ferro, S Kittner, H Mattle, J Olesen, and S Solomon for their invaluable collaboration and input.

References

1. Albers GW, Caplan LR, Easton JD, *et al*. Transient ischemic attack. Proposal for a new definition. *NEJM* 2002; **347**: 1713–16.
2. International Subarachnoid Aneurysm Trial (ISAT) Collaborative Group. International Subarachnoid Aneurysm Trial (ISAT) of neurosurgical clipping versus endovascular coiling in 2143 patients with ruptured intracranial aneurysms: a randomised trial. *Lancet* 2002; **360**: 1267–74.
3. International Study of Unruptured Intracranial Aneurysms Investigators. Unruptured intracranial aneurysms risk of rupture and risk of surgical intervention. *N Engl J Med* 1998; **339**: 1725–33.
4. Denier Ch, Labauge P, Brunereau L. Clinical features of cerebral cavernous malformations in patients with KRIT1 mutation. *Ann Neurol* 2004; **55**: 213–20.
5. Afidi S, Goadsby PJ. New onset migraine with a brain stem cavernous angioma. *J Neurol Neurosurg Psychiatry* 2003; **74**: 680–3.
6. Biousse V, Bousser MG. The myth of carotidynia. *Neurology* 1994; **44**: 993–5.
7. Burton BS, Syms MJ, Petermann GW, *et al*. MR imaging of patients with carotidynia. *AJNR* 2000; **21**: 766–9.
8. Mas JL, Henin D, Bousser MG. Dissecting aneurysm of the vertebral artery and cervical manipulation. *Neurology* 1989; **39**: 512–5.
9. Tzourio Ch, Benslamia L, Guillon B, *et al*. Migraine and the risk of cervical artery dissection: A case control study. *Neurology* 2002; **59**: 435–7.
10. Vahedi K, Chabriat H, Levy C, *et al*. Migraine with aura and brain MRI abnormalities in CADASIL. *Arch Neurol* 2004; **61**: 1237–40.
11. Singhal AB, Koroshetz WJ, Caplan LR. Cerebral vasoconstriction syndromes. In: *Uncommon causes of stroke* (eds Bogousslavsky J, Caplan LR). England: Cambridge University Press, 2001: 114–23.
12. Terwindt GM, Haan J, Ophoff RA, *et al*. Clinical and genetic analysis of a large Dutch family with autosomal dominant vascular retinopathy, migraine and Raynaud's phenomenon. *Brain* 1998; **121**: 303–16.
13. Vahedi K, Massin P, Guichard JP, *et al*. Hereditary infantile hemiparesis, retinal arterial tortuosity, and leukoencephalopathy. *Neurology* 2003; **60**: 657–63.

All other references are in The International Classification of Headache disorders. 2nd Edition. *Cephalalgia* 2004; **24** (suppl 1): 72–76.

25
Headache attributed to a substance or its withdrawal

S. D. Silberstein

The International Headache Society (IHS) previously grouped medication-induced headaches under the term 'headaches associated with substances or their withdrawal'.[1] The new IHS classification[2] calls them 'headaches attributed to a substance or its withdrawal' (Table 25.1).

Alcohol, food and food additives, and chemical and drug ingestion and withdrawal have all been reported to provoke or activate migraine in susceptible individuals.[3] Their association is often based on reports of adverse drug reactions and anecdotal data, and does not prove causality. Since headache is a complaint often attributed to placebo, a substance-related headache may occur as a result of expectation. The association between a headache and an exposure may be coincidental (occurring just on the basis of chance) or due to a concomitant illness or a direct or indirect effect of the drug, and may depend on the condition being treated. Headache can be a symptom of a systemic disease, and drugs given to treat such a condition will be associated with headache. Some disorders may predispose to substance-related headache, i.e. alone, neither the drug nor the condition would produce headache. A nonsteroidal anti-inflammatory drug (NSAID) may produce headache by inducing aseptic meningitis in susceptible individuals. Combinations such as alcohol and disulfiram may cause headache when the individual agents might not. The possible relationships between drugs and headache are outlined in Table 25.2.[3] Whether or not a drug induces a headache often depends on the presence or absence of an underlying

Table 25.1 Headache attributed to substance use or withdrawal

8.0 Headache attributed to a substance or its withdrawal
8.1 Headache induced by acute substance use or exposure
8.2 Medication-overuse headache (MOH)
8.3 Headache as an adverse event attributed to chronic medication
8.4 Headache attributed to substance withdrawal

Table 25.2 Drug and substance-related headache

A. Coincidental
B. Reverse causality
C. Interaction headache
D. Causal
1. Acute
a. Primary effect
b. Secondary effect

headache disorder. Headaches that are triggered by drug use are usually similar to the preexisting headache. When a new headache occurs for the first time in close temporal relation to substance exposure, it is coded as a secondary headache attributed to the substance. When a preexisting primary headache is made worse by substance exposure, there are two possibilities. The patient can either be given only the diagnosis of the preexisting primary headache or can be given both this diagnosis and the diagnosis of headache attributed to the substance.[2]

Headache induced by acute substance use or exposure (8.1)
(Tables 25.3A and 25.3B)

This group of headache disorders can be caused by (1) an unwanted effect of a toxic substance, (2) an unwanted effect of a substance in normal therapeutic use, and (3) experimental studies.

Headache, as an adverse event (AE), has been associated with many drugs, as well as placebo, often as a reflection of the very high prevalence of headache. A number of substances, such as nitric oxide (NO) donors and histamine, induce an immediate headache in normal volunteers and in migraineurs. Primary headache sufferers, in addition, can develop a delayed headache one to several hours after the inducing substance has been cleared from the blood. The drugs most commonly associated with acute headache can be divided into several classes.[4]

Vasodilators: Headache is a frequently reported AE of antihypertensive drugs, including the beta-blockers, calcium channel blockers (especially nifedipine), ACE inhibitors, and methyldopa. Nicotinic acid, dipyridamole, and hydralazine have also been associated with headache. The headache mechanism is uncertain.[5]

Nitric oxide donor-induced headache (8.1.1)

Headache is well-known as an AE of therapeutic use of nitroglycerin (GTN) and other NO donors. They may cause headache by activating the trigeminal vascular system. An immediate NO donor-induced headache (GTN headache), develops within 10 min after absorption of NO donor and resolves within

Table 25.3A Headache induced by acute substance use or exposure

8.1.1 Nitric oxide (NO) donor-induced headache

 8.1.1.1 Immediate NO donor-induced headache
 8.1.1.2 Delayed NO donor-headache

8.1.2 Phosphodiesterase (PDE) inhibitor-induced headache
8.1.3 Carbon monoxide-induced headache
8.1.4 Alcohol-induced headache

 8.1.4.1 Immediate alcohol-induced headache
 8.1.4.2 Delayed alcohol-induced headache

8.1.5 Headache induced by food components and additives

 8.1.5.1 Monosodium glutamate-induced headache

8.1.6 Cocaine-induced headache
8.1.7 Cannabis-induced headache
8.1.8 Histamine-induced headache

 8.1.8.1 Immediate histamine-induced headache
 8.1.8.2 Delayed histamine-induced headache

8.1.9 Calcitonin gene-related peptide (CGRP)-induced headache

 8.1.9.1 Immediate CGRP-induced headache
 8.1.9.2 Delayed CGRP-induced headache

8.1.10 Headache as an acute adverse event attributed to medication
used for other indications
8.1.11 Headache attributed to other acute substance use or exposure

Table 25.3B Headache attributed to acute substance use or exposure

Diagnostic criteria
A. Headache fulfilling criteria C and D
B. Acute use of or other acute exposure to a substance
C. Headache develops within 12 h of use or exposure
D. Headache resolves within 72 h after single use or exposure

1 h after release of NO has ended. A delayed NO donor-induced headache develops after NO is cleared from the blood and resolves within 72 h after a single exposure.[6]

Phosphodiesterase inhibitor-induced headache (8.1.2)

Phosphodiesterases (PDEs) are a large family of enzymes that break down cyclic nucleotides (cGMP and cAMP). PDE-5 inhibitors sildenafil and dipyridamole have been formally studied. The headache, unlike GTN-induced headache, is monophasic. In normal volunteers, it has the characteristics of tension-type headache, but in migraine sufferers, it has the characteristics of migraine without aura.[2]

Carbon monoxide-induced headache
(Warehouse workers' headache) (8.1.3)

Carbon monoxide-induced headache is typically mild. When carboxyhemoglobin levels are 10–20%, there are no associated symptoms; a moderate pulsating headache and irritability are present with levels of 20–30%; and severe headache with nausea, vomiting, and blurred vision occur when levels are 30–40%. When carboxyhemoglobin levels are higher than 40%, headache is not usually a complaint because of changes in consciousness.

Alcohol-induced headache (8.1.4)

Ethanol, alone or in combination with congeners (wine), can induce headache in susceptible individuals. There are two subtypes. Immediate alcohol-induced headache (8.1.4.1) develops within 3 h after ingestion of an alcoholic beverage. This headache (called 'cocktail headache') is due to a direct effect of the alcohol or alcoholic beverages. This headache is rarer than the other subtype, which is called delayed alcohol-induced headache (8.1.4.2) (previously 'hangover headache'). The attacks often occur after the blood alcohol level declines or reduces to zero.

In the United Kingdom, red wine is more likely to trigger migraine than white, while in France and Italy, white wine is more likely to produce headache than red. Headaches are more likely to develop in response to white wine if red coloring matter has been added. Migraineurs who believed that red wine (but not alcohol) provoked their headaches were challenged either with red wine or with a vodka mixture of equivalent alcoholic content. The red wine provoked migraine in 9/11 subjects, the vodka in 0/11. Neither provoked headache in other migraine subjects or controls.[7] It is not known which component of red wine triggers headache, and the study may not have been blinded to oenophiles.

The susceptibility to delayed alcohol-induced headache has not been determined. Some migraineurs suffer a migraine the next day after only modest alcoholic intake, while nonmigraineurs usually need a high intake of alcoholic beverages to develop delayed alcohol-induced headache.

Headache induced by food components
and additives (8.1.5)

This was previously called dietary headache. Chocolate, alcohol, citrus fruits, and cheese and dairy products are the foods that patients most commonly believe trigger their migraine, but the evidence that they do so is not persuasive.[8,9] Monosodium glutamate (MSG)[10] and aspartame, the active ingredient in Nutrasweet®, may cause headache in susceptible individuals.[11] Phenylethylamine, tyramine, and aspartame have been incriminated, but their headache-inducing potential is not sufficiently validated.

Monosodium glutamate-induced headache (Chinese restaurant syndrome) (8.1.5.1)

Monosodium glutamate can induce headache and the Chinese restaurant syndrome in susceptible individuals. The headache is typically dull or burning and nonpulsating, but it may be pulsating in migraine sufferers. It is commonly associated with other symptoms, including pressure in the chest, pressure and/or tightness in the face, burning sensations in the chest, neck, or shoulders, flushing of the face, dizziness, and abdominal discomfort.[10]

Aspartame, a sugar substitute, is an *o*-methyl ester of the dipeptide L-α-aspartyl-L-phenylalanine that blocks the increase in brain tryptophan, 5-HT, and 5-hydroxy-indoleacetic acid normally seen after carbohydrate consumption.[11] It produced headache in two controlled studies, but not a third [3]

Tyramine. Tyramine is a biogenic amine that is present in mature cheeses. It is probably not a migraine trigger.[3]

Phenylethylamine: Chocolate contains large amounts of β-phenylethylamine, a vasoactive amine that is, in part, metabolized by monoamine oxidase. The evidence to support it as a trigger is weak.[3]

Lactose intolerance is a common genetic disorder occurring in over two-thirds of African-Americans, native Americans, and Ashkenazic Jews, and in 10% of individuals of Scandinavian ancestry. The most common symptoms are abdominal cramps and flatulence. How lactose intolerance triggers migraine is uncertain.[3]

Chocolate: Chocolate is the food most frequently believed to trigger headache, but the evidence supporting this belief is inconsistent.[12] Chocolate is probably not a migraine trigger, despite the fact that many migraineurs believe that it triggers their headaches. It is the most commonly craved food in the United States. Women are more likely to have migraine than men, and they crave chocolate more than men. Sweet craving is a premonitory symptom of migraine and menses is often associated with an increase in carbohydrate and chocolate craving.[9,13]

Cocaine-induced headache (8.1.6)

Headache is common, develops immediately or within 1 h after cocaine use, and is not associated with other symptoms unless there is concomitant stroke or TIA.[14]

Cannabis-induced headache (8.1.7)

Cannabis use is reported to cause headache associated with dryness of the mouth, paresthesias, feelings of warmth, and suffusion of the conjunctivae.[15]

Histamine-induced headache (8.1.8)

Histamine causes an immediate headache in nonheadache sufferers and an immediate as well as a delayed headache in migraine sufferers. The mechanism is primarily mediated via the H_1 receptor because it is almost completely blocked by mepyramine.

The immediate histamine-induced headache develops within 10 min and resolves within 1 h after histamine absorption has ceased. The delayed histamine-induced headache develops after histamine is cleared from the blood and resolves within 72 h.[16]

Other substances

CGRP (8.1.9) has been reported to cause both immediate and delayed headache.

Headache as an acute adverse event attributed to medication used for other indications (8.1.10)

Nonsteriodal Antiflammatory Drugs

The NSAIDs, especially indomethacin, have been associated with headache. Mechanisms include aseptic meningitis (especially with ibuprofen) and reverse causality (ascribing a headache to a NSAID, when in fact it was a symptom of the disorder being treated).

Serotonin agonists

M-chlorophenylpiperazine, a metabolite of the antidepressant trazadone, can trigger headache by activating the serotonin (5-hydroxytryptamine [HT]) 2B and 2C receptors.[17] This may be the mechanism of headache induction during early treatment with selective serotonin reuptake inhibitors.

Medication-overuse headache (8.2)

Medication-overuse headache (MOH) was previously called rebound headache, drug-induced headache, and medication-misuse headache (Table 25.4). It is one of the most common causes of chronic daily headache (CDH). CDH refers to headache disorders experienced very frequently (15 or more days a month) and can be divided into primary and secondary varieties.[18] Secondary CDH has an identifiable underlying cause.[19–23] The second IHS classification[2] considers chronic migraine (CM), a complication of migraine. It is a primary variety of CDH, which is often mimicked by MOH. To diagnose CM requires the presence of migraine headaches on 15 or more days a month for more than 3 months without medication overuse. When medication overuse is present, the diagnosis is unclear until medication has been withdrawn and there has been no improvement. Medication overuse (i.e. MOH), is often the cause of CDH. These patients should be coded according to the antecedent migraine subtype (usually migraine without aura) plus probable CM plus probable MOH. If criteria for CM are still fulfilled two months after medication overuse has ceased, CM plus the antecedent migraine subtype should be diagnosed and the diagnosis of probable MOH discarded. If CM criteria are no longer fulfilled, the

Table 25.4   New IHS criteria for medication overuse[1]

8.2.6 Headache attributed to medication overuse
Diagnostic criteria
A. Headache present on >15 days/month fulfilling criteria C and D   Characteristics depend on drug

B. Regular overuse for >3 months of a medication
    Amount depends on drug
        Ergotamine, triptans, opioids, and combination analgesics >10 days/month
        Simple analgesics >15 days/month

C. Headache has developed or markedly worsened during medication overuse
D. Headache resolves or reverts to its previous pattern within 2 months after   discontinuation of overused medication

diagnosis should be changed to MOH plus the antecedent migraine subtype and the diagnosis of probable CM discarded.[2]

MOH (drug-induced CDH), or as Isler[24] has termed it, 'painkiller headache,' has been reported since the seventeenth century and reached epidemic proportions in Switzerland after the Second World War. In 1946, Horton and Macy were among the first physicians to identify the potential adverse effects of overusing symptomatic medications in the treatment of headache.[8] Wolfson and Graham published the first reports of ergotamine-induced headache in 1949. In 1951, Peters and Horton provided a theoretical explanation for the 'withdrawal rebound phenomena', based on the vascular activity of ergotamine. Thereafter, this phenomenon was virtually ignored in the literature until it was made prominent in the publications of Saper and Jones,[25] Wilkinson,[26] and Tfelt-Hansen and Krabbe.[27] In 1982,[28] Kudrow[29] discovered that withdrawing analgesics reduced the frequency of CDH and increased the effectiveness of prophylactic medication. In the same year, Isler[24] reported that analgesics and ergotamine, administered separately or in combination, could result in CDH. Dichgans and Diener[30] confirmed this observation. In 1999, Limmroth et al.[31] reported the first cases and the specific clinical features of drug-induced headache after the frequent use of zolmitriptan and naratriptan. MOH became a well-characterized disorder[1,9] and is a growing problem all over the world.

Patients with frequent headaches often overuse analgesics, opioids, ergotamine, and triptans.[32–37] Medication overuse may be both a response to and a consequence of chronic pain, or, in headache-prone patients, it may produce a CDH (MOH) accompanied by dependence on symptomatic medication.[38–41] In addition, medication overuse can make headaches refractory to preventive medication.[27,31,38,42–45] Although stopping the acute medication may result in the development of withdrawal symptoms and a period of increased headache, subsequent headache improvement usually occurs.[25,38–41] In American subspecialty centers, most patients with MOH are women who have a history of episodic migraine that has been converted into MOH as a result of medication overuse.[21,29,42,46–48] The headaches grow more frequent (over months to years) and the associated symptoms of photophobia, phonophobia, and nausea become less severe and less frequent than during typical migraine. Stopping the overused medication frequently results in headache improvement, although this may take days or weeks to occur.[43,49] Many patients remain improved after detoxification.

In population studies, less than one-third of CDH patients overuse medication.[50,51] Thus, medication overuse is not necessary for the development of CDH. Patients with episodic tension-type headache may also overuse acute medications and develop daily headaches. In chronic tension-type headache, in contrast to chronic migraine, most features of migraine are absent, as is prior or coexistent episodic migraine.[9]

Population-based studies report the prevalence rate of MOH to be 1–2%.[50,52] In European headache centers, 5–10% of the patients have MOH. One series of 3000 consecutive headache patients reported that 4.3% had MOH.[53] In American specialty headache clinics, most patients who present with CDH overuse acute medication.[9,24,50,51] Experience in the United Kingdom suggests that drug-associated headache is more common in Europe than the literature suggests. In the United States, over-the-counter analgesics are readily available and patients often consult multiple physicians who may not be aware of other analgesics that the patient is taking. In India, in contrast, medication overuse is less common.[54]

Diener and Tfelt-Hansen[55] summarized 29 studies including 2612 patients with chronic drug-induced headache. Migraine was the primary headache in 65% of patients, TTH in 27%, and mixed or other headaches (i.e. cluster headache) in 8%. Women had more drug-induced headaches than men (3.5 : 1; 1533 women, 442 men). The mean duration of primary headache was 20.4 years. The mean admitted time of frequent drug intake was 10.3 years in one study, and the mean duration of daily headache was 5.9 years. Results from headache diaries show that the number of tablets or suppositories taken daily averaged 4.9 (range 0.25–25). Patients averaged 2.5–5.8 different pharmacologic components simultaneously (range 1–14).[55]

Patients attending an outpatient neurology clinic in Austria reported taking, on an average, 6.3 different headache pain drugs.[56] Of these, 26.5% reported using both prescription and over-the-counter medications, 31.3% used over-the-counter medications only, and 27.7% used prescription drugs only. Acetaminophen (average dose 500 mg) was the most frequently used analgesic. Most patients attending a London migraine clinic used multiple medications.[57] Acetaminophen, again, was the most commonly used analgesic (34.9%), followed by aspirin (22.9%).

In a cross-sectional survey carried out in Tromsø in 1986–87, 19 : 137 men and women (aged 12–56 years) from the general population were asked about their drug use over the preceding 14 days. On an average, 28% of the women and 13% of the men had used analgesics. The most significant predictor of analgesic use was headache; a lesser association was found with infections. Drug use in women was associated with symptoms of depression, in men with sleeplessness. Higher drug use was associated with smoking and high coffee consumption, but not with frequent alcohol intake.[58]

In a representative sample of the Swiss population, 4.4% of men and 6.8% of women took analgesics at least once a week; 2.3% took them daily.[59] Analgesic dependency was more frequent than dependence on tranquilizers, hypnotics, and stimulating drugs in psychiatric inpatients in Switzerland.[60] In Germany, possibly 1% of the population take up to ten pain tablets every day.[61]

In the United States, 20.2% of a national sample survey of 20 468 individuals reported 'severe headache'; 62.6% of the women and 74.6% of the men used over-the-counter medications, while prescription drugs were used by 34.5% of the women and 21.3% of the men. Over-the-counter analgesic use was greater than prescription medication use among migraineurs as well as among those suffering from undefined severe headache.[62] Wang et al.[52] ascertained that significant risk factors for CDH included analgesic overuse (OR = 79), a history of migraine (OR = 6.6), and a Geriatric Depression Scale-Short Form score of 8 or higher (OR = 2.6). At follow-up, patients with persistent primary CDH had a significantly higher frequency of analgesic overuse (33% vs. 0%, $p=0.03$) and major depression (38% vs. 0%, $p=0.04$).

Granella et al.[63] looked for factors that were associated with the evolution of migraine without aura into CM. Risk factors included head trauma (OR 3.3), analgesic use with every attack (OR 2.8), and long duration of oral contraceptive use.

Scher et al.[64] described factors that predict CDH onset and remission in an adult population. They identified cases and controls in a population-based study of CDH and interviewed them on an average of two times in 11 months of follow-up. CDH was more common in women (OR 1.65 [1.3–2.0]), those previously married (OR 1.5 [1.2–1.9]), with obesity (BMI > 30) (OR 1.27 [1.0–1.7]), and those with less education. Obesity and baseline headache frequency were significantly associated with new-onset CDH. Other risk factors included high caffeine consumption, habitual daily snoring, and stressful life events.[65]

A random telephone survey of 24 159 households in Canada produced a sample of 1573 households with one or more eligible headache sufferers. Ninety percent of the IHS-diagnosed migraineurs reported using over-the-counter drugs and 44% reported using prescription drugs. In this sample, 1.5% of migraineurs had rebound headache resulting from ergotamine tartrate or analgesic overuse. Drug-induced rebound headache is a major public health problem in both the clinic and the community.[66]

Clinical features of MOH

Medication-overuse headache has not been demonstrated in placebo-controlled trials.[27,42,43,45] The actual dose limits and time needed to develop MOH have not been defined in rigorous studies. Clinical knowledge is derived from observing patterns of medication use in patients who have very frequent headaches. Because there may be large individual differences in susceptibility to MOH, anecdotal data must be generalized cautiously. Specific limits are necessary to prevent overuse. The frequency of days of use (treatment days, events) is as important as, if not more important than, the total monthly dose.[67]

Scholz et al.[68] studied simple analgesic consumption in patients with and without MOH. Patients with MOH consumed between 1200 and 1500 mg of analgesics a day.

Increased caffeine, but not codeine, consumption was correlated with the development of MOH. Barbiturate consumption was significantly higher in patients with MOH (60–500 mg a day; mean 160 mg a day) than in those without MOH (mean <60 mg a day). All of the triptans (sumatriptan, rizatriptan, naratriptan, and zolmitriptan), selective 5-HT$_1$ agonists that are effective in acute migraine treatment, have been reported to induce MOH.[69–72] Katsarava et al.[73] reported the first cases and the specific clinical features of MOH following the frequent use of zolmitriptan and naratriptan. All patients remained responsive to triptans. Six patients had never used triptans or ergotamine derivatives previously but developed drug-induced headache within six months of taking the drug. Four patients consumed 7.5–10 mg of zolmitriptan or 10–12 mg of naratriptan weekly. The weekly dosages necessary to initiate MOH with the centrally penetrant triptans may be lower than with ergotamines or sumatriptan and the time of onset might be shorter. Increasing attack frequency can be the first sign that MOH is developing. We recommend limiting the use of triptans to no more than three days a week (The IHS recommends <10 days/month).

Limmroth et al.[36] investigated pharmacologic features of MOH, such as the mean duration until onset, mean monthly intake frequencies, and mean monthly dosages, and specific clinical features of MOH following overuse of different acute headache drugs, with a special focus on newly approved triptans. All patients with tension-type headache as their primary headache developed a headache similar to chronic tension-type headache. The mean duration until onset of MOH was shortest for triptans (1.7 years), longer for ergots (2.7 years), and longest for analgesics (4.8 years). The mean monthly intake frequency was lowest for triptans (18 single doses per month), higher for ergots,[37] and highest for analgesics (114). Patients with migraine as their primary headache, however, developed different clinical features. Patients overusing ergots and analgesics typically experienced a daily tension-type headache. In contrast, patients with triptan-induced MOH were more likely to describe a daily migraine-like headache or a major increase in migraine frequency. Limmroth et al.[36] concluded that triptan overuse leads to MOH sooner and with lower dosages than ergots and analgesics. The study suggested that an increase in frequency of migraine attacks may be considered a triptan-specific form of MOH, which would then require a temporary discontinuation of the drug.

There are those who doubt the existence of drug-induced headache.[74] When Fisher[74] failed to find analgesic rebound headache in patients who were using analgesics for arthritis, he attempted to refute the concept. His work has been reinterpreted to suggest that headache-prone patients are especially vulnerable to the rebound phenomenon. Headache-prone patients often develop daily headaches if they are put on analgesics for a nonheadache indication.[75,76]

In addition to exacerbating the headache disorder, drug overuse has other serious effects. The overuse of acute drugs may interfere with the effectiveness of preventive headache medications. Prolonged use of large amounts of medication may cause renal or hepatic toxicity in addition to tolerance, habituation, or dependence. (Tolerance refers to the decreased effectiveness of the same dose of an analgesic, often leading to the use of higher doses to achieve the same degree of effectiveness. Habituation and dependence are, respectively, the psychological and physical need to use drugs repeatedly.)

Patients with MOH may develop psychological dependence, tolerance, and abstinence syndromes.[3] Medication overuse is usually motivated by a patient's desire to treat the headaches. However, some headache patients may overuse combination analgesics to treat their mood disturbance. Medication overuse rarely represents primary substance abuse. Medication overuse could result in resetting the pain control mechanisms in susceptible individuals, perhaps by enhancing on-cell activity, enhancing central sensitization through NMDA receptors, or blocking adaptive antinociceptive changes. Chronic opioid use has clearly been shown to activate RVM pain facilitation. Opioid-induced neurotoxicity may result in headache intractability by depleting inhibitory GABA interneurons.

Overuse is now defined by the IHS in terms of treatment days per month. It is crucial that treatment occurs both frequently and regularly, i.e. several days each week. For example the diagnostic criterion of use on 10 or more days a month (15 for simple analgesics) translates into 2–3 treatment days every week. Bunching treatment days and going for long periods without medication intake, as practiced by some patients, is unlikely to cause MOH. The amount of use that constitutes overuse depends on the drug. Ergotamine-overuse headache requires intake on 10 or more days a month on a regular basis for 3 or more months. The headache is often daily and constant. Triptan-overuse headache is usually frequent, intermittent, and migrainous. Triptan intake (any formulation) on 10 or more days a month may increase migraine frequency to that of chronic migraine. Evidence suggests that this occurs sooner with triptan overuse than with ergotamine overuse.[35,36]

Medication overuse is not the only cause of CDH (Table 25.5). Many patients develop chronic migraine or chronic tension-type headache without overusing medication, and others continue to have daily headaches long after the overused medication is discontinued. When a *new* headache occurs for the first time in close temporal relation to substance exposure, it is coded as a secondary headache attributed to the substance. This is true even if the headache has the characteristics of migraine, tension-type headache, or cluster headache. When a *preexisting* primary headache is aggravated in close temporal relation to substance exposure, there are two possibilities. The patient can either be given only the diagnosis of the preexisting primary headache or he can be given both this diagnosis and the diagnosis of headache attributed to the substance. A diagnosis of headache attributed to a substance usually becomes definite only when the headache resolves or greatly improves after exposure to the substance is terminated. In the case of MOH, an arbitrary period of two months after overuse cessation is now stipulated by the IHS; if the diagnosis is to be definite, improvement must occur in that time frame. Prior to cessation, or pending improvement within two months after cessation, the diagnosis of probable MOH should be applied. If improvement does not then occur within the two-month period, the MOH diagnosis is discarded.

Patients with a *pre-existing* primary headache who develop a new type of headache or whose migraine or tension-type headache is made markedly

Table 25.5 Chronic daily headache

Primary chronic daily headache
    Headache duration >4 h
        Chronic migraine (previously transformed migraine)
        Chronic tension-type headache
        New daily persistent headache
        Hemicrania continua
    Headache duration <4 h
        Cluster headache
           Paroxysmal hemicranias
        Hypnic headache
        Idiopathic stabbing headache
Secondary chronic daily headache
    Medication-overuse headache
    Posttraumatic headache
    Cervical spine disorders
    Headache associated with vascular disorders (arteriovenous malformation,
        arteritis [including giant cell arteritis], dissection, and subdural hematoma)
    Headache associated with nonvascular intracranial disorders (intracranial
        hypertension, infection [EBV, HIV], neoplasm)
    Other (temporomandibular joint disorder; sinus infection)

worse during medication overuse should be given the diagnosis of both the pre-existing headache and MOH. The headache associated with medication overuse often has a peculiar pattern shifting, even within the same day; from having migraine-like characteristics to having those of tension-type headache (i.e. a new type of headache). The diagnosis of MOH is clinically important, because patients rarely respond to preventive medications while they are overusing acute medications.

Headache as an adverse event attributed to chronic medication (8.3)

Headache can be due to a direct pharmacologic effect of medication, such as vasoconstriction producing malignant hypertension and headache, or to a secondary effect, such as drug-induced intracranial hypertension. The latter is a recognized complication of long-term use of anabolic steroids, amiodarone, lithium carbonate, nalidixic acid, thyroid hormone replacement, tetracycline, or minocycline. Regular use of exogenous hormones, typically for contraception or hormone replacement therapy, can be associated with increase in frequency or new development of headache or migraine (Table 25.6).

Table 25.6   Headache as an adverse event attributed
to chronic medication

Diagnostic criteria

A. Headache present on >15 days/month fulfilling criteria C and D
B. Chronic medication for any therapeutic indication
C. Headache develops during medication
D. Headache resolves after discontinuation of medication

Headache attributed to substance withdrawal (8.4)

The new IHS classification has specific criteria for caffeine-withdrawal headache, opioid-withdrawal headache, estrogen-withdrawal headache, and headache attributed to withdrawal from chronic use of other substances (Table 25.7).

Caffeine-withdrawal headache (8.4.1)

Stopping daily low-dose caffeine frequently results in withdrawal headache.[77] In a controlled study of caffeine withdrawal, 64 normal adults (71% women) with low-to-moderate caffeine intake (the equivalent of about 2.5 cups of coffee a day) were given a two-day caffeine-free diet and either placebo or replacement caffeine. Under double-blind conditions, 50% of the patients who were given placebo had a headache by day 2, compared with 6% of those given caffeine. Nausea, depression, and flu-like symptoms were very common in the placebo group. This study is relevant since caffeine is frequently used by headache sufferers for pain relief, often in combination with analgesics or ergotamine. The study is a model for short-term caffeine withdrawal, but does not demonstrate the long-term consequences of detoxification. In a community-based telephone survey of 11112 subjects in Lincoln and Omaha, Nebraska, 61% reported daily caffeine consumption, and 11% of the caffeine consumers reported symptoms upon stopping coffee.[78] A group of those who reported withdrawal symptoms were assigned to one of three regimes: abrupt caffeine withdrawal, gradual withdrawal, and no change. One-third of the abrupt-withdrawal group and an occasional member of the gradual-withdrawal group had symptoms that included headache and tiredness.

Table 25.7   Headache attributed to withdrawal from chronic
use of other substances

Diagnostic criteria

A. Bilateral and/or pulsating headache fulfilling criteria C and D
B. Daily intake of a substance other than those described above
    for >3 months, which is interrupted
C. Headache develops in close temporal relation to withdrawal of the substance
D. Headache resolves within 3 months after withdrawal

Estrogen-withdrawal headache (8.4.3) and headache attributed to withdrawal from chronic use of other substances (8.4.4)

Estrogen-withdrawal follows cessation of a course of exogenous estrogens (such as during the pill-free interval of combined oral contraceptives or following a course of replacement or supplementary estrogen) and can induce headache and/or migraine. It has been suggested, but without sufficient evidence, that withdrawal of the following substances may cause headache: corticosteroids, tricyclic antidepressants, selective serotonin reuptake inhibitors (SSRIs), NSAIDs (Table 25.7).

References

1. Headache Classification Committee of the International Headache Society. Classification and diagnostic criteria for headache disorders, cranial neuralgia, and facial pain. *Cephalalgia* 1988; **8**: 1–96.
2. Headache Classification Committee. The International Classification of Headache Disorders, 2nd Edition. *Cephalalgia* 2004; **24**: 1–160.
3. Silberstein SD. Drug-induced headache. *Neurol Clin N Amer* 1998; **16**: 107–23.
4. Olesen J, Tfelt-Hansen P, Welch KMA. In: *The headaches* (ed. Williams & Wilkins) 2nd edn. Philadelphia: Lippincott, 2000; 861–9.
5. Thomson Healthcare. *Physicians' desk reference*. 57th Ed. Montvale: Thomson Pdr, 2004.
6. Ashina M, Bendtsen L, Jensen R, *et al*. Nitric oxide-induced headache in patients with chronic tension-type headache. *Brain* 2000; **123**: 1830–7.
7. Littlewood JT, Glover V, Davies PT, *et al*. Red wine as a cause of migraine. *Lancet* 1988; 559.
8. Capobianco DJ, Swanson JW, Dodick DW. Medication-induced (analgesic rebound) headache: historical aspects and initial descriptions of the north american experience. *Headache: The Journal Of Head And Face Pain* 2001; **41**: 500–2.
9. Silberstein SD, Lipton RB, Goadsby PJ. Headache in clinical practice. Oxford: Isis Medical Media Ltd., 1998.
10. Schamburg HH, Byck R, Gerstl R, *et al*. Monosodium L-Glutamate: its pharmacology and role in the Chinese restaurant syndrome. *Science* 1969; **163**: 826–8.
11. Schiffmann SS, Buckley CE, Sampson HA, *et al*. Aspartame and susceptibility to headache. *N Engl J Med* 1987; **317**: 1181–5.
12. Scharff L, Marcus DA. The association between chocolate and migraine: a review. *Headache Quarterly* 1999; **10**: 199–205.
13. Amery WK, Waelkens J, Caers I. Dopaminergic mechanisms in premonitory phenomena. In: *The prelude to the migraine attack* (ed. Amery Wk, Wauquier A). London: Bailliere Tindall, 1986: 64–77.
14. Dhopesh V, Maany I, Herring C. The relationship of cocaine to headache in polysubstance abusers. *Headache* 1991; **31**: 17–19.
15. Elmallakh RS. Marijuana and migraine. *Headache* 1987; **27**: 442–3.
16. Krabbe AA, Olesen J. Headache provocation by continuous intravenous infusion of histamine, clinical results and receptor mechanisms. *Pain* 1980; **8**: 253–9.
17. Brewerton TD, Murphy DL, Mueller EA, *et al*. Induction of migraine like headaches by the serotonin agonist m-chlorophenylpiperazine. *Clin Pharmacol Ther* 1988; **43**: 605–9.
18. Silberstein SD, Lipton RB. Chronic daily headache including transformed migraine, chronic tension-type headache, and medication overuse. In: *Wolff's headache and other head pain* (ed. Silberstein SD, Lipton RB, Dalessio DJ). Seventh Ed. New York: Oxford University Press, 2001: 247–82.

19. Lake A, Saper J, Madden S, *et al.* Inpatient treatment for chronic daily headache: a prospective long-term outcome. *Headache* 1990; **30**: 299 (Abstract).
20. Brain WR. Some unsolved problems of cervical spondylosis. *Br Med J* 1963; **1**: 771–7.
21. Rapoport AM. Analgesic rebound headache. *Headache* 1988; **28**: 662–5.
22. Mathew NT. Chronic daily headache: clinical features and natural history. In: *Headache and depression: serotonin pathways as a common clue* (ed. Nappi G, Bono G, Sandrini G, Martignoni E, Micieli G). New York: Raven Press, 1991: 49–58.
23. Lake AE, Saper JR, Madden SF, *et al.* Comprehensive inpatient treatment for intractable migraine: a prospective long-term outcome study. *Headache* 1993; 55–62.
24. Isler H. Headache drugs provoking chronic headache: historical aspects and common misunderstandings. In: *Drug-induced headache* (ed. Diener HC, Wilkinson M). Berlin: Springer-Verlag. 1988: 87–94.
25. Saper JR, Jones JM. Ergotamine tartrate dependency: features and possible mechanisms. *Clin Neuropharmacol* 1986; **9**: 244–56.
26. Wilkinson M. Introduction. In: *Drug induced headache* (ed. Diener HC, Wilkinson M). Berlin: Springer Verlag. 1988: 1–2.
27. Tfelt-Hansen P, Aebelholt-Krabbe A. Ergotamine abuse. Do patients benefit from withdrawal? *Cephalalgia* 1981; **1**: 27–32.
28. Ala-Hurula V, Myllyla V, Hokkanen E. Ergotamine abuse: results of ergotamine discontinuation with special reference to the plasma concentrations. *Cephalalgia* 1982; **2**: 189–95.
29. Kudrow L. Paradoxical effects of frequent analgesic use. *Adv Neurol* 1982; **33**: 335–41.
30. Dichgans J, Diener HC. Clinical manifestations of excessive use of analgesic medication. In: *Drug-induced headache* (ed. Diener HC, Wilkinson M). Berlin: Springer-Verlag, 1988; 8–15.
31. Limmroth V, Kazarawa S, Fritsche G, *et al.* Headache after frequent use of new 5-Ht agonists zolmitriptan and naratriptan. *Lancet* 1999; **353**: 378.
32. Saper JR. Ergotamine dependency – a review. *Headache* 1987; **27**: 435–8.
33. Mathew NT, Kurman R, Perez F. Drug induced refractory headache – clinical features and management. *Headache* 1990; **30**: 634–8.
34. Katsarava Z, Muebig M, Fritsche G, *et al.* Clinical features of withdrawal headache following overuse of triptans in comparison to other antiheadache drugs. *Neurology* 2001; **57**: 1694–8.
35. Diener HC, Dahlof CG. Headache associated with chronic use of substances. In: *The headaches* (ed. Olesen J, Tfelt-Hansen P, Welch Kma). 2nd Ed. Philadelphia: Lippincott, Williams & Wilkins, 1999; 871–8.
36. Limmroth V, Katsarava Z, Fritsche G, *et al.* Features of medication overuse headache following overuse of different acute headache drugs. *Neurology* 2002; **59**: 1011–4.
37. Silberstein SD, Lipton RB. Chronic daily headache. In: *Headache* (ed. Goadsby PJ, Silberstein SD). Newton: Butterworth-Heinemann, 1997: 201–25.
38. Saper JR. Chronic headache syndromes. *Neurol Clin* 1989; **7**: 387–412.
39. Andersson PG. Ergotism: the clinical picture. In: *Drug induced headache* (ed. Diener HC, Wilkinson MS) Berlin: Springer, 1988; 16–19.
40. Rapoport Am, Weeks Re, Sheftell Fd, *et al.* The 'analgesic washout period': a critical variable evaluation in the evaluation of headache treatment efficacy. *Neurology* 1986; **36**: 100–1.
41. Baumgartner C, Wessly P, Bingol C, *et al.* Long-Term prognosis of analgesic withdrawal in patients with drug-induced headaches. *Headache* 1989; **29**: 510–4.
42. Mathew NT. Drug induced headache. *Neurol Clin* 1990; **8**: 903–12.
43. Saper JR. Ergotamine dependence. *Headache* 1987; **27**: 435–8.
44. Saper JR. Chronic headache syndromes. *Neurol Clin* 1990; **8**: 891–901.
45. Diamond S, Dalessio DJ. Drug abuse in headache. In: *The practicing physician's approach to headache* (ed. Diamond S, Dalessio DJ). 3rd Ed. Baltimore: Williams & Wilkins, 1982: 114–21.

46. Mathew NT, Reuveni U, Perez F. Transformed or evolutive migraine. *Headache* 1987; **27**: 102–6.
47. Diener HC, Dichgans J, Scholz E, *et al.* Analgesic-induced chronic headache: long-term results of withdrawal therapy. *J Neurol* 1984; **236**: 9–14.
48. Rasmussen BK, Jensen R, Olesen J. Impact of headache on sickness absence and utilization of medical services. *J Epidemiol Community Health* 1992; **46**: 443–6.
49. Mathew NT, Stubits E, Nigam MR. Transformation of episodic migraine into daily headache: analysis of factors. *Headache* 1982; **22**: 66–8.
50. Castillo J, Munoz P, Guitera V, *et al.* Epidemiology of chronic daily headache in the general population. *Headache* 1999; **39**: 190–6.
51. Scher AI, Stewart WF, Lipton RB. Is analgesic use a risk factor for chronic daily headache? *Neurology* 2001; **56**: A312. (Abstract).
52. Wang SJ, Fuh Jl, Lu SR, *et al.* Chronic daily headache in chinese elderly: prevalence, risk factors and biannual follow-up. *Neurology* 2000; **54**: 314–9.
53. Micieli G, Manzoni GC, Granella F, *et al.* Clinical and epidemiological observations on drug abuse in headache patients. In: *Drug-induced headache* (ed. Diener HC, Wilkinson M). Berlin: Springer-Verlag, 1988: 20–8.
54. Ravishankar K. Headache pattern in india: a headache clinic analysis of 1000 patients. *Cephalalgia* 1997; **17**: 143–4.
55. Diener HC, Tfelt-Hansen P. Headache associated with chronic use of substances. In: *The headaches* (ed. Olesen J, Tfelt-Hansen P, Welch KMA). New York: Raven Press Ltd, 1993: 721–7.
56. Schnider P, Aull S, Feucht M. Use and abuse of analgesics in tension-type headache. *Cephalalgia* 1994; **14**: 162–7.
57. Silberstein SD, Saper JR. Migraine: diagnosis and treatment. In: *Wolff's headache and other head pain* (ed. Dalessio DJ, Silberstein SD). Sixth Ed. New York: Oxford University Press, 1993: 96–170.
58. Eggen AE: The Tromsø study: frequency and predicting factors of analgesic drug use in a free-living population (12–56 Years). *J Clin Epidemiol* 1993; **46**: 1297–304.
59. Gutzwiller F, Zemp E. Der analgetikakonsum in der bevölkerung und socioökonomische aspekte des analgetikaabusus. In: *Das Analgetikasyndrom* (ed. Mihatsch MJ). Stuttgart: Thieme, 1986: 197–205.
60. Kieholz P, Ladewig D. Probleme des medikamentenmissbrauches. Schweis Arztezeitung 1981; **62**: 2866–9.
61. Schwarz A, Farber U, Glaeske G. Daten zu analgetikakonsum and analgetikanephropathie in der bundesrepublik. Offentiches gesundheitswesen 1985; **47**: 298–300.
62. Celentano DD, Stewart WF, Lipton RB, *et al.* Medication use and disability among migraineurs. *Headache* 1992; **32**: 223–8.
63. Granella F, Cavallini A, Sandrini G, *et al.* Long-term outcome of migraine. *Cephalalgia* 1998; **18**: 30–3.
64. Scher AI, Stewart WF, Ricci JA, *et al.* Factors associated with the onset and remission of chronic daily headache in a population-based study. *Pain* 2003; **106**: 89.
65. Scher AI, Lipton RB, Stewart W. Risk factors for chronic daily headache. *Cur Pain Headache Rep* 2002; **6**: 486–91.
66. Robinson RG. Pain relief for headaches. *Can Fam Physician* 1993; **39**: 867–72.
67. Saper JR. Headache disorders: current concepts in treatment strategies. Littleton: Wright-PSG, 1983.
68. Scholz E, Diener HC, Geiselhart S, *et al.* Drug-induced headache: does a critical dosage exist? In: *Drug-induced headache* (ed. Diener HC). Berlin: Springer-Verlag, 1988: 29–43
69. Catarci T, Fiacco F, Argentino C. Ergotamine-induced headache can be sustained by sumatriptan daily intake. *Cephalalgia* 1994; **14**: 374–5.
70. Diener HC, Haab J, Peters C, *et al.* Subcutaneous sumatriptan in the treatment of headache during withdrawal from drug-induced headache. *Headache* 1991; **31**: 205–9.

71. Gaist D, Hallas J, Sindrup SH, *et al*. Is overuse of sumatriptan a problem? A population-based study. *Eur J Clin Pharmacol* 1996; **50**: 161–5.
72. Bates D, Ashford E, Dawson R, *et al*. Subcutaneous sumatriptan during the migraine aura. *Neurology* 1994; **44**: 1587–92.
73. Katsarava Z, Limmroth V, Fritsche G, *et al*. Drug-induced headache following the use of zolmitriptan or naratriptan. *Cephalalgia* 1999; **19**: 414. (Abstract).
74. Fisher CM. Analgesic rebound headache refuted. *Headache* 1988; **28**: 666.
75. Bowdler I, Killian J, Gänsslen-Blumberg S. The association between analgesic abuse and headache—coincidental or causal. *Headache* 1990; **30**: 494.
76. Lance F, Parkes C, Wilkinson M. Does analgesic abuse cause headache de novo? *Headache* 1988; 61–2.
77. Silverman K, Evans SM, Strain EC, *et al*. Withdrawal syndrome after the double-blind cessation of caffeine consumption. *N Eng J Med* 1992; **327**: 1109–14.
78. Dews PB, Curtis GL, Hanford KJ, *et al*. The frequency of caffeine withdrawal in a population-based survey and in a controlled, blinded pilot experiment. *J Clin Pharmacol* 1999; **39**. 1221–32.

26 Headache attributed to trauma

M. J. A. Láinez

Background

Posttraumatic Headache (PTH) is one of the several symptoms of the postconcussive syndrome, usually the most frequent, and it may be accompanied by additional cognitive, behavioral, or somatic problems (Solomon 2001). Headache can start after brain, head, or neck injury and simulate the clinical characteristics of several primary headaches. Usually PTH is self-limited. Severe, moderate, and mild head injuries have been related to the beginning of new headaches. The mechanisms of headache are still poorly understood; biological, psychological, and social factors have been implicated. Similarly, the pathophysiology of the symptoms in individuals with postconcussive syndrome continues being a subject of some controversy ranging from neural damage to malingering (Keidel and Diener 1997).

The term *'whiplash'* commonly refers to symptoms and signs associated with a mechanical event such as a sudden acceleration and deceleration of the neck (in the majority of cases, due to a road accident). The clinical manifestations after whiplash include symptoms related to the neck, as well as somatic extracervical, neurosensory, behavioral, cognitive and affective disorders, the appearance, and mode of expression of which can vary widely over time. *Headache post-whiplash* (headache attributed to neck injury or whiplash) is usually accompanied by neck pain and has often a tensional or cervicogenic pattern. Whiplash is commonly evaluated in medico-legal practice (Bono *et al.* 2000). Several socio-demographic and crash-related factors, as well as a combination of specific musculoskeletal and neurological signs have been identified as predictive factors for a longer recovery.

Until now, *Acute posttraumatic headaches* might begin in less than 14 days after head or neck trauma and continue for up to 8 weeks post-injury (*Cephalalgia* 1988). Although onset proximate to the time of injury is the most common, any new headache type occurring within this period of time was referred to as an acute posttraumatic headache. Headache that develops longer than 14 days after was termed *delayed-PTH* or *late-acquired headache*. And, if such headaches persisted beyond the first two months post-injury, they were subsequently referred to as *Chronic posttraumatic headaches.*

There were no validation studies for the posttraumatic headache criteria of 1988 IHS Classification (*Cephalalgia* 1988) and when we looked at the literature there were very few publications. In Medline, between 1989 and 2001, only 67 references included the term PTH, 27 reviews, 25 case reports, and 15 originals. Only a small number of them, all retrospective studies, used IHS criteria (Weiss *et al.* 1991; Yamaguchi *et al.* 1992; Gfeller *et al.* 1994; Gilkey *et al.* 1997). For this reason, the new criteria are based not only on literature review, but also on clinical experience.

Posttraumatic Headache (PTH)

Clinical characteristics of PTH

A great variety of headache patterns has been described after head injury and may closely resemble primary headache disorders (mainly tension-type headache, cervicogenic headache, migraine with and without aura, cluster-like headache, and occipital neuralgia) (Hachinski 2000). Common headache pathways have been described for primary and post-traumatic headaches but, nowadays the pathogenesis of PTH is still not well-known (Martelli *et al.* 1999). Previous reviews about the clinical presentation of PTH revealed that tension-type headache was the most common variety (De Benedittis and De Santis 1983). In one of the first prospective studies, Hass followed-up 48 patients with PTH and the same number of controls with similar 'natural' or primary headache during 3 months after a traumatic event. According to previous IHS Criteria (*Cephalalgia* 1988), 75% of the patients with PTH had a tension-type headache, 21% had migraine without aura, and 4% had an unclassified headache (Hass *et al.* 1996). After this, other prospective studies but without control group, show that the headache pattern after head injury may be variable being tension-type, with cervicogenic and migrainous headaches being the most habitual ones (Bettuci *et al.* 1998; De Souza *et al.* 1999). Cluster-like headache, supraorbitary neuralgia, occipital neuralgia, exertional headache, and headache associated with sexual activity have been described sometimes in case reports. We conclude that PTH, with some of these patterns, could be possible.

Disorder definition

Mild, moderate, and severe head injuries can be associated with PTH. Clinical quantification of traumatic brain injury patients should be based on Admission Glasgow Coma Scale score (GCS), presence or absence of loss of consciousness and duration of unconsciousness (LOC), presence of posttraumatic amnesia (PTA), and any focal neurological findings. In 1988, the significance of the head trauma was related to at least one of the following conditions: presence of LOC, PTA longer than 10 min, or confirmatory signs of significant trauma (at least two of the following exhibit relevant abnormality: clinical neurological examination, X-ray of the skull, neuroimaging, evoked potentials, CSF examination, vestibular test, and neuropsychological testing).

When these conditions were not fulfilled, we talked about minor head trauma. We decided to define the *mild head trauma* (MHT) using similar criteria accepted by the majority of the medical community; MHT will not cause loss of consciousness or the LOC will be shorter than 30 min, and the trauma should cause symptoms and/or signs of *concussion* with GCS score ≥13. Headache, nausea, and dizziness are frequent symptoms after MTH and may continue for weeks or months after the trauma.

The relationship between severity of the injury and severity of the PTH has not been conclusively established. Moreover, there are some controversial data. Most studies suggest that PTH is *less* frequent when the head injury is *more* severe. For patients with symptoms after 6 months to several years, there is a strong probability that emotional, motivational, and premorbid personality factors could support these residual symptomatology (Yamaguchi 1992; Lanz and Bryant 1996).

After mild head injuries, laboratory and neuroimaging investigations are not usually needed. When GCS score is less than 13 in the emergency room immediately after head or neck trauma, LOC is longer than 30 min, there is PTA, neurologic deficits or personality disturbances, neuroimaging studies (CT Scan or MRI) are indicated. MRI (T1 weighted, T2 weighted, proton density, and gradient-echo sequence images) will be much more sensitive than CT scan in order to detect and classify minor brain lesions. Within one week of a head injury, only MRI can identify cortical contusions and lesions in the deep white matter of the cerebral hemispheres underdiagnosed by CT. MRI thus provides a sounder basis for diagnosis and treatment in patients suffering from late sequelae of cranial injuries (Voller *et al.* 2001). Other complementary studies (EEG, evoked potentials, CSF examination, vestibular function test) had been individually considered for patients with ongoing posttraumatic headaches.

There is no evidence that abnormalities of these other complementary explorations change the prognosis or contribute to treatment. Complementary studies will be considered on a case-by-case basis, or for research purposes.

Temporal relationship

The differentiation between a primary and a posttraumatic headache in some cases can be a difficult task. Patients who develop a new form of headache in close temporal relation to head or neck trauma, will be coded as a secondary headache. Patients who already have this type of headache which significantly worsens in close temporal relation to trauma, without evidence of a causal relationship between the primary headache and the other disorder, will receive only the primary headache diagnosis. However, if there is both, a very close temporal relation to the trauma and other good evidence that the particular kind of trauma has aggravated the primary headache, that is, if trauma in scientific studies of good quality has been shown to aggravate the primary headache disorder, the patient will receive the primary and the secondary headache diagnosis. In many cases of secondary headache, the diagnosis is definite only when headache resolves or greatly improves within a specified time after effective treatment or spontaneous remission of the causative disorder. In such cases, this temporal relation is an essential part of the evidence of causation.

It will be easy to establish the relationship between a headache and head or neck trauma when the headache develops immediately or in the first days after trauma has occurred (Cartlidge 1981). On the other hand, it will be very difficult when a headache develops weeks or even months after trauma, specially when the majority of these headaches have the pattern of tension-type headache; and the prevalence of this type of headache in the population is very high. Such late-onset posttraumatic headaches have been described in anecdotal reports but not in case-control studies (Nick and Sicard-Nick 1965; Cartlidge 1981). Evans's review demonstrated that headache presentation was highest within the first month (90%) after head or neck trauma, especially within the first week (71%) (Evans 1992). In other recent prospective studies, patients with a history of MHT have shown a usual beginning of post-concussion symptoms a week and a longer maintenance (32% after 1 year and 18% after 2 years) (Radanov *et al.* 1995; Sturzenegger *et al.* 1995; van der Naalt *et al.* 1999). In accordance with the new IHS Classification, acute PTH may develop within 7 days after head trauma or regaining consciousness following head trauma and resolve within 3 months. The reason to shorten this period has been to obtain more specificity even at the expense of less sensibility.

Headache resolution

After several months, some patients with the history of a mild head injury developed a daily headache. PTH is habitually a self-limited condition but, a minority of individuals may develop persistent headaches. After consensus, all chronic varieties of secondary headaches persist more than 3 months. Chronic PTH develops within 7 days after head trauma, regaining consciousness or memory and continues longer than three months. In the pathogenesis of chronic headaches, neurological, psychological, and legal factors have been implicated. Neurological factors should be implicated in the initial phase, psychological and socioeconomical factors (litigation and expectations for compensation) in the maintenance. Premorbid personality could contribute to development of chronic symptoms, affecting the adjustment to injury and the treatment outcome. Surprisingly, the risk of developing chronic disturbances seems to be also greater for mild-moderate head injuries.

Headache post-whiplash

Clinical characteristics of headache post-whiplash

Several prospective studies have shown the figures of prevalence and the patterns of headache post-whiplash clinical presentation. After the article of Evans in 1992, a lot of authors have followed different groups of patients with whiplash injury from several months to years (Evans 1992). For Foletti *et al.* 74% of 63 patients with headache and neck pain after whiplash showed characteristics of tension-type headache and around 10% of migraine with or without aura (Foletti and Regli 1995). Posttraumatic tension type was the most frequent type of PTH for Keidel *et al.* (85%) followed by cervicogenic (10%). The headache due to common whiplash was located occipitally (67%), was of dull-pressing or dragging character (77%), and lasted for an average of 3 weeks. In 80% of patients, headache post-whiplash showed remission within 6 months. Posttraumatic-migraine and cluster-like headache were observed in rare cases (Keidel 1997). In a new report, Pearce (2001) described the follow-up of 48 patients with headache 1 month after whiplash injury. Twenty-five of these 48 patients suffered a tension-type headache, only three (6%) fulfilled migrainous characteristics. Headache onset was maximum in the first 24 h after injury. Constant headaches disappeared within 3 weeks in 85% subjects (Pearce 2001). In a recent prospective study, Radanov *et al.* followed a cohort of 112 patients with a whiplash injury during 2.5 years. Thirty seven per-cent of patients had tension-type headache, 27% suffered from migraine, and 18% had cervicogenic headache. The rest were unclassified. In 104 (93%) neck pain was associated in time with headache (Radanov *et al.* 2001).

In conclusion, the occurrence of headache attributed to whiplash injury is around 80–90% with an early start after cervical trauma (usually within first 6 h). Headache has mainly an occipital localization (67%) with a dull or pressing charac-ter (77%). The pain is predominantly at evening and usually resolves in 3 or 4 weeks (Keidel 2000). Headache is associated with neck pain in the majority of the cases.

Disorder definition

The severity of neck injury is usually evaluated with the Quebec Classification. In 1995, a task force from Quebec, Canada, developed this classification to assist healthcare workers in making therapeutic decisions. The classification was applied to an inception cohort of patients presenting for emergency medical care following their involvement in a rear-end motor vehicle collision and following a rear-end motor vehicle collision.

The Quebec Whiplash Associated Disorders Task Force evaluates whiplash injury severity (neck pain, neck muscle contraction, neck mobility, and other additional symptoms presenting in the emergency medical care) and proposes five degrees that can be useful in prospective studies (WAD grades 0–IV). Grade 0 indicates no lesion, grades I and II refer a mild whiplash injury, and grades III and IV, a moderate and severe whiplash injury respectively (Bono *et al.* 2000; Hartling *et al.* 2001). An adequate multiparametric procedure is required to study WAD, which takes into account: the patient's principal details; an exact reconstruction of the event; descrip-tion and analysis of the signs and symptoms, with various complications and corre-lated dysfunctions; an objective neurological and neck–shoulder examinations; and a series of complementary instrumental tests (manual palpation, algometry, EMG, kinematic analysis of the cervical spine, neuro-psychological and psychological eval-uations), and evaluation of disability.

At this moment, there are no evidence that this subclassification would be useful to differentiate the patients with post-whiplash headaches.

Temporal relationship and headache resolution

After a long follow-up, prospective studies after mild whiplash injury have showed a high presence of headache, which can vary between 25 and 90% within few days after whiplash injury, between 12 and 44% within the first year and between 3 and 24% within 2–4 years. Only the studies of Kasch, Pearce, and Obelieniene had control groups. Especially interesting is the work of Diane Obelieniene *et al.* because the authors analysed the presence and duration of neck pain and headache, day to day, during the first 29 days after whiplash (Obelieniene *et al.* 1999). The majority of patients developed headache in the first 24 h after neck trauma and no patients developed a headache after more than 7 days; Because of this, we decided to apply the same time interval as in posttraumatic headache.

Litigation in posttraumatic headaches

In our increasingly litigious society, there is persistence of an attitude that posttraumatic headache and other injuries will either improve or disappear following resolution of claim. The role of litigation in the persistence of PTH is still discussed. Nowadays, the relationship between legal settlements and the temporal profile of chronic PTH is still not clearly established. In relation with this question it is important to carefully assess patients who may be malingering and/or seeking enhanced compensation.

Generally, there is no good evidence that litigation and economical expectation are associated with prolongation of headaches. However, the purpose of all specialists in medicine is that the medico-legal issues may be solved as soon as possible.

According to the reviews of Weiss and Evans, some patients improved when they were still involved in litigation and on the other hand, the resolution of litigation or compensation claims was not sufficient for headache resolution in another group of patients (Weiss *et al.* 1991; Evans 1992). For Packard, all fifty patients interviewed one year or more following a legal settlement continued to report persistent headache symptoms although other authors have posed that insurance and compensation systems have a large impact on recovery from posttraumatic and post-whiplash headaches (Cote *et al.* 2001). In a prospective, controlled inception cohort study, 210 victims of a rear-end collision from Lithuania were consecutively identified and followed by Obelieniene *et al.* Neck pain and headache were evaluated shortly after the accident, after 2 months and 1 year. One year later, there were no significant differences between the accident victims and the control group concerning frequency and intensity of these symptoms. They concluded that in a country where there is no preconceived notion of chronic pain arising from rear-end collision, insurance companies, or litigation, symptoms after an acute whiplash injury are self-limiting, brief, and do not seem to evolve to the so-called late whiplash syndrome (Obelieniene *et al.* 1999)

Conclusions

Posttraumatic headache is the most common postconcussive symptom and most frequent type of posttraumatic pain associated with mild head trauma. Tension-type headache is the usual presentation of PTH but other heterogeneous patterns can appear. Temporal diagnostic criteria have been reviewed and shortened with a view to gaining specificity. The definition of head injuries in mild, moderate, or severe cases will have treatment and prognostic implications. Long-term effect of litigation is still unclear. Medico-legal issues might be solved as soon as possible. Acceleration–deceleration injury or whiplash is also a frequent cause of neck pain and related headache. Quebec classification is useful to evaluate the severity of whiplash injury, with prognosis value. The pathogenesis of chronic symptoms is not known; neurological, psychological, and legal factors have been implicated. It is very important that we test the new criteria in clinical practice; it is the only way to improve them in the next version of the classification.

References

Bettuci D, Aguggia M, Bolamperti L, *et al.* Chronic posttraumatic headache associated with minor craneal trauma: a description of cephalalgic patterns. *Ital J Neurol Sci* 1998; **19**: 20–24.

Bono G, Antonaci F, Ghirmai S, *et al.* Whiplash injuries: clinical picture and diagnostic work-up. *Clin Exp Rheumatol* 2000; **18** (Suppl 19): S23–8.

Cartlidge NEF, Shaw V. Head injury, Saunders 1981.

Cote P, Cassidy JD, Carroll L, *et al.* A systematic review of the prognosis of acute whiplash and a new conceptual framework to synthesize the literature. *Spine* 2001; **26**: E445–58.

De Benedittis G, De Santis A. Chronic posttraumatic headache: clinical, psychopathological features and outcome determinants. *J Neurosurg Sci* 1983; **27**: 177–86.

De Souza JA, Moreira Filho PC, Jevoux Cda C. Chronic posttraumatic headache after mild head injuries. *Arch Neuropsiquiatr* 1999; **57**: 243–48.

Evans RW. The postconcussion syndrome and the sequelae of mild head injury. *Neurol Clin* 1992; **10**: 815–47.

Foletti G, Regli F. Characteristics of chronic headaches after whiplash injury. *Presse Med* 1995; **24**: 1121–3.

Gfeller JD, Chibnall JT, Duckro PN. Postconcussion symptoms and cognitive functioning in posttraumatic headache patients. *Headache* 1994; **34**: 503–7.

Gilkey SJ, Ramadan NM, Aurora TK, *et al.* Cerebral blood flow in chronic posttraumatic headache. *Headache* 1997; **37**: 583–7.

Hachinski W. Posttraumatic headache. *Arch Neurol* 2000; **57**: 1780.

Hartling L, Brison RJ, Ardem C, *et al.* Prognosis value of the Quebec: Classification of Whiplash-Associated Disorders. *Spine* 2001; **26**: 36–41.

Hass DC. Chronic posttraumatic headaches: classified and compared with natural headaches. *Cephalalgia* 1996; **16**: 486–93.

Headache Classification Committee of the International Headache Society. Classification and diagnostic criteria for headache disorders, cranial neuralgias and facial pain *Cephalalgia* 1988; **8** (Suppl 7): 1–96.

Headache Classification Subcommittee of the International Headache Society. The International Classification of Headache Disorders: 2nd edition *Cephalalgia* 2004; **24** (Suppl 1): 9–160.

Keidel M. In: *The headaches* (eds. Olesen J, Ftelt-Hansen P, Welch M). 2000; 763–70.

Keidel M, Diener HC. Posttraumatic headache. *Nervenarzt* 1997; **68**: 769–77.

Lanz S, Bryant RA. Incidence of chronic pain following traumatic brain injury. *Arch Phys Med Rehabil* 1996; **77**: 889–91.

Martelli MF, Grayson RL, Zasler ND. Posttraumatic headache: neuropsychological and psychological effects and treatment implications. *J Head Trauma Rehabil* 1999; **14**: 49–69.

Nick J, Sicard-Nick C. Late posttraumatic headache. Symptomatologic, physiopathological and therapeutic study. A propos of 240 cases. *Press Med* 1965; **73**: 2587–92.

Obelieniene D, Schrader H, Bovim G, *et al.* Pain after whiplash. a prospective controlled inception cohort study. *J Neurol Neurosurg Psychiatry* 1999; **66**: 279–83.

Packard RC. Posttraumatic headache: permanency and relationship to legal sttlement headache. *Headache* 1992; **32**: 496–500.

Pearce JM. Headaches in the whiplash syndrome. *Spinal Cord* 2001; **39**: 228–33.

Radanov BP, Di Stefano G, Augustiny KF. Symptomatic approach to posttraumatic headache and its possible implications for treatment. *Eur Spine J* 2001; **10**: 403–7.

Radanov BP, Sturzenegger M, Di Stefano G. Long-term outcome after whiplash injury. A 2-year follow-up considering features of injury mechanism and somatic, radiologic and psychosocial findings. *Medicine (Baltimore)* 1995; **74**: 281–97.

Solomon S. Posttraumatic headache. *Med Clin North Am* 2001; **85**: 987–96.

Sturzenegger M, Radanov BP, Di Stefano G. The effect of accident mechanisms and initial findings on the long-term course of whiplash injury. *J Neurol* 1995; **242**: 443–9.

van der Naalt J, van Zomeren AH, Sluiter WJ, *et al.* One year outcome in mild to moderate head injury: the predictive value of acute injury characteristics related to complaints and return to work. *J Neurol Neurosurg Psychiatry* 1999; **66**: 207–13.

Voller B, Auff E, Schnider P, *et al.* To do or not to do MRI in mild traumatic brain injury? *Brain Inj* 2001; **15**: 107–15.

Weiss HD, Stern BJ, Goldbert J. Post-traumatic migraine: chronic migraine precipitated by minor head or neck trauma. *Headache* 1991; **31**: 451–6.

Yamaguchi M. Incidence of headache and severity of head injury. *Headache* 1992; **32**: 427–31.

27 Duration of rebound headache in the treatment of substance-overuse headache: effects of prednisolone versus tricyclic antidepressants

H. Göbel, A. Heinze, and K. Heinze-Kuhn

Introduction

If taken too frequently, all effective migraine and headache drugs can lead to an increase in headache frequency and ultimately to permanent headache. Before the complete picture of 'medication-induced permanent headache' is reached, patients experience a continuous increase in the frequency of headache attacks and also an increase in the dosage needed to obtain relief. Medication-induced headache may also occur in cases of incorrect use of triptans. Reports in the literature about medication-induced headache in connection with the use of triptans have been known for several years.[1]

To avoid medication-induced permanent headache resulting from drugs for acute migraine therapy, it is essential to observe the most important rule regarding intake frequency for therapy of migraine attacks: *acute migraine drugs for treating migraine attacks must not be taken more frequently than 10 days a month.* In other words, on 20 days a month, no substances for treating migraine attacks should be taken. Observance of this rule ensures that no habituation effect takes place.

Our experience indicates that the quantity of the substances used and the frequency of intake on the 10 days do not play a relevant role.

To treat medication-induced headache, the procedure is to completely and abruptly discontinue the acute medication for a temporary period. The resulting 'rebound headache' typically occurs in a period of 5–10 days. Then the spontaneous permanent headache eases off. After this phase, the acute medication can be used again. Since triptans do not, strictly speaking, result in addiction, and since no withdrawal therapy is performed, we no longer speak of drug dependence and drug withdrawal, but of a 'drug holiday' and 'rebound headache'. Indeed, after this drug holiday, the patient can start taking the substances again.

Both for treatment and for final diagnosis of substance-overuse headache, successful discontinuation is necessary according to criterion D (IHS Code 8.2). We investigated the time course of the headaches after discontinuation of the acute medication (onset and duration) and compared the time course of the rebound headache when treated with either prednisolone or tricyclic antidepressants.

Methods

One hundred and sixty patients suffering from migraine according to IHS criteria who had developed a secondary substance-overuse headache were included in the evaluation. The patients were randomized into the individual treatment groups in the order they were admitted to hospital for inpatient treatment. After discontinuation of any acute headache treatment, pain intensity was documented by patients prospectively using a headache diary for a period of 30 days. The pain scale recorded pain intensity at hourly intervals for 24 h a day. The scale comprised four categories: 0 – no pain, 1 – slight pain, 2 – moderate pain, 3 – severe pain, and 4 – very severe pain. To arrive at a comprehensive measure of pain per day, the sum of the pain intensity scores for the 24 h of the day was calculated. Depending on randomization, 84 patients were treated with a 10-day-course of prednisolone and 76 with a tricyclic antidepressant. The tricyclic antidepressant was given in the form of 50 mg amitryptilin administered in the evening.

The prednisolone therapy consisted of 100 mg in the first three days, then 80 mg for a further two days, 60 mg for another two days, 40 mg for the next two days, 20 mg for the next two days, followed by complete discontinuation of prednisolone. Thus prednisolone was administered on a total of 11 days. After at least 3 headache-free days, the patient was allowed to resume acute headache medication if spontaneous migraine attacks occurred.

Results

Rebound headache occurred after 24–48 h following discontinuation of the acute medication (Fig. 27.1). It disappeared after a further 24–48 h.

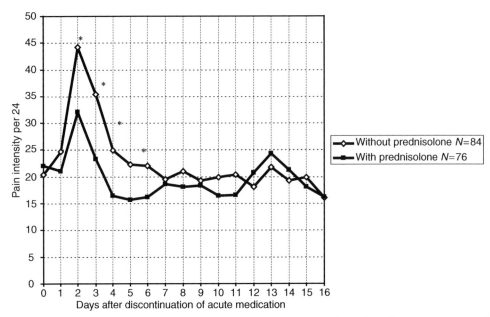

Fig. 27.1 Course of rebound headache intensity per day after discontinuation of overused acute medication. Treatment with or without prednisolone (*: *t*-test *p*<0.01).

Rebound headache was observed both in the group with prednisolone treatment and in the group without prednisolone. The maximal intensity of rebound headache was seen 48 h after discontinuation of acute headache treatment. Patients receiving prednisolone had a significantly lower rebound headache intensity and duration compared to patients treated with tricyclic antidepressant (*p*<0.01). The average duration of rebound headache was 3–5 days. After discontinuation of prednisolone treatment on day 11, a slight increase in headache was observed in the prednisolone group for two days, but then disappeared again spontaneously.

Conclusions

When headache due to overuse of acute medication is treated by discontinuing the medication previously taken continuously, headaches occur within 24–48 h.[1–7] These headaches are significantly shorter and less severe with accompanying prednisolone therapy. From the fifth day onward, the time course of the headache is largely stable. However, after discontinuation of prednisolone on day 11, a temporary slight increase in headache intensity is observed for about two days.

The second edition of the IHS Classification does not lay down any definitive headache phenotype for the rebound headache described, but it can be classified under code 8.4.4 – Headache attributed to withdrawal from chronic use of other substances.[8,9]

In the case of overuse of various acute medications, the second edition of the IHS Classification lays down diagnostic criteria (Codes 8.2.1–8.2.7) for the overuse phase. It seems advisable that the IHS criteria for substance-overuse headache should be revised in criterion D. The stated two months after which a drug holiday ought to have successfully proved a diagnosis of substance-overuse headache seems rather too long, since most patients experience only short-lived withdrawal symptoms—especially when treated. On the other hand, two months without treatment yet without improvement would seem an inappropriately long period for a patient to prove a chronic migraine.

References

1. Göbel H, Stolze H, Dworschak M, *et al*. Easy therapeutical management of sumatriptan-induced daily headache. *Neurology* 1996; **47** (1): 297–8.
2. Relja G, Granato A, Maria Antonello R, *et al*. Headache induced by chronic substance use: analysis of medication overused and minimum dose required to induce headache. *Headache* 2004; **44** (2): 148–53.
3. Fritsche G, Diener HC. Medication overuse headaches — what is new? *Expert Opin Drug Saf* 2002; **1** (4): 331–8.
4. Grazzi L, Andrasik F, D'Amico D, *et al*. Treatment of chronic daily headache with medication overuse. *Neurol Sci* 2003; **24** (Suppl 2): S125–7.
5. Eross E. Patient pages. Daily headaches due to medication overuse. *Neurology* 2003; **60** (10): E8–9.
6. Limmroth V, Katsarava Z, Fritsche G, *et al*. Features of medication overuse headache following overuse of different acute headache drugs. *Neurology* 2002; **59** (7): 1011–4.
7. Silberstein SD, Liu D. Drug overuse and rebound headache. *Curr Pain Headache Rep* 2002; **6** (3): 240–7.
8. Gobel H. Classification of headaches. *Cephalalgia* 2001; **21** (7): 770–3.
9. The International Classification of Headache Disorders: 2nd edition. *Cephalalgia* 2004; **24** (Suppl 1): 9–160.

28 Headache and spontaneous cervical artery dissections: time-course and follow-up

C. Lucas, M. Viallet, M. A. Mackowiak,
M. Girot, H. Hénon, and D. Leys

Background

Cervical artery dissection (CAD) account for up to one-fifth of ischemic strokes occurring before 45 years.[1,2] Headache is the initial symptom of dissection of the cervical artery in 60% patients and occur in 75% of them.[1,2] Pain is usually defined as ipsilateral throbbing headache or sharp pain located in the neck, jaw, pharynx, or face. Isolated pain may be a misleading symptom: sometimes pain mimics a migraine attack.[4,5] However, the relationship between CAD and migraine are complex and the course of headache in patients with CAD is not well-known.[3]

Aim of the study

The aim of this study was to evaluate the course of various types of headache in patients who had had spontaneous CAD.

Methods

We conducted a telephone interview with a structured questionnaire about existence and type of headache before and after the CAD in all consecutive patients hospitalized for spontaneous CAD in our stroke unit between 1998 and 2001, confirmed by a mural hematoma on MRI. We used χ^2 test with Yates correction or exact Fisher test when necessary to compare the data and Mann-Whitney U test for age.

Results

Forty-two patients had had a spontaneous CAD during this period. Twenty-two had had headache in the past: 7 isolated migraine without aura, 2 migraine without aura and episodic tension-type headache, 3 isolated migraine with aura, 2 migraine with aura and episodic tension-type headache, and 8 isolated episodic tension-type headache. Twenty-one (95.5%) improved their headache after the spontaneous CAD. Of 14 patients who were migraineurs, 13 (92%) had fewer migraine attacks after the CAD. Only 7 patients, without previous headache developed new headache after CAD: 3 migraine without aura, 3 episodic tension-type

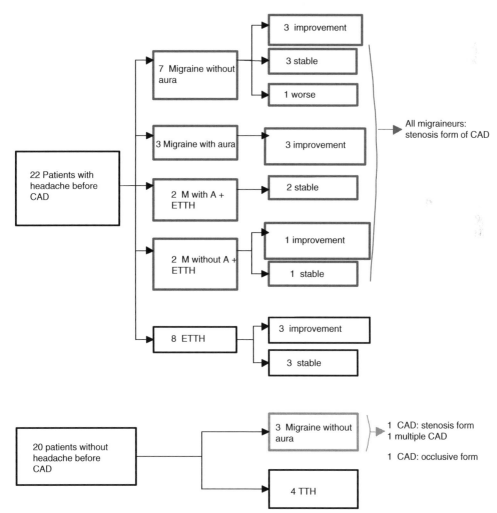

Fig. 28.1   Headache before and after CAD.

Table 28.1 Comparison of characteristics of CAD in migraineurs and nonmigraineurs

	Migraine before CAD	No migraine before CAD	P
N	14	28	
Male	6	13	0.826
Median age	44.5	43.5	0.59
Unique CAD	13	22	0.464
Multiple CAD	1	6	NS
Carotid artery D	6	17	0.273
Stenosis form	14	16	0.03*
Occlusive form	0	15	0.01
Aneurysm	6	1	0.03*
Dysplasia	3	2	0.197

NS: non significant. *$p < 0.05$.

headache, and one chronic tension-type headache (Fig. 28.1). We found that all migraineurs had had a stenosis form of CAD and that migraineurs before CAD had significantly more pseudo-aneurysm associated with CAD (Table 28.1). The patients who experienced increase of headache attacks frequency or severity after the CAD were significantly younger (Table 28.2).

Headache associated with cervicalgia was the first symptom of CAD in 19 (45.2%) patients. Headache associated with cervicalgia was present during the acute phase in 34 (80.9%) patients. Other symptoms during the CAD were TIA or ischemic stroke in 34 (80.9%) patients, Horner syndrome in 6 (26%).

Table 28.2 Characteristics of patients and CAD according to improvement of headache

	Improvement of headache	Increase of headache	P
N	34	8	
Male	16	3	0.92
Median age	44.5	38	0.04*
Unique CAD	5	0	0.56
Multiple CAD	30	5	0.07
Carotid artery D	17	6	0.38
Stenosis form	26	4	0.20
Occlusive form	9	5	0.18
Aneurysm	6	1	0.99
Dysplasia	5	0	0.56

*$p < 0.05$.

Conclusion

Most patients improved their preexisting headache after spontaneous CAD. Only a few patients developed a new headache after CAD.

References

1. Bogousslavsky J, Regli F. Ischemic stroke in adults younger than 30 years of age: cause and prognosis. *Arch Neurol* 1987; **44** (5): 479–82.
2. Bogousslavsky J, Pierre PH: Ischemic stroke in patients under age 45. *Neurol Clin* 1992; **10**: 113–14.
3. Leys D, Moulin TH, Stojkovic T, *et al.* for the Donald investigators: long term course of cervical-artery dissection. *Cerebrovasc Dis* 1995; **5**: 43–9.
4. Biousse V, D'Anglejean-Chatillon, Massiou H, *et al.* Head pain in non-traumatic carotid artery dissection: a series of 65 patients. *Cephalalgia* 1994; **14**: 33–6.
5. Shuaib A. Stroke from other etiologies masquerading as migraine stroke. *Stroke* 1991; **22**: 1068–74.

29 Hyperhomocysteinemia due to MTHFR C677T polymorphism as a possible link between stroke and migraine in young populations

P. Marchione, P. Giacomini, D. Fortini,
C. Vento, D. Samà, D. Corigliano, and G. Nappi

Background

Increased homocysteine levels are associated with various pathological conditions in humans, including stroke and cardiovascular disorders.[2] A recent study suggests that the MTHFR gene, causing mild hyperhomocysteinemia, may be a genetic risk factor for migraine.[4] Homocysteine acts as an excitatory amino acid in vivo and may influence the threshold of migraine headache. The aim of this study is to evaluate the prevalence of migraine in stroke patients with hyperhomocysteine due to MTHFR polymorphism.

Materials and methods

We enrolled 64 consecutive patients of 18–45 age range admitted to our Department with a first-ever stroke or TIA. All patients underwent a complete diagnostic algorithm for stroke in young people. Homocysteine serum dosage and genetic analysis of C667T polymorphism of MTHFR with standardized method have been performed in every patient as described.[3] Diagnosis of migraine was made according to 2003 IHS Criteria.[8] The frequency and relative association between hyperhomocysteinemia/MTHFR genotype and migraine in our population were evaluated using statistical package SPSS for Windows 2000 and the χ^2 test.

Results

Of the 64 stroke patients, 32 were men and 32 women. Mean age ± 2SD at first event was 33.5±2.3. A mild hyperhomocysteinemia (higher fasting values ranging from 16 to 100 µmol/L) was found in 27 patients (42.2%), 14 men and 13 women. Homozygousity for MTHFR C677T polymorphism was detected in all these patients. Prevalence of migraine in stroke patients with mild hyperhomocysteinemia was 66.6% ($p=0.02$, χ^2 test). According to 2004 IHS Criteria, migrainous infarction was excluded in these patients.[8] Migraine with aura (MWA) was more frequent (63%) than migraine without aura (MWO) (37%). We found a statistically significative association between MWA, stroke, and hyperhomocysteinemia/MTHFR homozygousity profile and female sex ($p=0.03$, χ^2 test) and between MWA and oral contraceptive therapy in female patients with stroke ($p=0.03$, χ^2 test) (Fig. 29.1).

Discussion

Hereditary hyperhomocysteinemia due to MTHFR C677T polymorphism is a well-known risk factor for juvenile stroke.[1,5,7,9] Recently, Kowa *et al.* found that

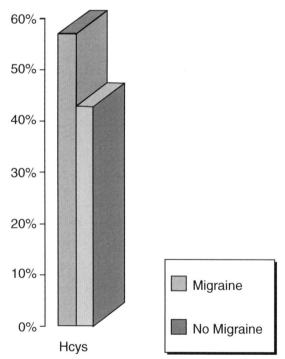

Fig. 29.1 Frequency of migraine in stroke patients with hyperhomocysteinemia.

homozygous C677T mutation in the MTHFR gene is a genetic risk factor for migraine.[4] An association between migraine and juvenile stroke has been suggested, particularly in women under 45 years and in subgroups of patients with MWA.[6] The main result of this study is the statistically significative association between migraine and mild hyperhomocysteinemia due to MTHFR C677T polymorphism in our stroke population. Despite the small size of the sample, we found that hereditary mild hyperhomocysteinemia is not a rare risk factor for stroke in young adults. Higher incidence of migraine in this subgroup of patients with juvenile stroke may account for a role of MTHFR C677T polymorphism in determining vascular risk in migraineurs. Particularly, the combination of sex, MWA, and other cerebrovascular risk factors identifies the patients with a higher ischemic risk. Oral contraceptive therapy in women with MWA may account for a higher risk of cerebrovascular disease in this subgroup of patients. These findings suggest a multifactorial etiology of ischemic stroke in migraineurs women under 45 years of age.[6] The association of several risk factors may influence the therapeutic strategies of secondary prevention.[1]

References

1. Boushey CJ, Beresford SAA, Omenn GS, *et al.* A quantitative assessment of plasma homocysteine as a risk factor for vascular disease: probable benefits of increasing folic acid intakes. *JAMA* 1995; **274**: 1049–57.
2. Clarke R, Daly L, Robinson K, *et al.* Hyperhomocysteinemia: an independent risk factor for vascular disease. *N Engl J Med* 1991; **324**: 1149–55.
3. Frosst P, Blom HJ, Milos R, *et al.* A candidate genetic risk factor for vascular disease: a common mutation in methylenetetrahydrofolate reductase. *Nat Genet* 1995; **10**: 111–13.
4. Kowa H, Yasui K, Takeshima T, *et al.* The homozygous C677T mutation in the methylenetetrahydrofolate reductase gene is a genetic risk factor for migraine. *Am J Med Gen* 2000; **96**: 762–4.
5. Madonna P, de Stefano V, Coppola A, *et al.* Hyperhomocysteinemia and other inherited prothrombotic conditions in young adults with a history of ischemic stroke. *Stroke* 2002; **33**: 51–6.
6. Milhaud D, Bogousslavsky J, van Melle G, *et al.* Ischemic stroke and active migraine. *Neurology* 2001; **57**: 1805–11.
7. Perry IJ, Refsum H, Morris RW, *et al.* Prospective study of serum total homocysteine concentration and risk of stroke in middle-aged British men. *Lancet* 1995; **346**: 1395–8.
8. Olesen J, Bousser M-G, Diener H, *et al.* for the International Headache Society. The International Classification of Headache Disorders. 2nd Edition. *Cephalalgia* 2004; **24** (Suppl 1): 1–160.
9. Verhoef P, Hennekens CH, Malinow MR, *et al.* A prospective study of plasma homocysteine and risk of ischemic stroke. *Stroke* 1994; **25**: 1924–30.

30 Posttraumatic headache in patients with mild traumatic brain injury

Y. Alekseenko and U. Luchanok

Introduction

Headache is the most common symptom of mild traumatic brain injury (MTBI). The diagnosis of MTBI is usually complicated, because the routine neurological examination of patients does not usually reveal any specific or informative changes. At the same time, the majority of MTBI symptoms including headache are mainly of a subjective character. There are some additional factors which can influence the clinical manifestations of MTBI and their development. Concomitant alcohol intoxication (AI) in patients with MTBI complicates the interpretation of symptoms as well as the distinction between traumatic and toxic effects. Therefore, the assessment of the main symptoms and history in such circumstances remains a challenge. To clarify the significance of some subjective posttraumatic disorders and to improve standard diagnostic protocols, we analysed the structure of the main clinical signs and the natural course of recovery in MTBI patients.

Patients and methods

This study involves 121 males with MTBI (aged 16–39) consequently admitted to the regional hospital in 2000–2003. The criteria for selecting patients with MTBI were as follows: (1) brief (min/s) loss or/and any alteration of consciousness (disorientation, confusion) at the time of the accident; (2) posttraumatic amnesia – several min/h; (3) physical symptoms (nausea, vomiting, dizziness, headache, vegetative disorders, etc); (4) absence of focal neurological deficit; (5) absence of skull fracture; (6) normal CT or MRI scan of the brain; (7) recovery preferably in 1–2 weeks (cerebral concussion, according to the national brain injury classification). All MTBI patients with significant concomitant neurological and therapeutical diseases were excluded from this study.

In 61 patients, the accident took place on the background of mild and moderate AI. AI in patients with MTBI was established on the basis of clinical features and blood alcohol concentration (0.5–1.5 g/L – mild AI; 1.5–3.0 g/L – moderate AI) at the moment of admission. In addition, the blood alcohol concentration was recalculated for the moment of the accident. The quantitative analysis (duration/intensity) of the main MTBI symptoms was carried out.

Results

Disorders of consciousness were observed in all MTBI patients at the time of the accident. Brief (several min/s) loss of consciousness was established in 93% of MTBI patients with AI compared to 53% of MTBI patients without AI ($p < 0.0001$). Alteration of consciousness (disorientation, confusion) at the time of the accident was registered mainly in MTBI patients without AI (7% and 47% accordingly; $p > 0.001$). MTBI patients with AI demonstrated a more extensive and frequent amnesia in comparison with MTBI patients without AI (anterograde amnesia – 67% and 36% accordingly; $p > 0.05$). Different combinations of consciousness and amnestic disorders were observed after the trauma and some of them were a challenge for interpretation and precise diagnosing. Only 40% of MTBI patients with AI were able to confirm such disturbances by themselves. The signs of head trauma (abrasions, bruises) as an indirect evidence of a probable brain injury were objectively observed in 95% of MTBI patients with AI compared to 72% of patients without AI.

Such symptoms as headache, dizziness, nausea, vomiting, fatigue, slight cognitive deficit, and some other autonomic disorders (orthostatic dysregulation and thermodysregulation) were the most common manifestations of MTBI. The above-mentioned constellation of symptoms persists in an acute period of trauma and is considered to be a base of the late post-concussive syndrome.[5] Besides, patients with MTBI demonstrate a wide variety of duration and intensity of such symptoms. MTBI patients with AI had less frequent vomiting (36% and 60% accordingly; $p < 0.05$) and demonstrated a relatively favorable recovery from subjective symptoms of autonomic dysfunction (4.0±2.1 and 5.6±2.8 days accordingly; $p < 0.01$), though the range of such clinical features may be wider than in patients without AI.

However, the headache was the most essential and cardinal complaint. The different types of headache were observed in all patients with MTBI. The structure of headache types was close to well-known and recently published data.[3] Posttraumatic headache, which is most often characterized as a tension-type headache manifests itself by a continuous holocephalic dull-pressing, dragging or pulling pain. Migraine-like headache was observed only in 4% of MTBI patients and mainly characterized as a pulsating and predominantly hemicranial pain. No significant differences in the spectrum of headache types in MTBI patients with or without concomitant AI were revealed. In all cases, the headache appeared just after the trauma and gradually decreased during the first or the second week after the accident. In 30% of all MTBI patients, the most intensive headache was observed on the next day after the trauma. It is noteworthy, that MTBI patients with concomitant AI were more quickly relieved of their headache in comparison with patients without AI (5.4±2.8 and 6.9±2.9 days accordingly; $p<0.05$). In general, no significant differences in the spectrum of clinical symptoms were observed between MTBI patients with mild and those with moderate AI.

Discussion

Many different terms were suggested to describe and define MTBI and several sets of diagnostic criteria are in use for this kind of brain injury.[3] That is why the assessment of clinical features, frequency, and development of some most significant symptoms in different patients' groups may be complicated.

Headache is one of the most common and informative symptoms in MTBI patients and it usually appears just after the trauma. At the same time, the signs and symptoms of MTBI can be precipitated by a mixture of brain injury, peripheral vestibular injury, and injury to the soft and bony tissue of the head or even neck and sometimes by other external influences including toxic effects of alcohol.[4] It is noteworthy that MTBI patients with AI demonstrated more extensive and frequent disorders of consciousness and amnesia in comparison with MTBI patients without AI. However, in MTBI patients with concomitant AI, a relatively favorable recovery from subjective symptoms of autonomic dysfunction and headache was observed. Concomitant mild and moderate AI seems to produce a complex dual effect on the spectrum of clinical symptoms of MTBI. AI seems to decrease the 'concussion threshold', simultaneously producing some neuroprotective influence on brain mechanisms and contributing to patients' recovery after the MTBI, though the spectrum of symptoms after the trauma may be wider. The character of such interrelation is strongly dependent on the AI degree. Thus, blood alcohol concentration should be taken into account. Moreover, the alcohol concentration should be calculated for the moment of the accident according to a special formula or a table.

According to up to date diagnostic protocols, headache is not an obligatory acute MTBI symptom, it is rather one of the physical signs which cannot be explained by a peripheral injury or some other causes and which may or may not persist for a varying length of time.[1,2] In case of headache appearing some time after the trauma, its interpretation as a MTBI symptom still remains controversial. Remote headache in patients with MTBI might to a greater extent be associated with the influence of additional factors and other mechanisms (psychological reactions to physical or emotional stress and other causes). Nevertheless, the headache combined with any period of consciousness loss at the time of the accident is the most important reason to apply to medical emergency departments. On the other hand, the headache is the most prominent indicator of a subjective recovery, which usually defines the terms of patients' disability and their returning to work.

Conclusion

Headache should be considered as a phenomenon graduated in intensity and duration, but at the same time as an obligatory sign of MTBI, and one of the most important. Although the character of headache in MTBI has no specific features, its evolution with the course of time is specific enough, taking into account other signs of the trauma. Concomitant mild and moderate AI seems to produce a dual effect on the spectrum of clinical symptoms of MTBI including headache. Posttraumatic amnesia and evidences of head trauma should be considered in MTBI diagnostic protocols.

References

1. Gerstenbrand F, Stepan CA. Mild traumatic brain injury. *Brain Injury* 2001; **15**: 95–7.
2. Kay T, Harrington DE, Adams R, *et al*. Report of the Mild Traumatic Brain Injury Committee of the Head Injury Interdisciplinary Special Interest Group of American Congress of Rehabilitation Medicine. Definition of mild traumatic brain injury. *J Head Trauma Rehabil* 1993; **8**: 86–7.
3. Keidel M, Ramadan NM. Acute posttraumatic headache. In: *The headache* (eds Olesen J, Tfelt-Hansen P, Welch KMA, eds). 2nd ed. Philadelphia: Lippincott Williams & Wilkins, 2000: 765–70.
4. de Kruijk JR, Twijnstra A, Leffers P. Diagnostic criteria and differential diagnosis of mild traumatic brain injury. *Brain Injury* 2001; **15**: 99–106.
5. Vos PE, Battistin L, Birbamer G, *et al*. EFNS guideline on mild traumatic brain injury: report of an EFNS task force. *Eur J Neurol* 2002; **9**: 207–19.

31
Posttraumatic headache attributed to mild head injury

L. J. Stovner, D. Mickeviciene, H. Schrader,
D. Obelieniene, D. Surkiene, R. Kunickas, and T. Sund

Introduction

Two studies on the postconcussion syndrome (PCS) have relatively recently been performed in Lithuania, one historical[1] and one prospective[2] cohort study, both with control groups. The present paper summarizes the results on headache in these studies, and discusses the results in relation to the relevant diagnoses of the International Classification of Headache Disorders (ICHD II): acute (5.1.2) and chronic (5.2.2) posttraumatic headache attributed to mild head injury.[3]

Patients and methods

Both studies were performed in Kaunas, Lithuania (University Hospital and the Red Cross Hospital). In the historical cohort study, 200 patients were identified by reviewing the charts of all consecutive patients who had been admitted in the emergency ward between 35 and 22 months earlier for a head trauma involving loss of consciousness (LOC) lasting < 15 min. In the prospective study, 300 patients with head trauma with LOC lasting < 15min were included consecutively. In both studies, duration of LOC (and in the prospective study also duration of amnesia) was assessed on the basis of witness descriptions. Exclusion criteria were any other major injury (defined as an injury requiring hospitalization). In the prospective study, patients with alcohol or drug abuse, other significant disease, previous concussion and abnormal neurological status at admission were also excluded. Due to limited availability of imaging, CT scans were performed in only 51 patients. No traumatic pathology was detected in these.

In both studies, patients answered self-report questionnaires sent by mail with questions about general health and detailed questions about headache and other symptoms attributable to the PCS (memory and concentration problems, dizziness, fatigue, etc). In the prospective study, the questionnaire was sent to the patients 7–14 days after the head trauma and then again after 3 months and after 1 year. The first questionnaire also included questions on headache and other symptoms before the concussion.

In both studies, a sex- and age-matched control person for each patient with concussion was identified from the charts. Inclusion criteria for the control person was a minor injury, not involving the head and neck, causing admission to the emergency ward not more than 2 weeks before or 2 weeks after the matching patient with concussion, and age maximally 3 years more or less than their matching patient. The controls received the same questionnaires as the patients.

Results

In the historical study, 131 of 200 (66%) answered the questionnaire, the mean interval being 28 months after the trauma. Of these, 60% were men (mean age 34 years) and 40% women (38 years). In the prospective study, 192 of 300 (64%), of which 66% were men of mean age 33 years and 34% women of mean age 38 years, answered the questionnaire at 12 months. The demographic status of the patients and the controls was not significantly different except that more controls were married in both studies.

Concerning headache at all during the last month, there was no significant difference (χ^2 test with Yates correction) after 3, 12, or 28 months. Frequent headache (>7 days/month) was nearly significantly more prevalent in the concussion group than in the controls ($P=0.053$) after 3 months (Table 31.1). Combining data from both studies ≥1 year after the concussion, no significant differences were found for any headache frequency (Fig. 31.1). Using the method described by Altman,[4] it can be calculated that with a combined sample size of 684, correcting for unequal sample sizes, there is an 80% chance of detecting a 10% increase in the proportion with headache 1 year after the trauma (i.e. from 61% in the control group to 71% in the concussion group) at a 0.05 probability level.

Headache right after the concussion is most reliably evaluated in the prospective study. 81% reported headache shortly after the trauma, 25% still had this headache when answering the first questionnaire after 2–3 weeks, this number being significantly higher than among controls. 11.5% still had headache after 3 months. Fifteen individuals (8%) reported headache both in the first questionnaire and again after 3 and 12 months. Eleven of these had headache also before the concussion, and the remaining four had headache 1–7 days per month.

Discussion

The main advantage of performing this study in Lithuania is that in this country few individuals expect persistent symptoms following a concussion,[5] and there is also very little possibility of financial compensation. A drawback was the limited

Table 31.1 Headache after concussion, and in controls

Time after trauma	Prospective cohort study						Historical cohort study		
	3 months			12 months			Mean 28 months		
Frequency of headache	Concussion (%) (n=200)	Controls (%) (n=210)	P^a	Concussion (%) (n=192)	Controls (%) (n=215)	P^a	Concussion (%) (n=131)	Controls (%) (n=146)	P^a
Headache during last month	131 (65)	125 (60)	0.25	124 (65)	138 (64)	0.98	80 (61)	89 (61)	0.92
No headache	69 (35)	85 (40)		68 (35)	77 (36)		51 (39)	57 (39)	
Headache									
1–7 days	89 (45)	97 (46)	0.053#	84 (43)	106 (49)	0.15#	50 (38)	55 (38)	0.95#
8–14 days	21 (11)	15 (7)		25 (13)	14 (7)		12 (9)	8 (6)	
>14 days	7 (4)	3 (1)		7 (4)	5 (2)		3 (2)	8 (6)	
every day	14 (7)	10 (5)		8 (4)	13 (6)		15 (12)	18 (12)	

$^a\chi^2$-test with Yates' correction, after concussion vs. controls.
#Frequent headache (>7 days per month) during the last month.

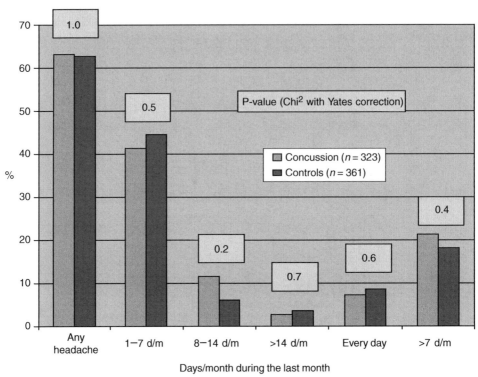

Fig. 31.1 Headache frequency ≥1 year after trauma (both studies combined).

availability of imaging which may have led to an underestimation of injury severity in some patients.

The data from the prospective study indicate that acute headache after mild head injury with LOC ≤15 min (ICHD-II diagnosis 5.1.2) is not only attributed to, but is probably causally related to the head trauma. As can be seen from Table 31.1, this effect is hardly detectable 3 months after the injury. The criterion in the ICHD-II classification limiting the duration of acute headache after mild head injury to 3 months therefore seems reasonable. At 12 months and later, there is no difference between the groups, neither with any headache or frequent headache. The power of the combined studies is sufficient to detect a ≥10% increase in the prevalence of headache. Headache was rather frequent also in the control group, in which the individuals had suffered from minor traumas not affecting the head or neck. We cannot, therefore, exclude other (psychological?) effects of a trauma, but headache as a late effect of the *head* trauma seems highly improbable. The validity of ICHD-II disorder 5.2.2 as a secondary disorder (i.e. caused by the head trauma) is therefore very low. This means that any headache occurring ≥3 months after a simple concussion with LOC <15 min, in most, if not all, patients is not related to the concussion. More studies are needed to evaluate headache occurrence after traumas with LOC of longer duration.

In conclusion, headache resulting from simple concussion with LOC <15 min usually lasts less than 3 months. Headache occurring 1 year or more after such a trauma is probably not causally related to the head trauma per se.

References

1. Mickeviciene D, Schrader H, Nestvold K, *et al*. A controlled historical cohort study on the post-concussion syndrome. *Eur J of Neurol* 2002; **9**: 581–7.
2. Mickeviciene D, Schrader H, Obelieniene D, *et al*. A controlled prospective inception cohort study on the postconcussion syndrome outside the medicolegal context. *Eur J of Neurol* 2004; **11**: 411–19.
3. The International Classification of Headache Disorders. 2nd Edition. *Cephalalgia* 2004; **24**: 1–160.
4. Altman DG. Practical statistics for medical research. London: Chapman & Hall, 1991: 441–76.
5. Ferrari R, Obelieniene D, Russell AS, *et al*. Symptom expectation after minor head injury. A comparative study between Canada and Lithuania. *Clin Neurol Neurosurg* 2001; **103**: 184–90.

32 Posttraumatic migraine secondary to organic lesions

A. M. Pascual, A. Salvador, R. Gil, and M. J. A. Láinez

Background

Posttraumatic Headache (PTH) is usually, one of the several symptoms of 'post-concussion syndrome' and therefore, may be accompanied by additional cognitive, behavioral, or somatic problems.[1,2] A variety of pain patterns may develop after head injury and may closely resemble primary headache disorders. Tension-type is the most common variety of PTH, followed by cervicogenic headache, migraine, and cluster-like headaches. Posttraumatic Migraine (PTM) represents approximately 8–10% of PTH.[3] Nowadays, the pathogenesis of PTH is still not well-understood. Common headache pathways and similar neurochemical changes have been implicated in Primary Migraine and Posttraumatic Migraine (PTM).[4,5] On the other hand, the current temporal criteria for PTH diagnosis are very restrictive in order to increase specificity. In accordance with the recent review of IHS Classification Criteria,[6] acute-PTH develops within 7 days after head trauma or regaining consciousness following head trauma and resolves within 3 months (Table 32.1).

Objectives

1. Discuss pathogenic implications of posttraumatic organic lesions as cause of migraine attacks.
2. Discuss the temporal diagnostic criteria of PTM.

Clinical cases

1. A man, thirty-two years old, without a clinical or family history of migraine, suffered severe left temporal head trauma associated to cortical-subcortical temporo-parietal hemorrhagic concussion. After cranial trauma, the patient was in

Table 32.1 Acute posttraumatic headache

5.1.1 Acute posttraumatic headache with moderate or severe head injury
   A. New headache appearing after head trauma and fulfilling B–D
   B. Head trauma with at least one of the following:
      1. Loss of consciousness >30 min
      2. Glasgow Coma Scale (GCS) <13
      3. Posttraumatic amnesia >48 h
      4. Imaging demonstration of a traumatic brain lesion
          (cerebral hematoma, brain contusion, or skull fracture)
   C. Headache occurs less than 7 days after head trauma or after regaining
       consciousness or memory
   D. Headache lasts <3 months after regaining consciousness or memory
5.1.2 Acute Posttraumatic Headache with mild head injury
   A. New headache appearing after head trauma and fulfilling B–D
   B. Head trauma with all the following:
      1. No loss of consciousness, or loss of consciousness of <30 min duration
      2. GCS ≥13
      3. Symptoms or signs diagnostic of concussion
   C. Headache occurs less than 7 days after head trauma or after regaining
       consciousness or memory
   D. Headache lasts <3 months after regaining consciousness or memory

coma for several days. When he recovered the level of consciousness, we proved he suffered a sensitive dysphasia and right hemiparesis. Brain MRI showed a porencephalic residual area. After rehabilitation, he recovered completely. Eight months later, the patient developed a new severe throbbing headache. Pain built in intensity over 45 min and lasted from 4 to 12 h without treatment. Pain was provoked by physical exercise and accompanied by nausea, photophobia, and phonophobia. Headache attacks repeated three or four times a year and were always preceded by symptoms of aura, consisting of transitory dysphasia and weakness of right extremities (the same symptoms presented during the head trauma). One or two tables of oral triptans (sumatriptan or rizatriptan) were effective in resolving the headache.

2. A twenty-year-old man, without a clinical or family history of migraine, suffered a mild fronto-parietal head trauma. At a time he was examined in the emergency department of our hospital. Head trauma did not cause alteration of the consciousness, posttraumatic amnesia, or positive neurologic findings. After 6 h of observation, the patient went home. One month later, he developed a new headache with clinical characteristics of migraine without aura. Initially, headache recurred twice or three times in a month, but after several months the pain became daily. After worsening of headaches, neuroimaging studies (MRI, CT scan) were performed and resulted normal. All preventive treatments (beta-blockers, calcium-antagonists, antidepressants, valproate topiramate, and botulinum toxin) were inefficient.

Following the trauma, the patient observed a small growing mass over the area of skull concussion on the parietal bone. Pressure over this area triggered the headache and the local injection of corticosteroids and anesthetics eliminated the pain completely for days. On several occasions, when we infiltrated the mass with placebo, the pain did not get relieved. Surgery resolved headache 2 years later. Pathologic examination showed a fibrotic tissue with small nerve fibers on the inside.

Discussion

Our case illustrates how in some cases both, central and peripheral 'sensitization' could be contributing mechanisms in PTM.[7-9] In patients without previous migraine and history of a recent mild head injury, the trigeminal neuron sensitization could also have a peripheral cause in relation with focal lesions.

In the first case, we think cortical residual lesion might origin a 'hyperexcitable region' that generates symptoms of aura and that, through some common headache pathways, activates brainstem and triggers headache. In our patient, curiously, all migraine attacks were provoked by important physical exercise and always preceded by transitory dysphasia and weakness of right extremities. We could discuss if a relative hypoperfusion over residual cortical lesion might be a precipitating factor for headache.

In the second, an abnormal stimulation of a regional nerve by a small neurofibroma could sensitize deeply nociceptive neurons and trigger headache through trigeminocervical complex. After head trauma, irritated unmyelinating fibers could arise from trigeminal ganglion or from upper cervical dorsal roots and cause interaction of nociceptors of trigeminocervical complex (upper cervical and occipital nerves) and trigeminovascular pathways. The uniformity of clinical presentation, the localization of the pain, the triggering mechanism, and the last response to the surgery suggest a significant relation with trauma. Peripheral trigger is demonstrated when migraine attacks disappeared completely after surgery.

It is easy to establish the relationship between a headache and head or neck trauma when the pain develops immediately or in the first days after trauma, but can be a very difficult task when a headache develops weeks or even months after trauma. Before the reviewed diagnosis criteria, acute PTH may begin before than 14 days after head trauma. After the new IHS Classification, acute PTH develops within 7 days and resolves within 8 weeks.[6] If headaches persist beyond the first 3 months post trauma, they are subsequently referred to as Chronic PTH (Table 32.2).

Nowadays, the current temporal criteria are very restrictive in order to increase the specificity.

In relation with this classification, our patients do not fulfill the temporal criteria for posttraumatic headache but in both, there is a strong evidence that the beginning of migraine is related with the head trauma. Due to this, we propose that when a causal relation can be clearly established, we could increase the temporal window for PTM.

Table 32.2   Chronic posttraumatic headache

5.2.1 Chronic Posttraumatic Headache with moderate or severe head injury

    A. New headache appearing after head trauma and fulfilling B–D

    B. Head trauma with at least one of the following:

        1. Loss of consciousness >30 min

        2. Glasgow Coma Scale (GCS) <13

        3. Posttraumatic amnesia >48 h

        4. Imaging demonstration of a traumatic brain lesion (cerebral hematoma, brain contusion, or skull fracture)

    C. Headache occurs less than 7 days after head trauma or after regaining consciousness or memory

    D. Headache lasts >3 months after regaining consciousness or memory

5.2.2 Chronic Posttraumatic Headache with mild head injury

    A. New headache appearing after head trauma and fulfilling B–D

    B. Head trauma with all the following:

        1. No loss of consciousness, or loss of consciousness of <30 min duration

        2. GCS ≥13

        3. Symptoms or signs diagnostic of concussion

    C. Headache occurs less than 7 days after head trauma or after regaining consciousness or memory

    D. Headache lasts >3 months after regaining consciousness or memory

Conclusions

PTM pathophysiology is still not well-known. In Primary Migraine, central and peripheral 'sensitization' mechanism have been recognized. In some cases of PTM, similar changes could be implicated. Trigeminal neuron sensitization could have a peripheral cause in relation with focal lesions after head trauma. On the other hand, the current temporal criteria for PTM diagnosis might be considered less restrictively when a causal evidence can be demonstrated between beginning headache and the head injury.

References

1. Solomon S. Post-traumatic headache. *Med Clin North Am* 2001; **85**: 987–96.
2. Keidel M, Diener HC. Posttraumatic headache. *Nervenarzt* 1997; **68**: 769–67.
3. Hachinski W. Posttraumatic headache. *Arch Neurol* 2000; **57**: 1780
4. Packard RC, Haw CP. Pathogenesis of PTH and migraine: a common headache pathway? *Headache* 1997; **37**: 142–52.
5. Martelli MF, Grayson RL, Zasler ND. Posttraumatic headache: neuropsychological and psychological effects and treatment implications. *J Head Trauma Rehabil* 1999; **14**: 49–69.

6. The International Classification of Headache Disorders: 2nd edition. Headache Classification Subcommittee of the International Headache Society. *Cephalalgia* 2004; **24** (Suppl 1): 9–160.
7. Malick A, Burstein R. Peripheral and central sensitization during migraine. *Funct Neurol* 2000; **15** (Suppl 3): 28–35.
8. Burstein R, Cutrer MF, Yarnitsky D. The development of cutaneous allodynia during a migraine attack. Clinical evidence for the sequential recruitment of spinal and supraspinal nociceptive neurons in migraine. *Brain* 2000; **123**: 1703–9.
9. Packard RC. The relationship of neck injury and posttraumatic headache. *Curr Pain Headache Rep* 2002; **6**: 301–7.

33
Discussion summary, the secondary headaches: Part I

P. J. Goadsby

The Secondary Headaches discussed in this poster session were those attributed to infection, vascular disorders, substance use, and trauma.

Headache associated with dissections of arteries of the neck were discussed. A poster on spontaneous dissections of the carotid and vertebral arteries were noted to be associated with neck pain, cervicalgia, in 45% of patients presenting to a stroke unit (Lucas). These dissections were diagnosed using MRI. Professor Bousser pointed out that a small percentage of dissections would be missed if formal angiography was not undertaken in cases where MRI/MRA were negative, and there was good clinical suspicion. Further discussion surrounded posters on headache in cerebral venous thrombosis (Cumurciuc) and subarachnoid hemorrhage as a presenting sign of cerebral venous thrombosis (Crassard). Twenty-five of 111 patients with cerebral venous thrombosis presented with headache alone. There were no distinguishing features of the headache and only a minority had had previous headache problems, notably migraine. There were no family history data. Remarkably, the presentation was of a few days of new headache. The cases highlighted cerebral venous thrombosis as a diagnostic possibility in New Daily Persistent Headache, using the term phenotypically.[1] Such patients need MRV, and Professor Bousser recommended initial treatment with heparin and a subsequent six-month course of warfarin. There are no clear controlled trials to guide this decision by evidence.

The second half of the discussion surrounded the headache after head injury. Discussants noted the shortening of the IHCD-2 criteria to requiring only 7 days from injury to headache onset.[2] A poster focusing on patients with mild traumatic brain injury noted how common headache was in the initial period (Alekseenko). All headaches had their onset within 24 h in this group. It was commented that brain injury should be disentangled from head injury, as in injury to extracerebral structures, since the two may not have the same consequences for headache (Legg). A poster exploring data from a cohort study of Lithuanians who had had head trauma involving loss of consciousness of less than 15 min was discussed in detail (Stovner). At 12 months, the brain injury cohort had the same occurrence of headache as the control group. It was pointed out that the control group had a high prevalence of headache, and that the study was powered for a 10% difference, whereas the difference may be smaller. Moreover, it is not clear if the genetic mix in the studied population is the same as that in Western societies, where chronic posttraumatic headache is well-recognized. Discussants agreed more work was required. It seems clear that some group of patients in Western countries have headache after head trauma, and that a high quality controlled prospective study was required in countries where the problem is common to try and understand the underlying issues.

There was some discussion on the level at which particular medicines should be labeled as causing medication overuse, i.e. how much is overused? In addition, it was agreed that the new ICDH-II phenotypic descriptions for medication overuse headaches may be incorrect.[2] An example was the phenotype of ergotamine-overuse headache that is described very much as tension-type headache, in contrast to that of triptans, which is described very much as migraine. The subcommittee (Silberstein) agreed to reconsider these criteria.

Acknowledgments

PJG is a Wellcome Trust Senior Research Fellow.

References

1. Goadsby PJ, Boes CJ. New daily persistent headache. *J Neurol Neurosurg Psychiatry* 2002; **72** (Suppl 6): ii6–9.
2. Headache Classification Committee of The International Headache Society. The International Classification of Headache Disorders. Second edition. *Cephalalgia* 2004; **24** (Suppl 1): 1–160.

Session V

The secondary headaches: Part II

34 Headache or facial pain attributed to disorders of cranium, neck, eyes, ears, nose, sinuses, teeth, mouth, or other facial or cranial structures

H. Göbel

Introduction

Since many headaches originate from the cervical, nuchal, or occipital regions or are localized there, disorders of the cervical spine and other structures of the neck and head have frequently been regarded as the commonest causes of headache. The objective of the second edition of the IHS classification is not to describe these headaches in all their forms; nor is it to pander to traditions, or to accept criteria which only permit 'knowing' by intuition that the headache is cervicogenic or caused by other structures of the head. The purpose is to define criteria that *uniquely* define this headache. This requires establishing a structural cause; not just believing in one. For example degenerative changes in the cervical spine can be found in virtually all people over 40 years of age. The localization of pain and the X-ray detection of degenerative changes have been plausible reasons for regarding the cervical spine disorders as the most frequent cause of headaches. However, large-scale controlled studies have shown that such changes are just as widespread among individuals who do not suffer from headaches. Spondylosis or osteochondrosis cannot therefore be seen as the explanation of headaches. A similar situation applies to other widespread disorders: chronic sinusitis, temporomandibular joint disorders, and refractive errors of the eyes. Without specific criteria, it would be possible for virtually any type of headache to be classified as *headache or facial pain*

Table 34.1 Classification of headache or facial pain attributed to disorders of cranium, neck, eyes, ears, nose, sinuses, teeth, mouth, or other facial or cranial structures according to the second edition of the IHS classification

---

11.1 Headache attributed to disorder of cranial bone
11.2 Headache attributed to disorder of neck

    11.2.1 Cervicogenic headache
    11.2.2 Retropharyngeal tendinitis
    11.2.3 Craniocervical dystonia

11.3 Headache attributed to disorder of eyes

    11.3.1 Acute glaucoma
    11.3.2 Refractive errors
    11.3.3 Heterophoria or heterotropia (latent or manifest squint)
    11.3.4 Ocular inflammatory disorders

11.4 Headache attributed to disorder of ears
11.5 Headache attributed to rhinosinusitis
11.6 Headache attributed to disorder of teeth, jaws, or related structures
11.7 Temporomandibular joint (TMJ) disorder
11.8 Headache attributed to other disorders of cranium, neck, eyes, ears, nose, sinuses, teeth, mouth, or other facial or cervical structures

---

attributed to disorder of cranium, neck, eyes, ears, nose, sinuses, teeth, mouth, or other facial or cranial structures, and this problem existed in the past. It is not sufficient merely to list manifestations of headaches in order to define them, since these manifestations are not unique.

For this reason, it has been necessary to identify strict specific operational criteria for cervicogenic headache and other causes of headache described in Chapter 11 of the second edition of the IHS classification. It has not been possible here to take account of diagnostic tests that are unconfirmed or for which quality criteria have not been investigated. Instead, the aim of the revised criteria is to motivate as a future task, the development of reliable and valid operational tests to establish specific causal relationships between headaches and cervicocranial disorders that are currently available only to a very limited extent.

Table 34.1 provides an overview of the structure of Chapter 11 of the second edition of the IHS classification.[1]

Headache attributed to disorders of cranial bone

The bone of the skull has limited sensitivity to pain because only a few nerve fibers enter it from the overlying periosteum. The periosteum is more pain sensitive, and skull lesions therefore produce headache chiefly by involving it. The lesions of the skull most likely to do this are those that are rapidly expansile, aggressively osteoclastic, or have an inflammatory component.

Most skull lesions are asymptomatic and are discovered as incidental findings on roentgenograms or other imaging procedures undertaken to investigate unrelated complaints. Relatively few skull lesions produce headache. Multiple myeloma often presents with bone pain anywhere in the body, and skull deposits are sometimes a source of such pain. Osteomyelitis produces spontaneous head pain because of its rapid evolution and its inflammatory component. Although most cases of Paget's disease of the skull are asymptomatic, remodelling of bone, by producing basilar invagination, may cause headache either through traction on the upper cervical nerve roots or by the production of cerebrospinal fluid pathway distortion with hydrocephalus.

Headache attributed to disorders of neck

Cervicogenic headache

The Headache Classification Committee saw no evidence for defining a specific, unique headache phenotype that would substantiate a cervical cause.[2–14] Neither do the diagnostic criteria of the Cervicogenic Headache International Study Group[11] specify any definitive pain phenotype, but only a very unspecific description with great scope for individual interpretation: Expressions such as 'usually', 'rather vague non-radicular nature', 'occasionally', 'episodes of varying duration', 'fluctuating', 'marginal effect' or 'not infrequent occurrence' do not permit an explicit operational definition of a specific pain phenotype. Moreover, both unilateral and bilateral headaches are known which can be attributed to disorders of the cervical spine. Among these are developmental anomalies of the craniovertebral junction and upper cervical spine, which frequently cause bilateral headaches. Acquired lesions of the craniovertebral junction and upper cervical spine, such as primary tumours (meningioma, schwannoma, and ependymoma), Paget's disease of the skull with secondary basilar invagination, osteomyelitis of the upper cervical vertebrae, and multiple myeloma of the skull base or upper cervical vertebrae may produce headache by erosion of the pain-sensitive structures or unilateral or bilateral traction on upper cervical nerve roots.

The diagnostic criteria for cervicogenic headache of the second edition of the IHS classification chart a clear diagnostic course to follow. Where headache of whatever kind is present, the doctor is to be called upon to detect a lesion, which is known or accepted to be a valid cause of headache on the basis of antecedent research. For cervicogenic headache to be a headache, there must be pain in the head, be it in the occiput or anywhere else. For it to be cervicogenic, there must be a cervical source. The cause may be substantiated by clinical, laboratory and/or imaging evidence. Known examples are tumor, fracture, and rheumatoid arthritis. Cervical spondylosis and osteochondritis are not accepted as valid causes, as studies have not confirmed that these cause headache. Similarly, increased pericranial tenderness or myofascial tender spots are not in themselves evidence of cervicogenic headache. Associated headaches should be coded under *tension-type headache*, if the diagnostic criteria for this are fulfilled.

For generally accepted headache causes, such as tumours, fracture, or upper cervical rheumatoid, there is no need to adduce evidence of the correlation between the headache cause and the headache. For dubious headache causes, however, the connection between the headache and the presumed cause must be shown on the basis of explicit criteria. It was decided not to state clinical diagnostic features such as movements, posture or tenderness, because such clinical features are neither reliable nor valid criteria for cervicogenic headache. Clinical signs acceptable for cervicogenic headache must have demonstrated reliability and validity. The future task is the identification of such reliable and valid operational tests. Clinical features such as neck pain, focal neck tenderness, history of neck trauma, mechanical exacerbation of pain, unilaterality, coexisting shoulder pain, reduced range of motion in the neck, nuchal onset, nausea, vomiting, photophobia, etc. are not unique to cervicogenic headache. They may be features of cervicogenic headache, but they do not define the relationship between the headache and the source of the headache.

Abolition of headache following diagnostic blockade of a cervical structure or its nerve supply using placebo or other adequate controls is the most powerful means of establishing a cervical source, but the critical aspect is that the diagnostic blocks must be controlled. A single injection of local anaesthetic proves nothing. Furthermore, abolition of headache means complete relief of headache, indicated by a score of zero on a visual analogue scale (VAS). Nevertheless, $\geq 90\%$ reduction in pain to a level of <5 on a 100-point VAS is acceptable as fulfilling criterion C2 of cervicogenic headache.

The diagnostic criteria for cervicogenic headache of the second edition of the IHS classification may appear 'general' but they are designed to be enabling without stipulating single or traditional methods of diagnosis. The criteria are general yet stringent. They deny traditional methods of diagnosis that lack reliability or validity, but they allow for methods yet to be discovered but which may prove to be reliable and valid. The criteria prohibit the use of unreliable, invalid, or untested tests; but permit tests provided that they have been shown to possess reliability and validity. Under those conditions, investigators must assess their tests, and if they can show that they are reliable and valid, they can be used to diagnose cervicogenic headache. The onus, however, is on the investigators. The classification does not provide a list of possible useful tests. The fact that there are only a limited number of such tests presently available is not the problem of the classification. The classification demands the appropriate quality of test used to define the connection with a disorder of the neck as the source of the headache. Without any further embellishment or elaboration, these criteria happen to be operational. They are strict and specific. They do not tolerate or indulge unproven tests. And they are open for any new research results and diagnostic tests showing reliability and validity.

Headache attributed to retropharyngeal tendonitis

Retropharyngeal tendinitis is a rare condition of unknown etiology for which specific headache characteristics are defined in the second edition of the IHS classification.

The disorder is characterized by the acute onset of upper cervical and occipital pain, aggravated by neck movements, especially extension, and accompanied by pain on swallowing and in the early stages, tenderness in the sides of the upper neck, mild to moderate fever, and often an increased erythrocyte sedimentation rate. The headache cause can be discovered by radiography. X-rays of the cervical spine show increased thickness of the C1-C4 prevertebral soft tissue, sometimes with calcification (computerized tomography may show this better); the symptoms and the prevertebral swelling subside over several days, though resolution may be accelerated with NSAIDs.

Headache attributed to craniocervical dystonia

Headache attributed to craniocervical dystonia is included in the classification[15-17] for the first time. Pain arising from *craniocervical dystonia* is either due to continuous contraction of muscles, or it may occur as a result of secondary irritation of neural structures, for example at the emergence of the occipital nerves, induced by muscular hyperactivity. If the condition persists for a long time, it may in some cases give rise to degenerative changes in the skeletal system of the cervical spine, mandibular joint, or dentition, which may cause additional local pain. The continuous contraction may lead to hypertrophy of the affected muscles. Dystonia is not a disease in itself, but a syndrome diagnosis. Dystonia is a syndrome characterized by continuous muscle contractions, which cause rotatory and repeated movements or abnormal postures. The involuntary movements may be phasal, tonic, or rhythmic and may occur to varying degrees and at various speeds. As in headache conditions, a distinction is made between primary (*idiopathic*) and secondary (*symptomatic*) forms. In recent decades, the focal dystonias occurring in the head and neck region have been described by various collective names (cranial, cervicofacial, oromandibular), which often have been used as synonyms. Certainly, there is no controversy about the distinction between *cranial dystonia* (blepharospasm, spasmodic dysphonia, mandibular, or lingual dystonia) and the *cervical dystonias* (torticollis). In view of the similarities between these two groups, it would seem sensible to use the term *craniocervical dystonia* (CCD). Under criterion B, the IHS classification lists as headache cause abnormal movements or defective posture of neck or head due to muscular hyperactivity. According to criterion D, the pain must disappear within 3 months after successful treatment. Treatment with botulinum toxin A is the therapy of first choice. Thus for the first time, it also acquires diagnostic significance within headache therapy.

Headache attributed to disorder of eyes

Most patients who present with head pain from ocular disorders have obvious signs (red eye), symptoms (decrease in vision), or history (eye trauma) that implicate the eye as the origin of pain.[18,19] Red eye with ciliary injection (dilated episcleral vessels radiating from the limbus); cloudy appearing cornea, dilated, unresponsive pupil, narrow-angle configuration in both eyes and marked elevation of intraocular pressure are typical signs of acute angle-closure glaucoma. They can easily be registered and defined as the headache cause.

Patients with headache attributable to refractive error or muscle imbalance constitute only a tiny percentage of all headache patients. True asthenopia requires a reasonable amount of visual effort. Simple clinical pointers provide evidence of the connection between headache cause and headache. In the case of refractive errors, headache is absent on awakening and aggravated by prolonged visual tasks at the distance or angle where vision is impaired. In cases of heterophoria or heterotropia, headache develops or worsens during a visual task, especially one that is tiring or is relieved or improved on closing one eye.

Ocular inflammation takes many forms and may be categorized variously by anatomic site (i.e. iritis, cyclitis, pars planitis, choroiditis), course (acute, subacute, chronic), presumed cause (infectious agents that are endogenous or exogenous, lens related, traumatic), or by type of inflammation (granulomatous, nongranulomatous). The last of these four categories is most useful in describing ocular causes of pain. Headache attributed to ocular inflammatory disorder is a new addition to the second edition of the IHS classification.

Headache attributed to disorder of ears

Headache attributed to disorder of the ears is experienced as fullness in the ear, throbbing, pressure, tenderness, phonophobia, burning, or itching. The pain may radiate to vertex and temples and may involve half of the head or even the global head. Pain intensity may vary from mild to quite severe. The character is described as dull, aching, or lancinating. Associated symptoms may be tinnitus, hearing loss, or vestibular disorders. Pathologic changes are often visible by examination, and manipulation may increase the pain intensity. Retroauricular or subauricular lymphadenitis is a possible marker of a pathologic situation and can increase pain and pressure. There is no unique headache phenotype, so here too the diagnosis is based on the detection of structural lesions in clinical investigation.

Headache attributed to rhinosinusitis

Acute sinusitis is characterized by acute inflammation symptoms of the nasal membrane and nasal sinuses and their vicinity.[20,21] Patients' complaints focus mainly on the nasal sinus that is primarily affected, but frequently several nasal sinuses are affected. In acute inflammation of the nasal sinuses, a purulent discharge into the nose is present. Headache also occurs simultaneously with the start of the nasal sinusitis. Preexisting headaches must not be attributed to the acute inflammation of the nasal sinus. Acute sinusitis typically occurs after an infection of the upper respiratory tract with rhinitis and swelling of the nasal mucous membrane. The result is obstruction of the orifices of the nasal sinuses with blockade of normal drainage and ventilation. Inflammation of the mucous membrane also disturbs the nasal ciliary action. This, too, causes a reduction in drainage. If an obstructive lesion is present in the region of the nasal cavity, normal drainage also is altered. The same applies to an obstruction of the middle meatus by nasal polyps. Maxillary sinusitis also may be caused by inflammations of dental origin, such as periapical abscesses or of iatrogenic origin as a result of dental surgery. Allergies, hypothyroidism, and cystic fibrosis also may favor the occurrence of sinusitis. The same applies to immune suppression and the existence of diabetes mellitus. Inflammation of the nose with swelling and blockade of sinus drainage may be due to nasotracheal intubation or nasogastral tube feeding. Traumatic impacts on the nasal sinus with fractures may also give rise to nasal sinusitis. Finally, hypertrophy of the adenoids or tonsils may induce nasal sinusitis as a result of reduced ventilation. Other conditions that are often considered to induce headache are not sufficiently validated as causes of headache. These include deviation of nasal septum, hypertrophy of turbinates, atrophy of sinus membranes, and mucosal contact. The last, however, is defined in the appendix as a new addition to the second edition of the IHS classification under A11.5.1 *Mucosal contact point headache*.

Migraine and tension-type headache are often confused with *Headache attributed to rhinosinusitis* because of similarity in the location of the headache. A group of patients can be identified who have all of the features of *Migraine without aura* and, additionally, concomitant clinical features such as facial pain, nasal congestion, and headache triggered by weather changes. None of these patients have purulent nasal discharge or other features diagnostic of acute rhinosinusitis. Therefore, it is necessary to differentiate *Headache attributed to rhinosinusitis* from so-called 'sinus headaches', a commonly-made but non-specific diagnosis. Most such cases fulfil the criteria for *Migraine without aura*, with headache either accompanied by prominent autonomic symptoms in the nose or triggered by nasal changes.

Headache attributed to disorder of teeth, jaws, or related structures

Dental disorders are *rarely* specific causes of headache. Dental disorders are primarily connected with *facial pain*, not with headache.[22-24] *Dentogenic inflammations* are most commonly found to give rise to mandibular and facial pain. Possible inflammatory diseases include parodontitis, periapical inflammations, pulpitis, osteomyelitis of the jaw, and osteitis. Other possible causes of *facial pain and headache* are root fragments impacted in the jaw, dental retention, inflammation-induced jaw cysts or acute odontogenous sinusitis. *Traumatic dental irritation*, for example especially an anterior tooth trauma, fractures of the lower jaw, upper jaw, or the middle part of the face and soft-tissue injuries may also result in *facial pain and headache*.

Headache or facial pain attributed to temporomandibular joint (TMJ) disorder

Temporomandibular pain is *extremely frequent* in the context of headache problems.[25] In view of the proximity to the temporomandibular joint, it is logical to assume that a disorder in this structure is the cause. In fact, however, it is *only in exceptional cases* that demonstrable organic disorders in the region of the temporomandibular joint give rise to headaches. Conversely, there are a number of patients who have *marked demonstrable disorders of the temporomandibular joint*, but who do *not* complain of facial pain and headache. When diagnosing headache and facial pain in cases of temporomandibular joint disorders, it is important to take account of the *clinical overlap with tension-type headache* in cases of *oromandibular dysfunction*.

Tension-type headache is *most frequently* responsible for temporomandibular pain. The crucial factor for *a diagnosis of headache* attributable to temporomandibular joint disorder is *that pain is localized in the jaw and the pain can be triggered by jaw movement and/or occlusion of the jaws*. However, there must also be *objective evidence of reduced freedom of movement, a grating sound, and tenderness under pressure*. An *intracapsular inflammation* due to a variety of conditions can also result in *jaw pain*. This also applies to a *disturbance of coordination* of the joint components necessary for the movement. Joint displacement on its own with irregularities in the region of the intracapsular structures is *not* usually accompanied by pain. It is not possible to give a specific headache phenotype, which means that clinical and apparatus-based investigation is of central importance for diagnosis.

References

1. The International Classification of Headache Disorders: 2nd edition. *Cephalalgia* 2004; **24** (Suppl 1): 9–160.
2. Aprill C, Axinn MJ, Bogduk N. Occipital headaches stemming from the lateral atlanto-axial (C1–2) joint. *Cephalalgia* 2002; **22** (1): 15–22.
3. Bogduk N. The neck. *Baillieres Best Pract Res Clin Rheumatol* 1999; **13** (2): 261–85.
4. Bogduk N. C2 ganglion can be injured by compression between the posterior arch of the atlas and the lamina of C2. *Spine* 1999; **24** (3): 308–9.
5. Bogduk N. Cervicogenic headache: anatomic basis and pathophysiologic mechanisms. *Curr Pain Headache Rep* 2001; **5** (4): 382–6.
6. Bogduk N. Diagnostic nerve blocks in chronic pain. *Best Pract Res Clin Anaesthesiol* 2002; **16** (4): 565–78.
7. Bogduk N. The anatomy and pathophysiology of neck pain. *Phys Med Rehabil Clin N Am* 2003; **14** (3): 455–72, v.
8. Bogduk N, Lord SM. Cervical spine disorders. *Curr Opin Rheumatol* 1998; **10** (2): 110–15.
9. Leone M, D'Amico D, Grazzi L, *et al*. Cervicogenic headache: a critical review of the current diagnostic criteria. *Pain* 1998; **78** (1): 1–5.
10. Sjaastad O. Reliability of cervicogenic headache diagnosis. *Cephalalgia* 1999; **19** (9): 767–8.
11. Sjaastad O, Fredriksen TA, Pfaffenrath V. Cervicogenic headache: diagnostic criteria. The Cervicogenic Headache International Study Group. *Headache* 1998; **38** (6): 442–5.

12. Vincent MB, Luna RA. Cervicogenic headache: a comparison with migraine and tension-type headache. *Cephalalgia* 1999; **19** (Suppl 25): 11–6.
13. Vincent MB, Luna RA, Scandiuzzi D, *et al.* Greater occipital nerve blockade in cervicogenic headache. *Arq Neuropsiquiatr* 1998; **56** (4): 720–5.
14. Wilk V. What of cervicogenic headaches? *Aust Fam Physician* 1998; **27** (10): 877–8.
15. Göbel H, Heinze A, Heinze-Kuhn K, *et al.* Botulinum toxin A in the treatment of headache syndromes and pericranial pain syndromes. *Pain* 2001; **91** (3): 195–9.
16. Göbel H, Heinze A, Heinze-Kuhn K, *et al.* Evidence-based medicine: botulinum toxin A in migraine and tension-type headache. *J Neurol* 2001; **248** (Suppl 1): 34–8.
17. Gupta AK, Roy DR, Conlan ES, *et al.* Torticollis secondary to posterior fossa tumors. *J Pediatr Orthop* 1996; **16** (4): 505–7.
18. Göbel H, TJ M. Ocular disorders. In: *The headaches* (eds J Olesen, P Tfelt-Hansen, KMA Welch). 2nd ed. Philadelphia: Williams & Willkins; 2000: 899–904.
19. Evans RW, Daroff RB. Expert opinion: monocular visual aura with headache: retinal migraine? *Headache* 2000; **40** (7); 603–4
20. Blumenthal HJ. Headaches and sinus disease. *Headache* 2001; **41** (9): 883–8.
21. Göbel H, RW B. Disorder of ear, nose, sinus. In: *The headaches* (eds J Olesen, P Tfelt-Hansen, KMA Welch). 2 ed. Philadelphia: Williams & Willkins; 2000. 905–912.
22. Ciancaglini R, Gherlone EF, Radaelli G. The relationship of bruxism with craniofacial pain and symptoms from the masticatory system in the adult population. *J Oral Rehabil* 2001; **28** (9): 842–8.
23. Ciancaglini R, Gherlone EF, Redaelli S, *et al.* The distribution of occlusal contacts in the intercuspal position and temporomandibular disorder. *J Oral Rehabil* 2002; **29** (11): 1082–90.
24. Sonnesen L, Bakke M, Solow B. Malocclusion traits and symptoms and signs of temporomandibular disorders in children with severe malocclusion. *Eur J Orthod* 1998; **20** (5): 543–59.
25. Ciancaglini R, Radaelli G. The relationship between headache and symptoms of temporomandibular disorder in the general population. *J Dent* 2001; **29** (2): 93–8.

35
Cranial neuralgias and central causes of facial pain

J. W. Lance

Pain in the head is mediated by afferent fibers in the trigeminal nerve, nervus intermedius, glossopharyngeal and vagus nerves, and the upper cervical roots via the occipital nerves. Impulses giving rise to the sensation of pain may be generated by compression or distortion of these nerves, and exposure to excessive heat or cold or other sources of irritation. Lesions of the central connections of sensory fibers can also cause pain referred to the distribution of the appropriate nerves.

Neural pain is referred to as neuralgia which may be constant or intermittent, and aching or stabbing in quality. Sometimes, its origin can be determined from the case history, physical signs, or imaging but in other cases, no cause may be apparent.

Trigeminal neuralgia

There is some difficulty in classifying trigeminal or glossopharyngeal neuralgia as primary or secondary because many, perhaps most, patients will be found to have an aberrant blood vessel impinging on the nerve and presumably responsible for their symptoms. Vascular decompression leads to rapid recovery of nerve conduction across the indented root.[1] For this reason, the term 'classical' has been preferred for those patients in whom a neuroma or similar identifiable cause has not been determined by imaging.

Classical trigeminal neuralgia

There is usually no clinically detectable sensory loss in classical trigeminal neuralgia so that other conditions, such as a tumor, must be considered if sensation is found to be impaired, in which case the condition is termed *symptomatic trigeminal neuralgia*.

The pain of classical trigeminal neuralgia is unilateral, brief, shock-like, and repetitive, limited to one or more divisions of the trigeminal nerve. It is evoked by trigger factors such as talking or chewing or by contact with trigger areas (commonly on the chin or nasolabial fold). The condition may remit and relapse. After a paroxysm, there may be a refractory period during which the condition cannot be precipitated.

Symptomatic trigeminal neuralgia

The character of the pain is the same as in classical trigeminal neuralgia but caused by a demonstrable structural lesion other than vascular compression. The association of trigeminal neuralgia with multiple sclerosis is classified and presented later in this chapter. There is no refractory period in symptomatic trigeminal neuralgia.

Fromm *et al.*[2] have described prodromal symptoms of pain resembling sinusitis or toothache that may precede the onset of typical trigeminal neuralgia by some days. Such pains may last for several hours and be triggered by jaw movements, or by hot or cold fluids, which may lead to unnecessary dental procedures.

Glossopharyngeal neuralgia

Classical glossopharyngeal neuralgia

Glossopharyngeal neuralgia is about 100 times less common than trigeminal neuralgia, and causes a similar type of lancinating pain in the ear, base of the tongue, tonsillar fossa, or beneath the angle of the jaw. The distribution is not only in the sensory area of the glossopharyngeal nerve but also those of the auricular and pharyngeal branches of the vagus nerve. It is provoked by swallowing, talking, or coughing. Of 217 cases reported by Rushton, Stevens and Miller,[3] 25 also had trigeminal neuralgia. Pain may predominate in the pharynx or in the ear, presenting as pharyngeal or otalgic forms of neuralgia. The ear on the affected side sometimes becomes red and painful.[4]

Symptomatic glossopharyngeal neuralgia

Glossopharyngeal neuralgia may be secondary to compression of the nerve by neoplasms, granulomas, or blood vessels. It is termed *Symptomatic Glossopharyngeal Neuralgia* when the cause is demonstrated by imaging.

Nervus intermedius neuralgia

Sensation from the external auditory canal and a segment of the external ear is mediated by the nervus intermedius, part of the facial nerve. Pain in the associated area of distribution may be experienced in geniculate herpes (Ramsay–Hunt syndrome).

It remains doubtful as to whether stabbing pains in the ear can ever be ascribed to the nervus intermedius or whether they represent the otalgic variation of glossopharyngeal neuralgia.

Superior laryngeal neuralgia

The superior laryngeal is a terminal branch of the vagus nerve. It can give rise to a rare disorder characterized by severe pain in the lateral aspect of the throat, submandibular region, and under the ear, brought on by swallowing, shouting, or turning the head. The pain may be constant or lancinating, triggered by pressure on the side of the throat. It may occasionally follow respiratory infections, tonsillectomy, or carotid endarterectomy. The diagnosis is confirmed by local anaesthetic block of the superior laryngeal nerve and the condition is relieved by neurectomy.

Nasociliary neuralgia

This is a rare condition which may be caused by a blow to the face or may occur spontaneously. Touching the outer surface of the nose causes a stabbing pain that radiates upwards to the midfrontal region. It is abolished by application of local anaesthetics to the nerve or into the nostril on the affected side.

Supraorbital neuralgia

Constant or jabbing pain is felt in the inner canthus of the eye and forehead in the distribution of the first division of the trigeminal nerve.[5] It is characterized by tenderness of the nerve to palpation in the supraorbital notch and is relieved by local anaesthetic blockade and subsequent ablation of the nerve by a radiofrequency probe or surgical section. Pain may be associated with diminished sensitivity to touch or pin prick in a frontal strip above the eyebrow.

Other terminal branch neuralgias

Injury or entrapment of other peripheral branches of the trigeminal nerve may cause constant or lancinating pain in the areas innervated by that nerve. Examples are neuralgias of the infraorbital, lingual, alveolar, and mental nerves.

Nummular headache

Pareja *et al.*[6] described a distinctive localized pain, the shape of a coin 2–6 cm in diameter, felt in the scalp as a continuous sensation which develops into a severe or stabbing pain on occasions. The underlying cause has not been established but presumably is neuralgia of a terminal twig of a trigeminal nerve branch. The condition is benign and may remit. The term nummular (as spelt in the paper cited) means coin-shaped.

Occipital neuralgia

Occipital neuralgia is characterized by an aching or paroxysmal jabbing pain in the area of distribution of the greater or lesser occipital nerves, usually accompanied by diminished sensation or dysaesthesia of the affected area. It may be accompanied by tenderness over the point where the nerve crosses midway between the mastoid process and the occipital protuberance, whereas the lesser occipital nerve crosses it about 4 cm behind the ear.

If the occipital pain is continuous and there is no impairment of sensation, it may be referred to pain from the atlantoaxial or C2–3 facet joints, from the posterior fossa, or even from the first division of the trigeminal nerve, the descending spinal tract of which converges with the C2–3 afferent fibers on second-order neurones in the upper three segments of the spinal cord. The distinction can often be made by assessing the response to infiltration of the tender area by a local anesthetic agent or blockade of the second cervical ganglion.[7] Caution must be exercised because the inadvertent injection of local anesthetics into the cerebrospinal fluid via an underlying long nerve root sleeve may lead to respiratory arrest.

Neck–tongue syndrome

Lance and Anthony[8] described an unusual syndrome affecting mainly children and young adults on sudden rotation of the neck. The patient experiences a sharp pain in the upper neck or occiput, which may be accompanied by numbness or tingling in these areas. At the same time, the ipsilateral half of the tongue becomes numb or feels as though it is twisting in the mouth. The explanation is that proprioceptive fibers from the tongue travel via communications from the lingual nerve to the hypoglossal nerve and thence to the second cervical root. Transient subluxation of the atlantoaxial joint can produce local pain by stretching the joint capsule and tongue symptoms by stretching the C2 ventral ramus, which contains proprioceptive fibers from the tongue.

External compression headache

A tight hat, a band around the head, the wearing of a protective helmet by construction workers, or the use of tight swimming goggles may induce headache.

Cold-stimulus headache

Headache attributed to external application of a cold stimulus

Exposure of the bare head to sub-zero temperatures or diving into cold water will cause headache from excessive stimulation of temperature-sensitive receptors in the face and scalp. Wolf and Hardy[9] induced pain by dipping the top of the head into cold water (<18°C) which reached a peak of 60 s and spread from the vertex to temples and occiput. The only areas of the body from which these authors could not provoke pain by exposure to cold were the ear lobes and the glans penis.

Headache attributed to ingestion or inhalation of a cold stimulus (ice cream headache)

Holding ice or ice cream in the mouth, or swallowing a cold food or drink as a bolus, may cause discomfort in the palate and throat. It may also refer pain to the forehead or temple by the trigeminal nerve and to the ears by the glossopharyngeal nerve.

A recent survey in Taiwan[10] of 8359 students found a 40.6% prevalence of ice cream headache. Students with migraine had a higher frequency of ice cream headache (55.2%) than those who did not suffer from headaches (29.1%). The location of ice cream headache correlated with the site of other habitual headaches. A negative report[11] concerning the relationship of migraine to ice cream headache was flawed by the ice cream used for the control group of students being 11°C colder than that used for the migrainous students.

The fact that ice cream headache is more common in migraine patients and is often referred to the part of the head afflicted by the patient's customary headache suggests that there may be a segmental disinhibition of central pain pathways in migraine patients, which is responsible for undue susceptibility to an afferent volley of impulses from the excitation of cold receptors in the oropharynx.

Constant pain caused by compression, irritation, or distortion of cranial nerves or upper cervical roots by structural lesions

The first division of the trigeminal nerve may be compressed in the orbit, the superior orbital fissure, cavernous sinus, or near the apex of the petrous temporal bone. When pain is present, it may be constant or stabbing in quality, often associated with sensory impairment in the appropriate area of distribution. Involvement of the nervus intermedius refers pain to the external auditory canal, the glossopharyngeal nerve to the base of the tongue and tonsillar fossa, and the vagus nerve to a region in or behind the ear. Facial pain around the ear or temple may result from invasion of the vagus nerve by lung carcinoma.[12]

Raeder's paratrigeminal neuralgia

The term Raeder's syndrome is applied to pain of trigeminal distribution, usually the ophthalmic division, in association with an ocular (post-ganglionic) sympathetic deficit comprising ptosis, miosis, and impairment of sweating over the medial aspect of the forehead but not elsewhere on the face.

Patients fall into two groups: those with episodic pain that we now recognize as cluster headache and those with aneurysms, neoplasms, inflammation, or trauma involving the internal carotid artery and impinging on the first division of the trigeminal nerve. Sjaastad et al.[13] distinguish the features of Raeder's syndrome from the superior orbital fissure syndrome of Tolosa and Hunt and the posterior cavernous sinus syndrome of Gradenigo. The concept of Raeder's syndrome has some localizing value but no more than that.

Gradenigo's syndrome

Lesions of the apex of the petrous temporal bone cause pain referred to the fronto-temporal region and ear in conjunction with a paralysis of the sixth cranial nerve, which runs across the bone at that point. Gradenigo's syndrome was originally described as a complication of middle ear infection but may also be found with tumors arising from or invading this area.

Optic neuritis

Pain in or behind the eye usually precedes impairment of vision by some hours or days in optic (retrobulbar) neuritis. The eyeball is usually tender to pressure and aches on eye movement. The characteristic visual field defect is a central scotoma. The optic fundi are usually normal to examination but swelling of the optic disc (papillitis) is observed if demyelination involves the nerve head. The pain and visual disturbance of optic neuritis usually responds rapidly to corticosteroids.

Ocular diabetic neuropathy

In diabetes mellitus, one or more of the ocular motor cranial nerves may become paralyzed, accompanied or preceded by pain in or around the affected eye. Pain may precede diplopia by up to 7 days. The third cranial nerve is most commonly involved, often with sparing of pupillary function, but the fourth and sixth cranial nerves are also susceptible.

Headache or facial pain attributed to herpes zoster

Acute herpes zoster

Herpes zoster is caused by reactivation of the varicella zoster virus, which is thought to lie dormant in the trigeminal, geniculate, and dorsal root ganglia after chicken pox infection in early life. The distribution of the rash and subsequent pain follows trigeminal distribution, mostly affecting the ophthalmic division. The rash may also involve the external auditory meatus, the soft palate, or the area supplied by the upper cervical roots. Paralysis of the third, fourth, or sixth cranial nerves, or a facial palsy may accompany the herpetic eruption. The combination of an herpetic rash in the external auditory canal and a facial palsy that results from invasion of the geniculate ganglion is known as *Ramsay–Hunt Syndrome*. An unpleasant burning pain often precedes the skin eruption by 2–4 days. Pain in the area of distribution of the first division of the trigeminal nerve may cause diagnostic difficulties when it appears several days before the rash or, on rare occasions, without any rash at all.

Post-herpetic neuralgia

Post-herpetic neuralgia has been defined as pain persisting 3 months or more after onset of the rash. The incidence of post-herpetic neuralgia is about 10% when all age groups are considered, but increases with age, reaching 50% by the age of 60 years. The pain is characteristic burning with occasional stabbing components and the lightest touch over the affected area may be felt as painful (allodynia).

The genesis of the pain is presumably related to a disturbance in the pattern of afferent impulses and the removal of some central inhibitory influence because pain usually persists after sectioning of the trigeminal nerve or medullary tractotomy.[14]

Tolosa–Hunt syndrome

Involvement of the superior orbital fissure by granuloma causes recurrent painful ophthalmoplegia (Tolosa–Hunt syndrome) that may be mistaken for ophthalmoplegic migraine and must be distinguished from other retro-orbital lesions such as intracranial aneurysms and sphenoid wing meningioma. It is probably identical with 'pseudo-tumor of the orbit'. The condition was described by Tolosa in 1954 and Hunt *et al.*[15] noted the responsiveness of the syndrome to steroid therapy. Although over 200 cases have been reported since then, few were with histological confirmation.

Painful ophthalmoplegia may be associated with Horner's syndrome and sensory impairment in the distribution of the first or second divisions of the trigeminal nerve. Paresis may occur with the onset of pain or within 2 weeks and resolves within 72 h when treated with corticosteroids, but persists for 8 weeks or so if untreated.

Diagnosis may be made by MR imaging. It is important to exclude other causes of similar symptoms. These are listed by Kline and Hoyt.[16] The major categories are vascular lesions such as aneurysms, tumors of various sorts, mucoceles, sarcoid, and Wegener's granulomatosis.

Ophthalmoplegic 'Migraine'

Recurrent attacks of migraine-like headache accompanied or followed by paresis of the third, fourth, or sixth cranial nerves has traditionally been considered as a variation of migraine. The fact that ophthalmoplegia may develop as long as 4 days after headache begins and that MRI often shows gadolinium uptake in the cisternal part of the affected cranial nerves has prompted thoughts of the condition being a recurrent demyelinating neuropathy.[17,18] The relationship between headache and neural involvement is unclear. The older concept of the ophthalmoplegia being the result of an ischemic neuropathy triggered by migrainous vasospasm has not been disapproved. As with Tolosa–Hunt syndrome, it is important to exclude compression of the cranial nerves caused by aneurysm or other space occupying lesions

Central causes of facial pain

Anaesthesia Dolorosa

This unpleasant and intractable condition consists of pain or other disagreeable sensations being experienced in a body area that is numb as the result of some deafferenting disease or procedure, comparable with a phantom limb.[19] It is as though central pain pathways, being deprived of their normal afferent input, discharge spontaneously to convey a false message of perceived pain to higher centers.

Central post-stroke pain

Pain and burning sensations in the face and scalp may be caused by central lesions involving the second-order trigeminal neurones (the quintothalamic tract), the ventrobasal nuclei of the thalamus or, less often, of the thalamo-cortical pathway. These pathways or nuclei may be damaged by vascular disease or multiple sclerosis and, less commonly, by syringomyelia or glioma. The pain often extends to the limbs and trunk on the affected side and diminished sensibility to pin prick and temperature can usually be detected over the painful half of the face or body. Touching the hypaesthetic area may evoke pain (allodynia).

Multiple sclerosis

Trigeminal neuralgia has been a symptom of multiple sclerosis in 1–8% of cases in reported series. From the other point of view, 2–3% of patients with trigeminal neuralgia have multiple sclerosis. In 80–90% of the documented cases, other symptoms of multiple sclerosis preceded the onset of trigeminal neuralgia by 1–29 years. In the remainder, the facial pain was the presenting symptom and other signs of multiple sclerosis followed 1 month–6 years later. Of patients with multiple sclerosis and trigeminal neuralgia, the pain becomes bilateral in 11–14% compared with 3–4% of patients with the idiopathic form. The pain is caused by a plaque of multiple sclerosis in the pons at the entry zone of the trigeminal nerve.

Persistent idiopathic facial pain (previously known as atypical facial pain)

By definition, this term embraces all of those patients whose symptoms do not fit in with a recognized pattern of headache or neuralgic symptoms. In practice, there is a distinctive group of patients with what might be called typical atypical facial pain, so that the term 'persistent idiopathic facial pain' is preferable. This commonly affects patients in their thirties or forties, women more often than men. The most common sites are in the nasolabial fold or on the chin overlying the lower gum. The pain is usually constant, fluctuating in intensity, and aching or boring in quality. It could be said that it bears the same relationship to 'lower-half headache' as tension headache does to migraine. It often starts after some apparently innocuous dental procedure or minor facial trauma.

I regard the condition as an organic syndrome of central origin for the following reasons:

1. The pain is remarkably similar in site and quality from patient to patient, and would be consistent with hyperexcitability of the trigeminal nerve, commonly the second division, or its central connections.
2. The most common sites of pain coincide with trigger points for trigeminal neuralgia.
3. The pain often starts after dental procedures, bringing up the possibility that some infection could be introduced at that time or that herpes simplex virus, a permanent resident in the second and third trigeminal divisions of many people, might be activated to involve central pain pathways and to set up a reaction akin to the neuralgia following herpes zoster.
4. Thermographic assessment of the facial circulation in nine of our patients with unilateral atypical facial pain demonstrated increased heat loss from the cheek of the affected side in 6 patients and from the orbit in 4.[20] This suggests a reflex vasodilator response to activity in the trigeminal system and supports the concept of an organic basis for this disorder.

Facial pain around the ear or temple may precede the detection of an ipsilateral lung carcinoma causing referred pain by invading the vagus nerve.[12] Eross *et al.*[21] warn that the clinical triad of a smoker suffering from periauricular pain who is found to have a high ESR should have a CT scan of the lung. Previously, refractory facial pain responds to effective treatment of the lung lesion.

Surgical measures do not usually help atypical facial pain and may make it worse. The regular administration of imipramine, amitriptyline, and dothiepin often eases the pain. I have also found baclofen useful in some instances.

Burning mouth syndrome

The complaint of a burning sensation in the mouth or tongue can be a symptom of a local or systemic disorder which responds to treatment of the underlying condition. When no medical, mucosal, or dental cause can be found, the condition is termed 'burning mouth syndrome'. It may be associated with subjective dryness, paraesthesia, and altered taste.[22] The pain may be confined to the tongue (glossodynia).

The syndrome affects predominantly women, increasing in prevalence with age, particularly following menopause. Many patients have symptoms of anxiety, depression, and personality disorders. The cause of the syndrome is unknown. One-third to one-half of patients improve spontaneously.

Treatment is unsatisfactory. Antidepressants and low dose clonazepam (mean 1 mg daily) have been employed but evidence of their effect is lacking.

Other cranial neuralgia or other centrally mediated facial pain

Sluder's sphenopalatine neuralgia

Sluder[23] reported 60 patients in whom symptoms and signs indicated a disturbance of the sphenopalatine ganglion. He described pain at the root of the nose, involving also the eye, jaws, teeth, and ear. On the affected side, he noticed diminished sensibility of the soft palate, a higher arch of the palate, and diminished taste sensation. Pain was relieved by application of 20% cocaine to the mucosa overlying the sphenopalatine ganglion.

Sluder cited examples of a woman aged 27 with episodes of such pain recurring from 3 times weekly to once every 3 months (which may have been 'facial migraine'), patients with pain accompanying respiratory infections and one whose pain extended down the arm and leg. The International Headache Society Classification Committee considered this condition to be a synonym for cluster headache, but it appears more likely to be a collection of facial pains of differing aetiology.

Vail's Vidian neuralgia

Vail[24] considered that many of the cases described by Sluder had pain arising from the Vidian nerve rather than the sphenopalatine ganglion and ascribed the cause to inflammation of the sphenoid sinus. He described 31 cases, 28 of whom were female, between 24 and 59 years of age. The attacks often came on between 2 and 3 a.m. suggesting that many of these patients may have had migraine or cluster headache. The diagnosis, like that of Sluder's neuralgia, is of historical interest only.

Eagle's syndrome

Pain in the upper pharynx radiating to the ipsilateral ear and made worse by swallowing was reported by Eagle in 1937 to be related to an elongated styloid process.[25] He later reported 200 cases, claiming that approximately 4% of people with a long styloid process suffer from facial/pharyngeal pain. I remain sceptical as we have not seen a convincing example in our clinic.

Points for discussion

Problems in the classification of cranial neuralgias for discussion are:

(a) Are the terms classical and symptomatic trigeminal neuralgia appropriate?
(b) Is nummular headache acceptable as a terminal brand neuralgia of the trigeminal nerve?
(c) Should simple terms such as 'ice cream headache' take preference over more specific but pedantic terms such as 'headache attributed to ingestion or inhalation of a cold stimulus'?
(d) Are we satisfied that ophthalmoplegic 'migraine' is a demyelinating neuropathy?
(e) Is there any more information about the cause and treatment of 'burning mouth syndrome'?
(f) Is Eagle's syndrome sufficiently validated to accept in classification?
(g) What were Sluder and Vail describing in the papers cited? Can we ignore them now?

References

1. Love S, Coakman HB. Trigeminal neuralgia: pathology and pathogenesis. *Brain* 2001; **124**: 2347–60.
2. Fromm GH, Graff-Radford SB, Terrence CF, *et al.* Pre-trigeminal neuralgia. *Neurology* 1990; **40**: 1493–5.
3. Rushton JG, Stevens JC, Miller RH. Glossopharyngeal (vagoglossopharyngeal) neuralgia. A study of 217 cases. *Arch Neurol* 1981; **38**: 201–5.
4. Lance JW. The red ear syndrome. *Neurology* 1996; **47**: 617–20.
5. Caminero AB, Pareja JA. Supraorbital neuralgia: a clinical study. *Cephalalgia* 2001; **21**: 216–23.
6. Pareja JA, Caminero AB, Serra J, *et al.* Nummular headache: a coin-shaped cephalgia. *Neurology* 2002; **58**: 1678–9.
7. Bogduk N. Greater occipital neuralgia. In: *Current therapy in neurological surgery* (ed. Long DM). Toronto, BC Decker, Saint Louis, CV Mosby 1985: 175–80.
8. Lance JW, Anthony M. Neck-tongue syndrome on sudden turning of the head. *J Neurol Neurosurg Psychiat* 1985; **43**: 97–101.
9. Wolf S, Hardy JD. Studies on pain. Observations on pain due to local cooling and on factors involved in the 'cold pressor' effect. *J Clin Invest* 1941; **20**: 521–33.
10. Fuh JL, Wang S-J, Lu S-R, *et al.* Ice-cream headache – a large survey of 8359 adolescents. *Cephalalgia* 2003; **23**, 977–81.
11. Bird N, MacGregor A, Wilkinson MIP. Ice-cream headache – site, duration and relationship to migraine. *Headache* 1992; **32**: 35–8.
12 Schoenen J, Broux R, Moonen G. Unilateral facial pain as the first symptom of lung cancer. *Cephalalgia* 1992; **12**: 178–9.
13. Sjaastad O, Elsas T, Shen J-M, *et al.* Raeder's syndrome: 'anhidrosis', headache and a proposal for a new classification. *Funct Neurol* 1994; **9**: 215–34.
14. Portenoy RK, Duma C, Foley KM. Acute herpetic and postherpetic neuralgia; clinical review and current management. *Ann Neurol* 1986; **20**: 651–61.
15. Hunt WE. Tolosa-Hunt syndrome: one cause of painful ophthalmoplegia. *J Neurosurg* 1976; **44**: 544–9.

16. Kline LB, Hoyt WF. The Tolosa-Hunt syndrome. *J Neurol Neurosurg Psychiat* 2001; **71**: 577–82.
17. Lance JW, Zagami AS. Ophthalmoplegic migraine: a recurrent demyelinating neuropathy? *Cephalalgia* 2001; **21**: 84–5.
18. Mark AS, Casselman J, Brown D, *et al.* Ophthalmoplegic migraine: reversible enhancement and thickening of the cisternal segment of the oculomotor nerve on contrast-enhanced MR images. *Am J Neuroradiol* 1998; **19**: 1887–91.
19. Bowsher D. Central pain: clinical and physiological characteristics. *J Neurol Neurosurg Psychiat* 1996; **61**: 62–9.
20. Drummond PD. Vascular changes in atypical facial pain. *Headache* 1988; **28**: 121–3.
21. Eross EJ, Dodick DW, Swanson JW, *et al.* A review of intractable facial pain secondary to underlying lung neoplasms. *Cephalalgia* 2003; **23**: 2–5.
22. Zakrzewska JM. Burning mouth. In: *Pain research and clinical management* (ed. Zakrzewska JM, Harrison SO). 14th ed. *Elsevier Science* 2002: 367–380.
23. Sluder G. The syndrome of sphenopalatine ganglion neurosis. *Am J Med Sci* 1910; **140**: 868–78.
24. Vail HH. Vidian neuralgia. *Ann Otol Rhinol Laryngol* 1932; **41**: 837–56.
25. Montalbetti L, Ferrandi D, Pergami P, *et al.* Elongated styloid process and Eagle's syndrome. *Cephalalgia* 1995; **15**: 80–93.

36 Headache diagnosis in systemic mastocytosis

S. Ashina and M. Ashina

Introduction

Mastocytosis is a clonal disorder of mast cells in both children and adults.[1] It is characterized by overproliferation, accumulation, and activation of the mast cells in different tissues.[1] Mast cell hyperplasia can be restricted to the skin (cutaneous mastocytosis), or may also involve extracutaneous organs (systemic mastocytosis) such as skeleton, bone marrow, gastrointestinal tract, liver, spleen, lymph nodes, and the CNS. Prevalence or incidence of the disease is unknown and is probably difficult to determine because of the underdiagnosis of the systemic disease without the cutaneous manifestation.[2] Occurrence of cutaneous mastocytosis has been estimated in 0.1–0.8% of patients visiting dermatology and allergy clinics.[3] Headache is the most frequent neurological complaint in systemic mastocytosis.[1,4] We report a case of the systemic mastocytosis associated with frequent headaches.

Case story

A 47-year-old female was presented at the Danish Headache Center. She was diagnosed with systemic mastocytosis and referred from the Department of Dermatology for the evaluation of frequent headaches. Patient's mastocytosis-related symptoms included: skin lesions (urticaria pigmentosa), pruritus, dyspepsia, and diarrhea. The patient has had skin lesions for the past 20 years, and diagnosis of systemic mastocytosis was verified by skin biopsy 9 months ago and colon biopsy 7 months ago. She had a history of frequent episodes of headache since puberty. Both the patient's mother and daughter suffer from migraine without aura. At the admission, she was taking a H2-receptor blocker (cimetidine), two H1-receptor blockers (cetirizine and hydroxyzine), and a SSRI (citalopram), and was receiving ultraviolet A therapy for the skin lesions. The neurological examination was normal except known monocular temporal hemianopsia due to previous retinal detachment. Cimetidine caused partial relief of the headaches, i.e. reduction in the

Table 36.1 Percentages of headache characteristics in a patient with systemic mastocytosis during the 6-week period

Localization	Bilateral: 100%			
Quality	Pressing: 100%			
Severity		Mild: 70%	Moderate: 15%	Severe: 15%
Nausea	None: 89%	Mild: 11%	Moderate: 0%	Severe: 0%
Photophobia	None: 11%	Mild: 74%	Moderate: 15%	Severe: 0%
Phonophobia	None: 93%	Mild: 7%	Moderate: 0%	Severe: 0%

Amount of used analgesics prior to treatment with montelukast (g/6 weeks): 22 g of acetaminophen.

number of severe attacks. After the first consultation, the patient was instructed to complete a diagnostic headache diary[5] for the next 6 weeks. At the second visit, patient's headaches were diagnosed according to International Headache Society (IHS) Classification criteria.[16] Patient experienced headache for 27 days in a 6-week period. Nineteen percent of her headaches fulfilled criteria for migraine without aura and 81% for frequent episodic tension-type headache (Table 36.1). CT-scan of the head did not demonstrate any lesions in the brain. A daily dose of 10 mg of montelukast (Singulair®, MSD), a specific D_4 leukotriene receptor antagonist, was then prescribed. During the 11 weeks of treatment, headache frequency was reduced to 2 episodes of headache fulfilling criteria for infrequent, episodic, tension-type headache. The effect of the drug was already observed in the first week of the treatment. Unfortunately, montelukast was discontinued after approximately 3 months of treatment because of reported side effects (swelling and pain in finger joints). However, it is unclear whether these symptoms were side effects or manifestation of symptoms of systemic mastocytosis. The symptoms remained after discontinuation of the drug for a few months. Patient began to complain of headaches again. Unfortunately, the patient did not complete the diagnostic headache diary after stop of montelukast treatment. During the interview, she reported that frequency of her headaches gradually increased to 8 episodes per month in the following 3-month period. Eighty percent of her headaches were tension-type-like headaches (bilateral, pressing, associated with mild photophobia) and 20% of her headaches were migraine-like (without aura, throbbing, associated with nausea, photophobia and aggravated by physical activity). Patient is being followed at the Danish Headache Center.

Discussion

It has been reported that headache in systemic mastocytosis has heterogenic presentation.[1] It may be a mild frontal, dull headache; a headache with migraine characteristics; and a headache associated with autonomic symptoms such as rhinorrhea and lacrimation.[1,4] However, headaches in systemic mastocytosis have never been classified according to IHS criteria.[6] In our patient, we describe two types of headaches: tension-type-like and migraine-like (migraine without aura).

The pathophysiological mechanisms of headache in patients with systemic mastocytosis are unknown. Mast cells might be involved in neurogenic inflammation by releasing histamine and leukotrienes, which may lead to the immune cell infiltration and sensitization of sensory neurons.[7] Mediators of mast cells may be involved in pathophysiology of migraine.[8,9] Moreover, it is believed that release of inflammatory mediators from mast cells may be responsible for development of headache in systemic mastocytosis.[1,10] In an open-label study[8] of 17 patients with migraine, it has been shown that a specific leukotriene receptor antagonist, montelukast, may be effective as preventive treatment.

Our observation suggests that both tension-type-like and migraine-like headaches in systemic mastocytosis may be due to peripheral sensitization induced by release of histamine and leukotrienes from mast cells. The reduced headache frequency by treatment with montelukast in the patient with systemic mastocytosis suggests that leukotriene antagonists may be effective in the treatment of headaches associated with this disorder.

Conclusions

We report two types of headache in a patient with systemic mastocytosis: tension-type-like and migraine-like headaches. Mediators of mast cell, histamine, and leukotrienes, may be involved in development of frequent episodes of headache in patients with systemic mastocytosis and a specific D_4 leukotriene receptor blocker, montelukast, may be tried as preventive treatment.

Reference

1. Castells M, Austen KF. Mastocytosis: mediator-related signs and symptoms. *Int Arch Allergy Immunol* 2002; **127**: 147–52.
2. Kumar S, Moody P. Mastocytosis. *Pediatr Rev* 2001; **22**: 33–4.
3. Golkar L, Bernhard JD. Mastocytosis. *Lancet* 1997; **349**: 1379–85.
4. Scully RE, Mark EJ, McNeely WF, *et al.* Case records of the Massachusetts General Hospital. Weekly clinicopathological exercises. Case 7–1992. A 57-year-old man with a 20-year history of episodic headache, flushing, hypotension, and occasional syncope. *N Engl J Med* 1992; **326**: 472–81.
5. Russell MB, Rasmussen BK, Brennum J, *et al.* Presentation of a new instrument: the diagnostic headache diary. *Cephalalgia* 1992; **12**: 369–74.
6. Headache Classification Committee of the International Headache Society. The International Classification of Headache Disorders. 2nd edition. *Cephalalgia* 2004; **24** (Suppl 1): 1–160.
7. Raja SN, Meyer RA, Ringkamp M, *et al.* Peripheral neural mechanisms of nociception. In: *Textbook of pain* (eds Wall PD, Melzack R). 4th ed. Churchill Livingstone, 1999: 11–84.

8. Sheftell F, Rapoport A, Weeks R, *et al.* Montelukast in the prophylaxis of migraine: a potential role for leukotriene modifiers. *Headache* 2000; **40**: 158–63.
9. Krabbe AA, Olesen J. Headache provocation by continuous intravenous infusion of histamine. Clinical results and receptor mechanisms. *Pain* 1980; **8**: 253–9.
10. Valent P, Akin C, Sperr WR, *et al.* Diagnosis and treatment of systemic mastocytosis: state of the art. *Br J Haematol* 2003; **122**: 695–717.

37
Polycythaemia: a cause of secondary headache?

A. H. Aamodt, A. Waage, and L. J. Stovner

Introduction

Headache is a common symptom in conditions with polycythaemia and elevated haemoglobin levels.[1] There are some observations indicating that elevated haemoglobin values/polycythaemia may induce headache by increasing blood viscosity. In one recent population-based study, headache prevalence seems to be related to haemoglobin levels.[2] This paper summarizes relevant reports in the literature and proposes diagnostic criteria for headache caused by polycythaemia.

Polycythaemia is a common term for conditions with increased red cell mass, usually divided into polycythaemia vera and secondary polycythaemia. Haemoglobin concentration and haematocrit are both indirect measures of red cell mass and commonly substitute for the more cumbersome radio isotope methods. High haemoglobin concentration can also be generated by the combination of low normal plasma volume and high normal red cell mass (relative polycythaemia). Most maintain their individually normal haemoglobin value throughout life, 2.5% of these by definition being above the upper normal range.

Epidemiology

The association between headache and haemoglobin was analysed in a cross-sectional study where 2385 women aged 20–55 years responded to a headache questionnaire and had blood samples for measuring haemoglobin and ferritin.[2] In the multivariate analyses, adjusting for age and education, there was a linear trend of decreasing prevalence of headache ($P = 0.02$) and migraine ($P = 0.01$) with decreasing haemoglobin. In particular, migraine was less likely among women with low haemoglobin (values < 11.5 g/dL) (OR = 0.4, CI 0.2–0.9). As demonstrated in Fig. 37.1, there was a slight tendency to increasing prevalence of headache with increasing haemoglobin values. However, the number of persons with deranged haemoglobin levels was low. Totally, only 21 women had haemoglobin levels

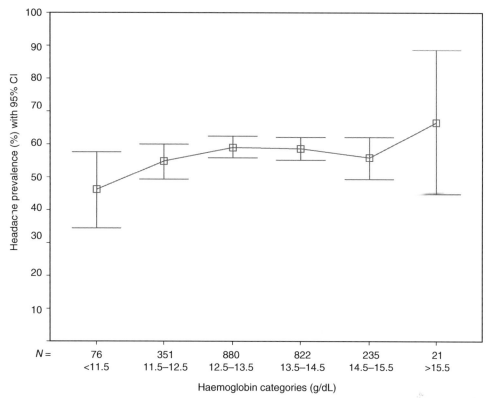

Fig. 37.1   One year prevalence of headache with 95% confidence interval (CI) related to haemoglobin values.

above the reference limit at 15.5 g/dL. There was no correlation between headache prevalence and ferritin.

Polycythaemia vera

In this myeloproliferative disorder, polycythaemia vera headache is reported by almost half of the patients.[1,3,4] In one study, 37% of the patients sought medical attention primarily because of headache.[5] The headache prevalence in patients with polycythaemia vera seems to correlate well with the height of the haematocrit,[5] which is a major determinant of blood viscosity. The headache is thought to be caused by hyperviscosity, which induces disturbed microcirculation by increasing resistance for flow and circulatory transport.[3,4,6] The red cell deformability seems to be decreased and there may be an increase in the intrinsic aggregability of the blood. The high haematocrit and the low flow may facilitate red cell aggregation. The levels of leucocytes and thrombocytes are often elevated and probably also contribute to increased viscosity by the increased likelihood of their adhesion to the vascular endothelium. The leucocytes may also impede microcirculation due to their low deformability.[6]

There are few reports about the clinical characteristics of the headache in polycythaemia vera, but a migraine-like or painful, generalized 'fullness' in the head has been described.[5] The headache responds well to treatment with phlebotomy which reduces the haematocrit and increases the cerebral blood flow towards normal levels.[3–6] With haematocrit in the upper reference limit, a reduction of 6 units (i.e. from 49 to 43) will lower the viscosity by 30% and increase the cerebral blood flow by 50% at low shear rates.[3] The leucocyte and platelet count is not affected by phlebotomy.[1]

Secondary erythrocytosis

In secondary polycythaemia, the red cell mass is increased by enhanced stimulation of red cell production, either due to hypoxia or aberrant production or response to erythropoietin. Although primary and secondary polycythaemia are entirely different disorders, the patients' symptoms may be quite similar.[1]

In chronic mountain sickness, which occurs in people living at high altitude, headache is a common symptom and is thought to be caused by both hypoxia and elevated haemoglobin values.[7] Increased viscosity due to the elevated haemoglobin values and hypoxia reduces oxygen delivery to the tissues, and in the brain this may alter the levels of various neurotransmitters. In an epidemiologic study, a high prevalence of headache, in particular migraine, was found among people residing at high altitude compared to a similar population at sea level. The frequency of migraine attacks was associated with haemoglobin levels.[7]

Familial erythrocytosis is defined as at least two family members having polycythaemia without any signs of polycythaemia vera or secondary causes. Erythrocytosis may be severe with haemoglobin levels of more than 20 g/dL. Headaches are commonly present.[1]

Headache has also been observed in anaemic renal failure patients after treatment with recombinant human erythropoietin (rHuEpo).[8] It seems to occur more frequently with higher doses of rHuEpo and more rapid rises in haemoglobin.[8] The reason for rHuEpo-induced headache may be increased blood viscosity or increased blood pressure.[8,9] However, headache after treatment with rHuEpo has also been reported in patients with well-controlled blood pressure.[9] The headache resolved with reduced dosages or when the treatment was stopped.[8,9] The main site of erythropoietin production is in the kidney and liver, but erythropoietin and its receptors are also produced in the central nervous system. Therefore, one may also speculate that erythropoietin induces headache by a direct effect in the central nervous system. According to available evidence, rHuEpo does not cross the blood brain barrier, but rHuEpo is found to stimulate NO synthase activity.[10] It may be that rHuEpo induces headache via increased NO-production.

Conclusion

Headache related to polycythaemia seems to be well-documented. However, further research is needed about the headache characteristics and the levels of haemoglobin which may cause headache. We recommend that headache caused by polycythaemia should be included in the chapter 'Headache attributed to disorder of homeostasis' in 'The International Classification of Headache Disorders'. The diagnostic criteria proposed are:

A. Headache, no typical characteristics known, fulfilling criteria B–D
B. Evidence of polycythaemia vera or secondary erythrocytosis with haemoglobin levels above the reference limit
C. Headache develops within 2 months after onset of the disorder
D. Headache resolves within 3 months after normalization of haemoglobin levels

References

1. Beutler E. Polycythaemia. In: *Williams hematology* (eds Beutler E, Lichtman MA, Coller BS, Kipps TJ, Seligsohn U) 6th ed. New York: McGraw-Hill, *Inc* 2001; **61**: 689–701.
2. Aamodt AH, Borch-Iohnsen B, Hagen K, *et al*. Headache related to haemoglobin and ferritin. The HUNT Study. *Cephalalgia* 2004; **24**: 758–62.
3. Newton LK. Neurologic complications of polycythaemia and their impact on therapy. *Oncology* 1990; **4**: 59–64.
4. Ickenstein GW, Klotz JM, Langohr HD. Kopfsmertz bei Polycythaemia vera. Klassifikation eines Kopfsmerzes bei Stoffwechselstörungen. *Schmerz* 1999; **13**: 279–82.
5. Silverstein A, Gilbert H, Wasserman L. Neurologic complications of polycythaemia. *Ann Intern Med* 1962; **57**: 909–16.
6. Wassermann LR, Berk PD, Berlin NI, eds. Polycythaemia vera and the myeloproliferative disorders. 1st ed. Philadelphia: W.B. Saunders Company, 1995.
7. Arregui A, León-Velarde F, Cabrera J, *et al*. Migraine, polycythaemia and chronic mountain sickness. *Cephalalgia* 1994; **14**: 339–41.
8. Abraham PA. Practical approach to initiation of recombinant human erythropoietin therapy and prevention and management of adverse effects. *Am J Nephrol* 1990; **10** (Suppl 2): 7–14.
9. Cheng IKP, Cy C, Chan MK, *et al*. Correction of anemia in patients on continous ambulatory peritoneal dialysis with recombinant erythropoietin twice a week: a long term study. *Clin Nephrol* 1991; **35**: 207–212.
10. Buemi M, Cavallaro E, Floccari F, *et al*. The pleiotropic effects of erythropoietin in the central nervous system. *J Neuropathol Exp Neurol* 2003; **62**: 228–36.

38

Discussion summary, the secondary headaches: Part II

J. Olesen

The new entity cerebral venous sinus stenosis has been diagnosed in patients with the new persisting headache and increased intracranial pressure by lumbar puncture. In such patients, a stenosis of one or both of the transverse sinuses has been demonstrated. In the experience of Professor Diener, some of these cases were cured by balloon dilatation while, in others, it was not possible to dilate the sinus. The syndrome is still too new to give further details about clinical characteristics and treatment results. Once it is better established, it may have to be moved to Chapter 6 – since it is probably in most cases a consequence of previous cerebral venous sinus thrombosis. Spontaneous low pressure headache was another important condition discussed at length. Immediately after lumbar puncture, the headache has the typical characteristics, but this may not be so in patients who have had headache for 3 or 4 years. Such cases are seen in Headache Centers. They have originally received one or maybe two blood patches without sufficient result and have afterwards suffered from orthostatic headache. In some of these patients, a constant headache independent of body position becomes more and more prevalent and some patients even lose the orthostatic component. Meningeal enhancement is a good sign of spontaneous low pressure, but it is neither 100% specific nor 100% sensitive. Patients with typical orthostatic headache without dural enhancement and patients with dural enhancements without orthostatic headache are known. The demonstration of a leak is best done by a lumbar contrast injection and CT myelography, by MR demonstration of the actual leak or isotope leakage demonstrated by scintigraphy. These tests are, however, successful only in approximately 50% of the patients. A poster from Paris presented a pragmatic approach to these headaches consisting of simply giving blood patch without any further investigations. After one blood patch (most of the patients had previously had a blood patch), 90% had immediate relief but 9 of 30 patients relapsed within days or weeks. However, a second blood patch gave relief in 6 out of 9 so that only 7 patients remained who were not cured by two blood patches. The side effects of blood patch were discussed, because reports have suggested that persistent lumbar pain may not be a rare feature after blood patch. However, none of the participating Centers, each having a considerable experience, have had problems with persisting lumbar pain except a single case observed at the Danish Headache Center.

In this section was also a poster demonstrating an inverse relationship between headache and hematocrit. It was suggested that polycythemia may be a cause of headache and later suggested that venesection is an effective treatment for such a headache.

Cervicogenic headache has been redefined in the second edition of the Headache Classification, but the new diagnostic criteria for cervicogenic headache were criticized on grounds that they were too difficult to fulfil. It was said that practitioners today do not have the evidence requested in the criteria and thus were not able to diagnose cervicogenic headache. Professor Göbel pointed out, however, that in all the patients where a clear structural abnormality was present in the cervical spine, there was enough evidence to classify patients. The uncertainty related to patients with no clear objective findings. Professor Diener pointed out that a study in his department, presently still ongoing, had demonstrated significant amounts of headache after cervical disk operations as compared to patients after lumbar disk operations. This had substantiated the existence of cervicogenic headache, but only in patients with clear pathology. The chairman of the classification committee, Jes Olesen, pointed out that simply having tender spots in the neck was not enough for a diagnosis of cervicogenic headache. Such patients should be treated as tension-type headache. The merit of the new classification system and the diagnostic criteria is that the syndrome can now be studied in a meaningful fashion. Criteria previously proposed by Sjaastad give no meaning, because they simply describe a number of features that can be present and are wide open for individual interpretation. Future research will focus on the new criteria and could suggest that these criteria are too tight or too loose.

The new chapter on headache attributed to psychiatric disorder was generally well-received. However, it was pointed out that migraine patients who are evaluated by rating scales often fill out items because of their migraine that would result in a score suggesting depression without the patient actually being depressed. Even with that factor taken into account, there is no doubt about the highly significant comorbidity between migraine with aura, migraine without aura, and depression. It was underlined that multiple sets of criteria in the appendix are for research and cannot be applied in the routine clinical situation because of lack of evidence. An issue that generally creates uncertainty if not confusion is that, for all secondary headaches, probable means that there is no treatment evidence of their existence, i.e. that criterion D is not fulfilled. For the primary headaches, probable means that one of the criteria describing the headache is not fulfilled. It is not possible to give a diagnosis of probable cervicogenic headache because the headache does not meet one of the criteria except for criterion D. Another difficult point was the question of chronic postxxx headache. This was only recognized for chronic post bacterial meningitis headache and for chronic posttraumatic headache, because evidence was not sufficient for other entities. However, the classification committee strongly suspects that there will be many other causes of chronic postxxx headache and encourages the Headache Community to do more research in this field. A question addressed the so-called nummular headache. This is a coin-shaped headache located at a particular spot of the cranium. Strictly localized headaches suggest the presence of a bony lesion or another organic lesion, and always warrants imaging studies. Nummular headache is reserved for patients where no such lesion is found. The condition is described in the appendix and merits further study.

Session VI

Practical implementation and research

39
Algorithms and simplified approaches to headache diagnosis

R. B. Lipton and M. E. Bigal

....

Migraine remains a substantially under-diagnosed and under-treated condition. Prior reports have divided barriers to migraine diagnosis and treatment as follows: 1. Under-recognition of migraine by headache sufferers themselves; 2. Under-consultation among migraine sufferers who need medical care; 3. Failure to diagnose all who consult; 4. Failure to initiate appropriate therapy among all who are diagnosed; 5. Lack of on-going assessment of the benefits of treatment. Screening tools and simplified approaches to headache diagnosis may help address these barriers to care. In this chapter, we review the issue of screening for migraine and describe the development of ID-Migraine, a three-item primary care tool intended to support diagnosis. In addition, we present algorithms that may facilitate the diagnosis of migraine in clinical practice.

Screening migraine

Effective application of diagnostic screening and disability tools might increase recognition of migraine, encourage consultation, and facilitate appropriate care from the time of the first visit. In primary care settings, such tools might increase the speed and efficiency of headache diagnosis, target patients who need treatment, and provide an outcome tool.

Screening tests must be safe, cost-effective, and acceptable to patients as well as healthcare providers. In general, potential screening tests can be classified into four different groups: tests based on measurements in blood or other tissues (i.e. cholesterol determinations, pap smears, genetic tests), physiologic or functional tests (i.e. stress testing for coronary artery disease), anatomic imaging tests (CT or MRI), and questionnaire-based screening (i.e. questionnaires for migraine, secondary headache, dementia, or depression). The healthcare context (i.e. the reason for testing), not the nature of the test itself, determines whether it is a screening test.

The goal of screening for symptomatic disorders is to detect and treat current disability in people not receiving care, not just to prevent future disability.

For migraine headaches, screening for symptomatic disease may prove beneficial because the disorder is under-recognized and under-treated. An ideal screening instrument for migraine should be brief and easy to use. It should have operating characteristics that would make it useful in the primary care setting where most patients consult. Specifically, it should have sufficient sensitivity to detect patients in need of treatment, and sufficient specificity and positive predictive value to ensure that relatively few patients who do not have migraine screen positive for it. Validation studies should be conducted in the setting of the intended use, using a clinical evaluation on the gold standard.

Recently, a three-item migraine screener (ID-Migraine) was found to be a valid and reliable screening instrument for migraine headaches in the primary care (See Fig. 39.1). The first phase of its development study involved 563 patients presenting for routine appointments at 26 primary care practice sites – the setting of intended use of ID-Migraine. Eligible subjects were those reporting the occurrence of at least two headaches in the previous 3 months. Each subject completed a self-administered screening questionnaire that consisted of nine questions referring to the severity and nature of headache pain, the presence of associated migraine symptoms, and the extent to which the headaches resulted in disability. Study subjects then underwent independent diagnostic evaluations performed by headache specialists. Based on the specialists' clinical judgment and/or the International Criteria for Headache Disorders (ICHD), a gold-standard diagnosis of migraine was made. Results of the gold-standard diagnostic evaluation were then compared with

---

Do you have **headaches** that limit your ability to work, study, or enjoy life?

Do you want to talk to your healthcare professional about your headaches?

Please answer these questions and give your answers to your healthcare professional.

During the last 3 months, did you have the following with your headaches:

1. You felt nauseated or sick to your stomach
   ( ) Yes   ( ) No

2. Light bothered you (a lot more than when you don't have headaches
   ( ) Yes   ( ) No

3. Your headaches limited your ability to work, study, or do what you needed to do for at least one day
   ( ) Yes   ( ) No

Fig. 39.1 The ID-Migraine (with permission).

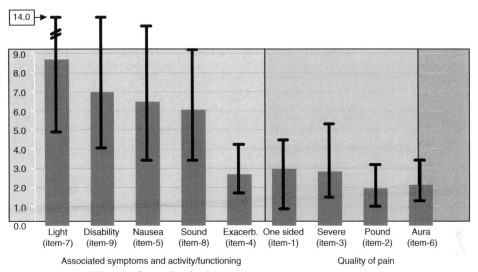

Fig. 39.2 Odds ratio for individual migraine screening items.

those of a nine-item screener, and the diagnostic sensitivity and specificity of each item was computed. Logistic regression was used to identify those screener items that were most strongly associated with a gold-standard migraine diagnosis (Fig. 39.2). These identified items, were strongly and independently associated with migraine. Those items were disability (missing 1 or more days in the previous 3-months due to headache), nausea, and photophobia.

Individuals who indicated that they had two of three of these features were said to screen positive for migraine. In addition, a test–retest reliability was assessed in a study involving 121 patients. The three-item ID-Migraine screener had a sensitivity of 0.81, a specificity of 0.75, and a positive predictive value of 93% using an IHS-based clinical diagnosis as the gold standard. Test–retest reliability was good (Kappa coefficient of 0.68). The excellent performance characteristics of the three-item ID-Migraine suggest it as a simple method for increasing the recognition of migraine in the primary care setting. Important principles include validation studies in the setting of intended use, assessment of validity against a clinical gold standard, and assessment of reliability. In addition, instruments must be designed to meet the needs of the intended user; for the primary care doctor, these include brevity and ease of use.

Algorithms to headache diagnosis

Headache diagnosis using the ICHD-2 (2004) should proceed in an orderly fashion. In this discussion, we assume that only one headache disorder is present. If multiple headache disorders occur together, the conceptual process needs to be repeated for each headache type.

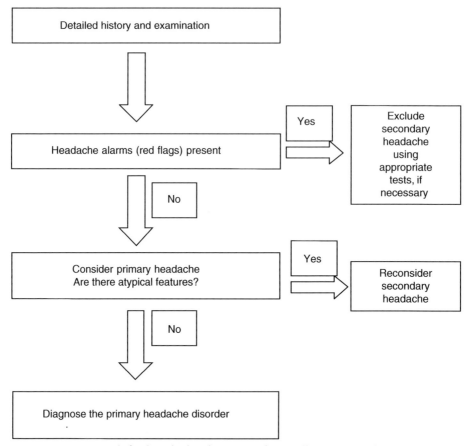

Fig. 39.3 Approach for headache diagnosis (from Silberstein *et al.* 2001).

The first step is to distinguish between primary and secondary headaches. The approach is to spot 'red flags' that suggest the possibility of secondary headache (Fig. 39.3), to conduct the workup indicated by those red flags (Table 39.1) and thereby diagnose or exclude secondary headache disorder that is present.

In the absence of secondary headache, the clinician proceeds to diagnosing a primary headache disorder. Discussing the diagnostic criteria of primary headaches is beyond the scope of this chapter.

Once secondary headache is excluded by clinical history and physical examination or by appropriate investigation, the next step is to divide the primary headaches into three groups, based on average monthly frequency and duration of the attacks. We divide headaches into syndromes of short duration (<4 h) and syndromes of long duration (≥4 h). Long-duration headache attacks are further divided into episodic (<15 attacks per month) or chronic daily headache (≥15 headache days per month) based on headache days (Fig. 39.4).

Table 39.1 Red flags in the diagnosis of headache (modified from Silberstein *et al.* 2001)

Red flag	Consider	Possible investigation(s)
Sudden-onset headache	Subarachnoid hemorrhage, bleed into a mass or AVM, mass lesion (especially posterior fossa)	Neuroimaging Lumbar puncture (after neuroimaging evaluation)
Worsening-pattern headache	Mass lesion, subdural hematoma, medication overuse	Neuroimaging
Headache with systemic illness (fever, neck stiffness, cutaneous rash)	Meningitis, encephalitis, Lyme disease, systemic infection, collagen vascular disease, arteritis	Neuroimaging Lumbar puncture Biopsy Blood tests
Focal neurologic signs, or symptoms other than typical visual or sensory aura	Mass lesion, AVM, collagen vascular disease	Neuroimaging Collagen vascular evaluation
Papilledema	Mass lesion, pseudotumor, encephalitis, meningitis	Neuroimaging Lumbar puncture (after neuroimaging evaluation)
Triggered by cough, exertion, or Valsalva	Subarachnoid hemorrhage, mass lesion	Neuroimaging Considerer lumbar puncture
Headache during pregnancy or postpartum	Cortical vein/cranial sinus thrombosis Carotid dissection Pituitary apoplexy	Neuroimaging
New headache type in a patient with		
Cancer	Metastasis	Neuroimaging, lumbar puncture
Lyme disease	Meningoencephalitis	Neuroimaging, lumbar puncture
HIV	Opportunistic infection, tumor	Neuroimaging, lumbar puncture

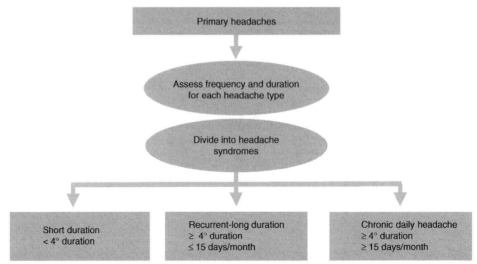

Fig. 39.4 Approach to the primary headaches.

Headaches of shorter duration (Fig. 39.5)

For shorter duration primary headache of low or high frequency, headaches are further classified first based on associated symptoms and then based on the presence or absence of triggers. If the pain has a trigeminal distribution and attacks are associated with autonomic features, consider a trigeminal autonomic cephalgia (3). These include episodic (3.1.1) and chronic (3.1.2) cluster headache, episodic (3.2.1) and chronic (3.2.2) paroxysmal hemicrania, and SUNCT syndrome (3.3). All these headaches are associated with autonomic features. Based on triggers, consider whether it is triggered or not by coughing (Primary cough headache, 4.2), straining or Valsalva maneuver or by exertion (Primary exertional headache, 4.3), sexual activity (Primary headache associated with sexual activity, 4.4), or sleep (hypnic headache, 4.5). If the headache is neither triggered nor associated with autonomic features, consider primary stabbing headache (4.1), trigeminal neuralgia (13.1), or tension-type headache (2) of short duration (30 min to 4 h).

Headaches of long duration and low-to-moderate frequency (Fig. 39.6)

Low-to-moderate frequency headaches of long duration include migraine (1) and episodic tension-type headache (2.1 and 2.2). In contrast to migraine, the main pain features of TTH are bilateral location, nonpulsating quality, mild-to-moderate intensity, and lack of aggravation by routine physical activity. The pain is not

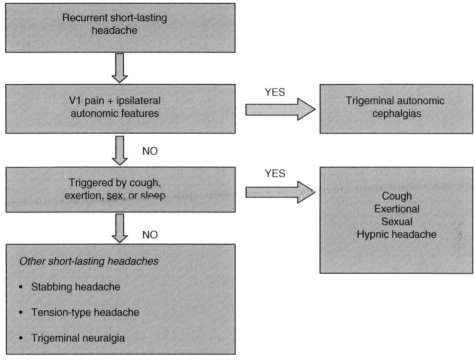

Fig. 39.5 Approach to short-duration headaches.

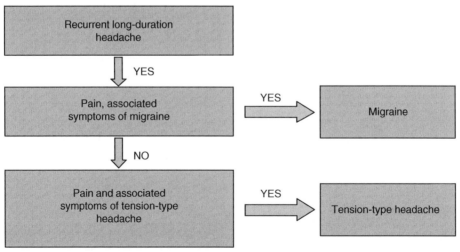

Fig. 39.6 Approach to long-duration recurrent headaches.

accompanied by nausea, though just one of photo- or phonophobia does not exclude the diagnosis. Migraine attacks may be unilateral and throbbing, and are usually moderate or severe and aggravated by physical activity. More important, in contrast to TTH, migraine sufferers have at least one of the following: nausea or vomiting; photophobia and phonophobia.

Headaches of long duration and high frequency (Fig. 39.7)

High-frequency headaches of long duration include chronic migraine (1.5.1), chronic TTH (2.3), new daily-persistent headache (4.8), and hemicrania continua (4.7).

Abrupt transition from no headache to daily headaches suggests a diagnosis of new daily-persistent headache. More than 15 days of migraine per month indicates chronic migraine, while more than 15 days of tension-type headache per month

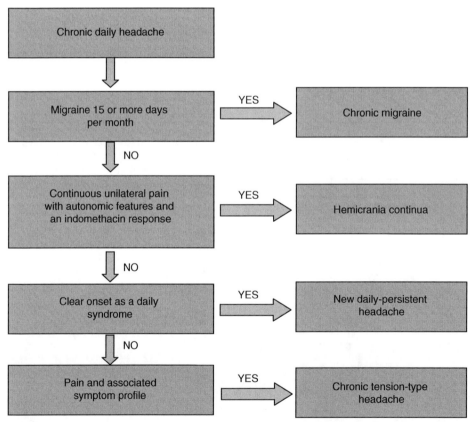

Fig. 39.7 Approach to long-duration chronic daily headaches.

suggests CTTH. In a patient with more than 15 TTH per month with some migraine attacks superimposed, the ICHD-2 would recommend diagnosing both CTTH and migraine. Alternatively, the diagnosis of transformed migraine would be applied by several clinicians, an entity not recognized by the ICHD-2. Finally, if there is continuous unilateral pain with occasional exacerbations eventually associated with autonomic features, a diagnosis of hemicrania continua (4.7) may be established.

The approach to differential diagnosis and the precise criteria for each disorder are presented elsewhere. We hope that these algorithms help neurologists and clinicians generate useful differential diagnoses based on ICHD-2.

Suggested Reading

1. Ameri A, Bousser MG. Cerebral venous thrombosis. *Neurol Clin* 1992; **10**: 87–111.
2. Bassi P, Bandera R, Loiero M, *et al*. Warning signs in subarachnoid hemorrhage: a cooperative study. *Acta Neurol Scand* 1991; **84**: 277–81.
3. Bigal ME, Lipton RB, Cohen J, *et al*. Epilepsy and migraine. *Epilepsy Behav* 2003 Oct; **4** (Suppl 2): 13–24.
4. Bigal ME, Rapoport AM, Lipton RB, *et al*. Chronic daily headache in a tertiary care population. Correlation between The International Headache Society Diagnostic Criteria and Proposed Revisions of Criteria for Chronic Daily Headache. *Cephalalgia* 2002; **22**: 432–8.
5. Calandre L, Hernandez-Lain A, Lopez-Valdes E. Benign Valsalva's maneuver-related headache: an MRI study of six cases. *Headache* 1996; **36**: 251–3.
6. Dodick DW, Brown RD, Britton JW, *et al*. Nonaneurysmal thunderclap headache with diffuse, multifocal, segmental and reversible vasospasm. *Cephalalgia* 1999; **19**: 118–23.
7. Dodick DW, Wijdicks EF. Pituitary apoplexy presenting as a thunderclap headache. *Neurology* 1998; **50**: 510–11.
8. Evans MI, Krivchenia EL. Principles of screening. *Clin Perinatol* 2001; **28**: 273–8.
9. Evers S, Wibbeke B, Reichelt D, *et al*. The impact of HIV infection on primary headache. Unexpected findings from retrospective, cross-sectional, and prospective analyses. *Pain* 2000; **85**: 191–200.
10. Forsyth PA, Posner JB. Headaches in patients with brain tumours: a study of 111 patients. *Neurology* 1993; **43**: 1678–83.
11. Garg RK. Recurrent thunderclap headache associated with reversible vasospasm causing stroke. *Cephalalgia* 2001; **21**: 78–9.
12. Headache Classification Committee of the International Headache Society. Classification and diagnostic criteria for headache disorders, cranial neuralgias and facial pain. *Cephalalgia* 1988; **8** (Suppl 7): 1–96.
13. Headache Classification Committee of the International Headache Society. The International Classification of Headache Disorders. *Cephalalgia* 2004; **24**: 1–160.
14. Landtblom AM, Fridriksson S, Boivie J, *et al*. Sudden onset headache: a prospective study of features incidence and causes. *Cephalalgia* 2002; **22**: 354–60.
15. Linet MS, Celentano DD, Stewart WF. Headache characteristics associated with physician consultation: a population-based survey. *Am J Prev Med* 1991; **7**: 40–6.
16. Linn FHH, Wijdicks EFM. Causes and management of thunderclap headache: a comprehensive review. *The Neurologist* 2002; **8**: 279–89.
17. Lipton RB, Amatniek JC, Ferrari MD, *et al*. Migraine. Identifying and removing barriers to care. *Neurology*. 1994; **44** (Suppl 4): 63–8.
18. Lipton RB, Dodick D, Sadovsky R, *et al*. A self-administered screener for migraine in primary care: The ID Migraine (TM) validation study. *Neurology* 2003 Aug 12; **61** (3): 375–82.

19. Lipton RB, Lowenkopf T, Bajwa ZH, *et al.* Cardiac cephalgia: a treatable form of exertional headache. *Neurology* 1997; **49**: 813–6.
20. Lipton RB, Stewart WF, Simon D. Medical consultation for migraine: results from the American Migraine Study. *Headache* 1998; **38**: 87–96.
21. Maizels M, Saenz V, Wirjo J. Impact of a group-based model of disease management for headache. *Headache* 2003 Jun; **43** (6): 621–7.
22. Mathew NT. Transformed or evolutional migraine. *Headache* 1987; **27**: 305–6.
23. Scelsa SN, Lipton RB, Sander H, *et al.* Headache characteristics in hospitalized patients with Lyme disease. *Headache* 1995; **35**: 125–30.
24. Silberstein SD, Lipton RB, Dalessio DJ. Overview, diagnosis and classification of headache. In: *Wolff's headache and other facial pain* (eds Silberstein SD, Lipton RB, Dalessio DJ). New York, Oxford, 2001: 6–26.
25. Silberstein SD. Practice parameter—evidence-based guidelines for migraine headache (an evidence-based review): Report of the Quality Standards Subcommittee of the American Academy of Neurology for the United States Headache Consortium. *Neurology* 2000; **55**: 754–62.
26. Weiss NS. Application of the case-control method in the evaluation of screening. *Epidemiol Rev* 1994; **16**: 102–8.
27. Woolf SH, Di Guiseppi CG, Atkins D, *et al.* Developing evidence-based clinical practice guidelines: lessons learned by the US Preventive Services Task Force. *Annu Rev Public Health.* 1996; **17**: 511–38.

40 National and international action plans for improving headache diagnosis

T. J. Steiner

Headache disorders are ubiquitous, common, and disabling. Migraine alone, according to the World Health Organization (WHO), is nineteenth in the list of all causes of years of healthy life lost to disability (YLDs).[1] There are huge consequential financial costs.[2,3]

Effective healthcare can alleviate much of this illness burden. The problem is that it depends not only on the existence of efficacious therapies, which we have, but also on the allocation of healthcare resources to deliver them to those who need them. There is good evidence that this need is not well met. A consensus conference in 1998[4] concluded that migraine – the best-recognized headache disorder – is under-diagnosed and under-treated throughout the world.

This paper concentrates on under-diagnosis as perhaps the single most important factor in under-treatment. Improving headache diagnosis is the essential first step to closing the large gaps between the healthcare that is provided for headache and what is needed.

ICHD-II

My starting premiss is that The International Classification of Headache Disorders, 2nd edition (ICHD-II),[5] perfect or not, sets out the best diagnostic criteria we have. It is the product of working groups whose members are experts from all over the world, who have brought together, over years, all the evidence known in the world, and who have filled the gaps in this evidence with their immeasurable experience. My secondary premiss, and the conclusion of the syllogism, is that the best must be used everywhere and that, therefore, these criteria must be used everywhere if the diagnosis of headache disorders is to be made accurately throughout the world as the necessary basis of effective treatment. Furthermore, if this is true in secondary (specialist) care, it must be true in primary care also.

So, at least in part, actions to improve the diagnosis of headache – wherever they are put into effect – must encompass the promotion of ICHD-II. When ICHD-II is scrutinized with this object in mind, problems do become apparent. ICHD-II will, inevitably, be found to contain faults and errors arising from incomplete knowledge. It incorporates a number of compromises made necessary in the quest for consensus, some of which satisfy nobody. And it depends from time to time on somewhat arbitrary criteria. All of these, taken together, arguably render ICHD-II suboptimal as the basis for international standardization.[6]

We can accept that ICHD-II is imperfect without losing sight of its qualities, and without letting opportunity of acting 'pass away before we [can] free ourselves of doubt'.[7] Not only is it the best we have, but it is the best we are likely to have for some time. I intend, for this paper, to acknowledge these issues and, whilst not dismissing them, set them aside. Instead I will consider others that we may reasonably do something about.

The PCP in Peru

The challenge may be expressed as follows: *if* ICHD-II sets out the diagnostic criteria that *must* be used in the clinic because they are the best, how do we get it into the routine clinical practice of the primary care physician in Peru?

Peru came into my mind for no better reason than alliteration. When it did, the primary care physician (PCP) in Peru seemed to perfectly encapsulate the realities of this challenge. I shall refer to the PCP in Peru as the notional target of proposed action plans throughout this paper.

Dismantling barriers

ICHD-II occupies 160 pages to cover thirteen categories of headache disorder. They include, depending upon exactly what is considered to be a diagnostic entity, some 200 of them. They are described in English, and the classification is published in a specialist journal. It is fair to say that these aspects of ICHD-II erect substantial barriers to its use by the PCP in Peru as an instrument that might improve his diagnosis of headache disorders.

How might these be dismantled?

First, ICHD-II needs translating. Some 20 languages were achieved for the first edition but worldwide usage depends on availability in many, many more. The key agencies, the International Headache Society (IHS) and World Headache Alliance (WHA) in particular, need to prioritize languages by their usage, and then support the member national societies of IHS to do the work. However, if the task of translation is left wholly to national societies, there will be no penetration wherever there is no society, which is most of the world. IHS needs also to work with other agencies, such as the pharmaceutical industry and WHO, both of whom have an interest in seeing this done.

Second, ICHD-II needs distributing. Successful and widespread distribution requires more money and better networks than IHS commands. Again there is need to prioritize regions and work with national societies, and again the pharmaceutical industry can help and should wish to, given that they have good distribution networks in many countries. It is also possible to use the Global Campaign[8] (more about which is discussed later) as it develops regional initiatives.

Third, ICHD-II needs simplifying. It has far, far too many entities for the practising physician because, of course, it is serving the purposes of everybody. Even specialists will not use most of the diagnostic categories in daily practice which still need to be classified. Unfortunately for the nonspecialist, and particularly the PCP in Peru, ICHD-II gives no prominence to those that are common or important. In addition, as a diagnostic aid it works backwards!

I believe the IHS classification subcommittee needs to prepare a 'core version' of ICHD-II, to which national or regional groups can add according to local variation. For example, Box 40.1 lists a set of nine diagnostic entities, all of them primary headache disorders. In the Western world at least, if every PCP becomes familiar with and can correctly diagnose each of these, the lives of their headache patients will be transformed.

Box 40.2 contains another set of eleven headaches, nine secondary and two neuralgias, making twenty in all. If PCPs master these as well, they will probably have done all that they should. The reason for this is that the law of diminishing returns always applies to improvements in doctors' clinical skills: the marginal benefit to patients is large with the first unit of improvement but falls off rapidly with each further unit thereafter (Fig. 40.1).

I need to explain what is meant by 'working backwards'. It is the thinking behind the *Reader's Digest Reverse Dictionary*.[9]

The PCP, in Peru or elsewhere, is not given the diagnosis of which he can then check the features in ICHD-II; what he is given is a presenting complaint, as in Box 40.3. There is no way, except through familiarity with it, that ICHD-II will lead the PCP from this presenting complaint to the correct diagnoses (which are 2.2 *Frequent*

Box 40.1   Core set of nine primary headache disorders

1.1 Migraine without aura
1.2 Migraine with aura

    1.2.1 Typical aura with migraine headache
    1.2.3 Typical aura without headache

2.1 Infrequent episodic tension-type headache
2.2 Frequent episodic tension-type headache
2.3 Chronic tension-type headache

    3.1.1 Episodic cluster headache
    3.1.2 Chronic cluster headache

Box 40.2 Core set of nine secondary headache disorders and two cranial neuralgias

5.2.1 Chronic posttraumatic headache attributed to moderate or severe head injury
6.4.1 Headache attributed to giant cell arteritis
7.1.1 Headache attributed to idiopathic intracranial hypertension
7.4.1 Headache attributed to increased intracranial pressure or hydrocephalus caused by neoplasm
7.4.2 Headache attributed directly to neoplasm
8.1.3 Carbon monoxide-induced headache
8.2 Medication-overuse headache
8.4.3 Oestrogen-withdrawal headache
11.2.1 Cervicogenic headache
13.1.1 Classical trigeminal neuralgia
13.8 Occipital neuralgia

episodic tension-type headache giving way to 2.3 *Chronic tension-type headache*—the history of cancer has no temporal relationship).

Simplification therefore means reversing the manner of use: in other words, developing ICHD-II-based diagnostic pathways or algorithms. This seems to me something of a priority if ICHD-II is to reach the PCP anywhere, let alone in Peru. Should these be computerized? They can be once developed, but I do not think they

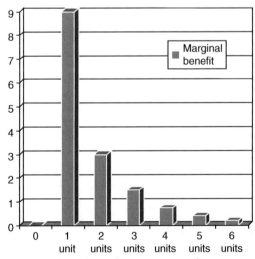

Fig. 40.1 Expected marginal benefit to patients from improving doctors' skills (arbitrary units).

Box 40.3 A presenting complaint of headache

- Female, 55 years old
- Two-year history of moderate generalized headache in episodes, initially monthly on average but occurring with increasing frequency, with phonophobia but no other associated symptoms
- Continuous headache for the last 4 months with occasional mild nausea rather than phonophobia
- Breast cancer 5 years ago, treated with mastectomy, radiotherapy, and tamoxifen
- Physical examination otherwise normal

---

should be developed so they can only run on computers. The crucial message for IHS has to be: *Always keep in mind the primary care physician in Peru.*

Stepping back — and forward

Let me take a step back from ICHD-II. National and international action plans for improving headache diagnosis must acknowledge three prerequisites for accurate diagnosis:

- the patient must recognize that a medical problem exists, and present to the doctor;
- the doctor must recognize that a medical problem exists, and listen to the patient;
- the doctor must have the knowledge and skill to diagnose.

ICHD-II addresses only the third of these, and only in a limited way. A much broader set of activities is required to tackle the first two and the remainder of the third. Essentially, this calls for global delivery of education. This is the realm of the Global Campaign referred to earlier.

The three major nongovernmental international headache organizations, WHA, HIS, and the European Headache Federation (EHF), believe that through a formal collaboration with WHO, harnessing its experience, know-how, contacts, and resources, they can open doors, address problems, and propose and test potential solutions in parts of the world that cannot otherwise be reached. Joint action by these four groups will take the form of a Global Campaign formally entitled *Reducing the Burden of Headache Worldwide* but branded more simply as *Lifting The Burden.*[10]

Partnership in action

Ultimately the Campaign entails setting priorities and finding, region by region, effective and affordable solutions to the headache problem as it exists locally, achievable with locally available resources, and within a defined term. The Campaign's central pillar is that the healthcare solution for headache in most areas of the world will be *education*. This should begin with awareness of headache as a medical problem and extend to correct recognition and diagnosis and the principles of management and avoidance of mismanagement of the common headache disorders.

The Campaign will proceed in three phases. The first of these is to know the size of the headache problem in all regions of the world. WHO calls this 'information for better decisions',[11] and it will be achieved by bringing out all of the available worldwide evidence of the burdens attributable to headache and by setting up studies where the evidence is lacking or of poor quality. The second is to exploit this evidence, using it to persuade others that headache manifestly should have higher priority for treatment. These others will include healthcare providers, people directly affected by headache, and the general population. They will also include governments and other health service policy makers with influence over change.

The third is proof of concept, through what WHO calls 'demonstrational projects'. The Campaign will set priorities, not simply identifying the countries or communities with greatest need but having sensible regard for where action can achieve results. It will work with local policy makers and other key stakeholders to plan and implement healthcare services for headache that are appropriate to local systems, resources, and locally-assessed needs. Within these projects, better diagnosis and better care will be fostered again through education. They will be paid for through more efficient use of resources, avoidance of wastage in mismanagement, and reductions in consequential financial costs.

All of this will have to be proved on the ground in each project. This will mean measuring the effect of change in terms of reduced headache burden in the population, and the costs before and after – a challenge in itself.

Conclusions

Better classification of headache disorders enables better description of them, better understanding of them, and better diagnosis of them – all prerequisites for better management of a set of disabling neurological disorders. ICHD-II is one support in a scaffold upon which national and international action plans for improving headache diagnosis can be and are being erected. It requires adaptation for some purposes, but it is adaptable.

The Global Campaign is a ready vehicle for many of these plans.

References

1. World Health Organization. *The World Health Report 2001*. WHO, Geneva.
2. Fishman P, Black L. Indirect costs of migraine in a managed care population. *Cephalalgia* 1999; **19**: 50–57.

3. Steiner TJ, Scher AI, Stewart WF, *et al.* The prevalence and disability burden of adult migraine in England and their relationships to age, gender and ethnicity. *Cephalalgia* 2003; **23**: 519–27.
4. American Association for the Study of Headache, International Headache Society. Consensus statement on improving migraine management. *Headache* 1998; **38**: 736.
5. International Headache Society Classification Subcommittee. The International Classification of Headache Disorders, 2nd edition. *Cephalalgia* 2004; **24** (Suppl 1): 1–160.
6. Gupta VK. Bureaucratisation of migraine. *Lancet Neurol* 2004; **3**: 396.
7. Descartes R. Principles of human knowledge. In: *The meditations and selections from the principles* (ed. Transl Veitch J) repr 1988. Open Court, Illinois, 1991: 130.
8. Steiner TJ. Lifting the burden: the global campaign against headache. *Lancet Neurol* 2004; **3**: 204–5.
9. The Reader's Digest Association Ltd. *Reader's digest reverse dictionary*. Reader's Digest, London 1989.
10. Lifting The Burden, at www.liftingtheburden.org (or www.l-t-b.org).
11. World Health Organization. *Mental health global action programme (mhGAP)*. WHO, Geneva 2002.

41
ICHD classification research

M. B. First

The first edition of the International Classification of Headaches was established in order to introduce needed precision in the definition of the various types of headaches by assuring 'reasonably low inter-observer diagnostic variability'. (Introduction to Classification and Diagnostic Criteria for Headache Disorders, Cranial Neuralgias, and Facial Pain, 1988, p 10). By a number of measures, the first edition of the IHS Classification has been quite successful: (1) the use of these criteria in articles is virtually mandatory for acceptance in international journals; (2) the great majority of evidence-based treatments for headache were developed using the first edition of the classification; (3) the principles of the classification have altered clinical practice (e.g. new criteria such as aggravation of headaches by physical activity are being put to use in daily practice); and (4) the classification has been translated into 20 different languages. However, despite evidence for its widespread use in headache research (a Medline search looking for 'IHS' yielded over 780 articles), only a relatively handful (around 30) consisted of research focused on the classification itself.

In the Preface to the second edition of the International Classification of Headache Disorders (ICHD-2), Olesen asks for 'the headache community at large and headache researchers in particular [to] support the use of the ICHD-2'. (Preface, International Classification of Headache Disorders, Second Edition, 2004, p 9). An important factor contributing to the support of a classification by its intended user base is the development of evidence documenting its reliability, its validity, and its clinical utility. Certainly one of the most important factors facilitating the widespread acceptance of the Diagnostic and Statistical Manual of Mental Disorders, Third Edition (DSM-III), the first medical classification to adopt diagnostic criteria, was the results of its general field trials indicating improved reliability as compared to earlier editions of the DSM that did not employ diagnostic criteria.[1] This chapter describes the type of studies on the classification itself that is likely to be useful both in eliciting support for the classification by the research and clinical communities as well as generating data that will help lay the groundwork for the next iteration of the headache classification.

Classification research focusing on diagnostic reliability

The reliability of the headache classification is the extent to which users can agree on headache diagnoses when applied to subjects with headache presentations. Although an invalid classification can be used reliably, the validity of a classification is limited by the extent that it can be used reliably, i.e. if a system is totally lacking in reliability, it cannot be used validly. However, if reliability is only fair (as it often is in diagnostic classifications), there can be some validity but that validity is limited.

Typically a headache diagnosis is made by a clinician after interviewing the patient, doing a physical examination and obtaining routine laboratory tests, reviewing chart notes and old records, and sometimes speaking to other informants. The reliability of the headache classification can be determined by having two or more clinicians examine a series of cases and independently make diagnostic judgments. It is important to understand that there are many possible components that can contribute to reliability problems, technically referred to sources of variance.

Information variance

This source of unreliability occurs when clinicians base their diagnoses on different sets of information. For example, a patient may report to one clinician that he has never had any migraines preceded by an aura, whereas when discussing his symptoms with a second clinician, he remembers having had several migraines associated with an aura, thus resulting in a diagnostic disagreement between the two clinicians (i.e. migraine without aura vs. typical aura with migraine headaches). It should be noted that information variance is not only caused by patients changing their stories over time. Sometimes patients provide different clinical information because of differences in interviewing techniques. For example, perhaps the first clinician above simply asked the patient if the headache was preceded by an aura without adequately explaining to the patient what he meant by aura. Whereas the second clinician went into a lengthy description of an aura, providing different examples, one of which resonated with the patient.

Interpretation variance

This source of unreliability occurs when clinicians are presented with the same clinical information but interpret its significance differently. For example, many criteria sets include a requirement for a certain level of pain intensity (e.g. migraine require the pain to be moderate to severe, whereas tension headaches are required to be of mild to moderate severity). In order to decide whether or not this criterion is met, clinicians must listen to the patient's description of his or her headache pain and then interpret from this description whether the intensity of the pain is mild, moderate, or severe. If one clinician interprets the pain to be of 'moderate' severity and the other interprets the same description to be of 'mild' severity, then a diagnostic disagreement could result.

Criterion variance

This source of unreliability results from two clinicians using two different sets of criteria (or in the absence of operationalized criteria, two different definitions of headache type). For example, two clinicians making headache diagnoses using the two different editions of the International Classification of Headache Disorders could end up with different diagnoses by virtue of their relying on different definitions for the headaches.

Occasion variance

This results from true changes in clinical status that may occur over time, presenting the two evaluators with different clinician presentations. Occasion variance does not contribute to unreliability since it does not represent diagnostic disagreement but true change.

By providing very specific operationalized criteria, the ICHD-II is likely to improve diagnostic disagreement by reducing both criterion variance and interpretation variance. Criterion variance is reduced by providing physicians and researchers with a widely available set of operationalized definitions. As long as physicians use these definitions to guide their headache diagnoses (as opposed to their own potentially idiosyncratic definitions of the various types of headache), diagnostic agreement is likely to improve. The ICHD-II classification also reduces interpretation variance in a number of ways. First of all, the IHS definitions have been designed to be very precise in their specification of required headache frequencies, durations, and symptom counts. This is in contrast with the previous headache classification, namely classification of the Ad Hoc Committee of the National Institute of Health which used terms such as 'commonly', 'often', and 'frequently', all of which required much more clinical judgment in interpreting what was intended. Furthermore, the ICHD-II provides additional notes and comments alongside the diagnostic criteria to further clarify the intention of the diagnostic criteria. Although the ICHD-II definitions will have less impact on information variance (since this mostly reflects discrepancies in the available information used by the clinician), the ICHD-II may indirectly have an impact by increasing the likelihood that the assessment procedure itself is standardized (e.g. via the development of structured interviews[2] and computerized structured records[3]). These structured assessment procedures, based on the IHS criteria, reduce information variance by insuring that clinical information about the patients is gathered in a more uniform way.

Empirical studies designed to determine diagnostic reliability have three potential goals: (1) to establish improved reliability of diagnoses using operationalized definitions as compared to diagnoses made without using IHS criteria (i.e. 'practice-as-usual'); (2) to establish levels of achievable reliability and to compare reliability across the different parts of the classification; and (3) to identify specific problematic criteria responsible for poor reliability with the goal of guiding future revisions. As noted above, a crucial factor in the widespread acceptance of the DSM-III was the establishment of adequate system-wide reliability.[1] In subsequent editions of the DSM, data reanalyses and field trials comparing the reliability of specific criteria sets were used to determine which among the alternative sets of criteria should be adopted. (See example in ref. [4].)

There are two basic designs for reliability studies: *joint reliability* and *test–retest reliability*. In studies using a joint reliability design, different raters each apply the diagnostic criteria to the same clinical information and their resulting diagnoses are compared. The clinical evaluation can be done live in a group setting (in which one rater conducts the clinical assessment while the other raters observe and optionally ask questions) or a group of raters can make diagnoses based on videotaped evaluations, chart material, or case vignettes. Studies determining test–retest reliability involve two (or more) completely independent evaluations of the patient on two different occasions. When designing a test–retest reliability study, it is important that the interval between evaluations be sufficiently long so that the results of the second evaluation are not unduly influenced by the patient's memory of the first evaluation but not so long as to have the disease course change (e.g. the number of headaches occurring during the interval since the first evaluation could legitimately result in a different diagnosis for the second evaluation).

Joint reliability studies are much more commonly carried out because of their lower cost – only one clinical evaluation per patient is required as compared to two or more for a test–retest design. However, test–retest designs are generally considered to be a more rigorous test of reliability because they are more closely approximate to the real-life application of the diagnostic criteria in clinical settings. It should be noted that reliability assessed using a test–retest design is typically lower than that obtained using a joint design because the joint design eliminates information variance (since all raters are by design presented with the identical set of clinical information). Therefore, when comparing results of reliability studies, it is important to note whether the statistics were collected using a test–retest vs. joint design.

There have been several reliability studies of the IHS criteria, some examining general reliability of headache diagnoses on consecutive series of patients,[2,5,6] and others focusing on a particular diagnosis (for example see ref. [7]). Although reasonably good reliability has been demonstrated (e.g. with kappas ranging from 0.65 to 1.0), all of the studies used a joint reliability design and the three studies that focused on consecutive patients used chart material or videotaped case material, rather than 'live' patients.

Classification research focusing on diagnostic validity

While improving the reliability of the diagnosis of headache is an important and necessary goal, the ultimate goal of a classification is to be *valid*, i.e. ideally that the concepts and categories embodied in the classification reflect the true state of nature. Unfortunately, our current understanding of the etiology and pathophysiology of headache leaves us with a lack of any gold standard for the diagnosis of headache.

In the absence of a gold standard for determining whether a patient's headache diagnosis is 'correct', what standard should be used for setting the diagnostic thresholds that are a necessary component of operationalized criteria? For example, many criteria sets consist of lists of symptoms in which some subset is required (e.g. 2 out of a list of 6 symptoms), or set a minimum requirement for the number of headaches or their duration.

Several alternatives to a gold standard are available when trying to develop criteria sets that are maximally valid. One method employed in the development of criteria sets for the DSMs is to use clinical diagnosis as standard, setting diagnostic thresholds in order to best replicate the clinician's judgment of whether or not a particular diagnosis is present. For example, the diagnosis of migraine requires that at least two out of a list of four characteristic qualities be present (e.g. unilateral location, pulsating quality, moderate or severe pain intensity, and aggravation by or avoidance of physical activity). The diagnostic threshold (which in the IHS criteria was set as a result of expert consensus) could be empirically set by determining which number of symptoms best corresponds with an independently assigned clinical diagnosis of migraine.

Another alternative is to maximize agreement with an external validator, that is an associated feature of the headache diagnosis that is extrinsic to the operationalized definition itself. Examples of external validators include treatment response, level of disability, correlation with biological markers, family history, and future course. For example, to increase the validity of the distinction between migraine and tension-type headaches, one could set the parameters in the definition of migraine to maximize treatment response to those medications known to preferentially treat migraine vs. tension-type headaches.

Classification research focusing on clinical utility

The clinical utility of a classification is the extent to which the classification assists clinical decision makers in fulfilling the various functions of a classification.[8] These functions include assisting clinicians in conceptualizing diagnostic entities, communicating clinical information, utilizing categories in clinical practice (e.g. for differential diagnosis), choosing effective interventions to improve clinical outcomes, and predicting future clinical management needs. Classification research can examine the extent to which each of these goals is being realized by examining usage issues, the impact of the classification on clinical decision making, and its impact on clinical outcomes.

Empirical research into usage can focus on the extent to which the classification is being used by its target populations (i.e. headache specialists, neurologists, and general practitioners) and the extent to which it meets the needs of the target population. This can be measured by administering surveys assessing usage and user acceptability, reviewing clinical records to determine the extent to which the classification is being applied to the diagnostic process, and conducting field trials in which users are asked to apply the operationalized criteria to cases and then evaluate its acceptability (e.g. ease of use, goodness of fit). Two surveys of headache specialists were conducted to assess their usage of IHS criteria. One survey[9] asked the specialists to review four case vignettes of headache patients and to assign a diagnosis, and were also asked to rank IHS criteria along with other features commonly used in the diagnosis of headache in order of importance. They found that the specialists often diagnosed the cases incorrectly (e.g. only 14.7% of respondents correctly diagnosed the migraine case) and that there was no difference in ranked importance for the IHS criteria as compared with the non-IHS criteria. The second survey[10] also asked members of the American Headache Society to rate the importance of IHS and non-IHS diagnostic criteria, and indicated that one-third of the respondents use additional non-IHS criteria and de-emphasizes certain IHS criteria.

Impact on clinical decision making and on clinical outcomes can be measured by determining whether clinicians are more likely to make 'correct' treatment decisions (according to established practice guidelines) if the classification is used (as compared to diagnostic assessments made without using the IHS definitions). Similarly, specific outcome variables (e.g. reduction in headache frequency, severity, disability) can be assessed by comparing the outcomes of patients diagnosed using the ICHD-II to 'treatment-as-usual' (i.e. not using the ICHD-II).

Conclusions

Now that the ICHD-II is available, research is needed that focuses on aspects of the classification itself, including reliability, validity, and clinical utility. Although the IHS classification has been widely embraced by the research community, surveys indicate that a substantial proportion of clinicians continue to use non-IHS criteria in clinical practice. Although there are many possible reasons for this, research establishing the reliability, validity, and clinical utility of the ICHD-II may encourage wider acceptance in the clinical community.

References

1. Spitzer R, Forman J, Nee J. DSM-III field trials: I. Initial interrater diagnostic reliability. *Am J Psychiatry* 1979; **136**: 815–17.
2. Granella F, D'Alessandro R, Manzoni G, *et al*. International Headache Society Classification: interobserver reliabiltiy in the diagnosis of primary headaches. *Cephalalgia* 1994; **14** (1): 3–4.
3. Gallai V, Sarchielli P, Alberti A, *et al*. Application of the 1988 International Headache Society diagnostic criteria in nine Italian headache centers using a computerized structured record. *Headache* 2002; **42** (10): 1016–24.
4. Widiger T, Cadoret R, Hare R, *et al*. DSM-IV antisocial personality disorder field trial. *J Abnorm Psychol* 1996; **105** (1): 3–16.
5. Wynkoop T, McCoy K, Dean R. Diagnostic agreement in the classification of headache using Ad Hoc Committee and IHS criteria. *Int J Neuroscience* 1996; **85** (3–4): 285–90.
6. Leone M, Filippini G, D'Amico D, *et al*. Assessment of International Headache Society diagnostic criteria: a reliability study. *Cephalalgia* 1994; **14** (4): 280–84.

7. van Suijekom J, de Vet H, van den Berg S, *et al*. Interobserver reliability of diagnostic criteria for cervicogenic headache. *Cephalalgia* 1999; **19** (9): 767–8.
8. First M, Pincus H, Levine J, *et al*. Using clinical utility as a criterion for revising psychiatric diagnoses. *Am J Psychiatry* 2004; **161** (6): 948–54.
9. Marcus D, Nash J, Turk D. Diagnosing recurring headaches: IHS criteria and beyond. *Headache* 1994; **34** (6): 329–36.
10. Nash J, Lipchik G, Holroyd K, *et al*. American Headache Society members' assessment of headache diagnostic criteria. *Headache* 2003; **43** (1): 2–13.

42
Application of ICHD 2nd edition criteria for primary headaches with the aid of a computerized, structured medical record: some considerations

P. Sarchielli, M. Pedini, A. Alberti, and G. Capocchi

Introduction

Diagnostic requirements for primary headaches in the new Classification System ICHD-II appear to be improved and certainly represent an evolution of the previous criteria included in the first edition of IHS Classification.[1,2] Modifications to the previous criteria are based on the clinical and pathophysiologic acquisitions of the last 15 years. Among the changes to migraine diagnostic requirements in the ICHD second edition, the most important one is the introduction of the diagnostic subtype of 1.5.1 *Chronic migraine* among the complications of migraine for those rare patients who fulfil the diagnostic criteria for migraine on 15 or more days a month for at least three months without overusing medications.

For tension-type headache, the terms 'infrequent' and 'frequent' tension-type headache were introduced in the new classification to indicate: episodic tension-type headache attacks occurring < 1 day per month (<12 days per year), and ≥1 day per month and <15 days per month for at least 3 months (≥12 days and <180 days per year), respectively. When the patient has an attack >15 days per month for at least a three-month period (>180 days per year), the diagnosis is the same as in the previous classification. The subdivision of tension-type headache attacks with or without the association with pericranial tenderness estimated on manual palpation has remained unchanged. Causal factors which defined the fourth digit of the old IHS Classification were instead eliminated.

In Group 3 *Cluster headache and other trigeminal autonomic cephalalgias*, paroxysmal hemicrania was subdivided into two groups: episodic paroxysmal hemicrania and chronic paroxysmal hemicrania. Short-lasting unilateral neuralgiform headache with conjunctival injection and tearing (SUNCT) was included in this group. Hemicrania continua was expected to be included in this group, for the presence of autonomic symptoms and responsiveness to indomethacin, but was moved to the other primary headache disorders group.

All the primary headache types in their episodic forms are defined as probable attacks fulfilling all but one of criteria A–D for 1.1 *Migraine without aura* (code: 1.6.1), *Migraine with aura* (new code 1.6.2), *Infrequent episodic tension-type headache* (code: 2.4.1), *Frequent episodic tension-type headache* (code: 2.4.2), and *Cluster headache* (3.1), respectively, in the case in which they are not attributed to another disorder.

For chronic migraine and chronic tension-type headache, the term probable is limited to the cases in which there is a concomitant medication overuse. In these cases, the default rule in the new classification is to classify both the probable chronic migraine or probable chronic tension-type headache and probable medication-overuse headache. When these criteria for chronic migraine are still fulfilled two months after medication-overuse withdrawal, the diagnosis of chronic migraine or chronic tension-type headache is accepted and that of probable medication over-use is discarded.

It is necessary and fundamental to verify the applicability of the new criteria in terms of sensitivity and specificity for transfer to the clinical practice.

In this regard, our research group, immediately after publication of the ICHD-II classification, developed a computerized, structured medical record based exclusively on the proposed new classification system for primary headaches. This computerized system examines all the diagnoses of primary headaches on the basis of the variables needed to fulfil their mandatory criteria. This is very difficult to obtain in particular cases without having the support of a computerized device.

Methods

The program, developed with the help of an expert (MP), is called 'IHS Diagnostic Criteria for Primary Headaches' version 2.0 ITA, and is strictly based on the ICHD-II operational diagnostic criteria for primary headaches. Details of the computerized record are reported in the paper 'Diagnostic Criteria for Primary Headaches of ICHD 2nd Edition 2004: Electronic Clinical Sheets ver. Int. W. 2.0®'

by Mauro Pedini, Andrea Alberti, Giovanni Mazzotta, Paola Sarchielli, published in this volume.

The clinical sheets relative to 200 consecutive patients attending our headache center in 2004 were examined and included all items needed to make a diagnosis of one of the primary headache disorders according to the new ICHD classification. Only trained clinicians recorded data on the clinical sheets, having worked for many years with patients affected by headache, and were well experienced, from a theoretical point of view, with the new ICHD-II criteria.

We tested the computerized structured record by entering and analysing all 200 of the above cases of primary headaches and the corresponding output diagnoses, with particular regard to the new entities introduced: diagnoses of probable migraine with and without aura, probable frequent and infrequent tension-type headache, chronic and probable chronic migraine, and finally, probable tension-type headache.

Results and discussion

The software was able to furnish a single diagnosis in 82% of the cases, while in 15% of these, the output diagnoses were multiple (up to 4), and in many cases were of 'probable forms'. In the remaining 3% of the cases, the diagnosis was 14.1 *Headache not elsewhere classified*, because they did not fit into any of the existing chapters of primary headaches and the headache was not attributable to another disorder. The introduction of 'probable subtypes' for the episodic and chronic forms necessitates, therefore, a careful reexamination of these definitions and will lead to suggestions for overcoming possible drawbacks in the diagnosis that, however, is ultimately entrusted to the clinician.

We present three examples for consideration regarding the mandatory criteria for the diagnosis of primary headaches. For each case, we will provide the input variables and output diagnoses, as well as the fulfilled mandatory criteria:

Case 1

Variables	
No. of previous attacks	>10
Days with headache/month	8
Period of observation	2 months
Duration of attacks	10 h
Pain location	Unilateral
Intensity of pain	Moderate
Quality of pain	Pressing
Aggravation by or causing avoidance of routine physical activity	No
Accompanying symptoms	Phonophobia
Increased tenderness of pericranial muscles	Yes
Exclusion of a secondary headache	Yes

The output diagnoses are:

Diagnoses	Diagnostic criteria		
	A	B	C
Probable frequent episodic tension-type headache 2.4.2	Episodes fulfilling all but one of criteria A–D for 2.2 *Frequent episodic tension-type headache*	Episodes do not fulfil criteria for 1.1 *Migraine without aura*	Not attributed to another disorder
Probable infrequent tension-type headache 2.4.1	Episodes fulfilling all but one of criteria A–D for 2.1 *Infrequent episodic tension-type headache*	Episodes do not fulfil criteria for 1.1 *Migraine without aura*	Not attributed to another disorder
Probable migraine without aura	Episodes fulfilling all but one of criteria A–D for 1.1 *Migraine without aura*	Not attributed to another disorder	

This case has three probable output diagnoses. From a clinical point of view, we assume the described cases should be coded as probable frequent episodic tension-type headache, because we have 8 days with headache/month with the characteristics of frequent episodic tension-type headache. However, the period of observation is only 2 months, so we could not exclude theoretically the criteria of probable infrequent tension-type headache, which are also fulfilled, because episodes satisfy all but one of the criteria A–D for '2.1 *Infrequent episodic tension-type headache.*'

The definition of probable infrequent tension-type headache implies, in fact, that if criterion A in all its components is not fulfilled including the frequency <1 day per month on average, which defines infrequent tension-type headache, we have also fulfilled all the mandatory criteria for the diagnosis of probable frequent headache.

To avoid this drawback, we propose changing the criteria for infrequent tension-type headache as follows:

A. Headache episode occurring on <1 day per month on average (<12 days per year) for a period of >3 months and lasting from 30 min to 7 days.
B. At least 10 episodes fulfilling criterion A.
C. Headache has at least two of the following characteristics:

    1. bilateral location
    2. pressing/tightening (nonpulsating) quality
    3. mild or moderate intensity

    4. not aggravated by routine physical activity such as walking or climbing stairs

D. both of the following:

    1. no nausea or vomiting (anorexia may occur)
    2. no more than one of phonophobia or photophobia

E. not attributed to another disorder

According to these modified criteria, the diagnosis of probable infrequent headache will be excluded. It will remain, therefore, the differential diagnosis between probable episodic tension-type headache and probable migraine without aura. This possibility is underscored in the comment to '2.4 *Probable tension-type headache*'. Patients meeting one of these sets of criteria may also meet the criteria for one of the subforms of '1.6 *Probable migraine*'. In such cases, all other available information should be used by the clinician to decide which of the alternatives is the more likely.

Another interesting example concerns a case of chronic daily headache, which evolved from a previous case of episodic migraine without aura and lost some of the characteristics of typical migraine attacks, including the occurrence and severity of accompanying symptoms.

This is reported here:

Case 2

Variables	
No. of previous attacks	> 10
Days with headache/month	23
Period of observation	> 3 months
Duration of attacks	4 h
Pain location	Bilateral
Intensity of pain	Severe
Quality of pain	Pulsating
Aggravation by or causing avoidance of routine physical activity	Yes
Accompanying symptoms	Phonophobia
Increased tenderness of pericranial muscles	No
Medication overuse	Yes
Exclusion of a secondary headache	Yes

The output diagnosis given by the software is:

	Diagnostic criteria	
Diagnosis	A	B
Probable migraine without aura 1.6.1	Episodes fulfilling all but one of criteria A–D for 1.1 *Migraine without aura*	Not attributed to another disorder

This is the only possible diagnosis with our software because all but one of criteria A–D are fulfilled for migraine without aura; specifically, criterion C, referring to accompanying symptoms, is not satisfied. No diagnostic item is available, in this specific case, to furnish information regarding its chronic state, although headache lasts 23 days/month and the period of observation is ≥3 months. The classification, in fact, rigorously states that, for giving the diagnosis of probable chronic migraine (probable because we have a medication overuse), all the mandatory criteria for migraine without aura have to be fulfilled.

This observation is not a rare occurrence in the clinical practice and should prompt reflection on the possible implications that the rigorous criteria for migraine without aura will have, in the near future, on studies concerning the classification of patients with chronic daily headache according to the new classification ICHD-II. This problem regarding the impossibility of classification also extends to chronic tension-type headache, which satisfies all but one of the ICHD-II criteria both in the presence and absence of medication-overuse. Even for chronic tension-type headache, it was not foreseen that one or more criteria may not be satisfied, and the definition of probable chronic tension-type headache is limited exclusively to the forms that fully satisfy all the criteria for chronic tension-type headache but for which there is simultaneous fulfilment of criterion B for any of the subforms of '8.2 Medication-overuse headache'.

As a last example, we bring to your attention another case of tension-type headache, which became more frequent in a period of observation of <3 months:

Case 3

Variables	
No. of previous attacks	38
Days with headache/month	19
Period of observation	2 months
Duration of attacks	1 h
Pain location	Bilateral
Intensity of pain	Moderate
Quality of pain	Pressing
Aggravation by or causing avoidance of routine physical activity	No
Accompanying symptoms	Phonophobia
Increased tenderness of pericranial muscles	No
Medication overuse	No
Exclusion of a secondary headache	Yes

Two output diagnoses given by the computerized system are surprisingly: probable infrequent tension-type headache and probable frequent tension-type headache because, for both forms, all but one (criterion A) of the diagnostic criteria are fulfilled and therefore what we stated for the previously reported Case 1 is also valid.

In reality, the diagnosis should be *Headache not elsewhere classified* 14.1, because the diagnosis for chronic tension-type headache cannot be given due to the lack of fulfilment of two of criteria A–D as better shown here:

	Diagnostic criteria for chronic tension-type headache				
Diagnosis Headache	A	B	C	D	E
not elsewhere classified 14.1	Headache occurring on ≥15 days per month on average for >3 months and fulfilling criteria B–D *This criterion is not fulfilled*	Headache lasts for hours or may be continuous *This criterion is not fulfilled*	Headache has at least two of the following charac- teristics: 1. Bilateral location 2. Pressing/ tightening 3. Mild or moderate intensity 4. Not aggravated by routine physical activity *This criterion is fulfilled*	Both of the following: 1. No more than one of photophobia, phonophobia, or mild nausea 2. Neither moderate or severe nausea nor vomiting *This criterion is fulfilled*	Not attributed to another disorder *This crite- rion is fulfilled*

The diagnosis of headache not elsewhere classified would result if modifications were made to the criteria for probable frequent and infrequent tension-type headache.

The same is also true when the period of observation is >3 months.

According to the actual ICHD-II classification, again, the two diagnoses of probable frequent and infrequent tension-type headache will be given by the computerized system, which will disappear if modifications of the criteria for both forms were made according to our suggestions.[3] In this case, again, headache not elsewhere classified will be the most appropriate because the lack of criteria specific for chronic tension-type headache fulfilling all but one of criteria A–D is not foreseen by the classification and the term probable is reserved for chronic tension-type headache, which satisfies all criteria for chronic tension-type headache in the presence of medication overuse.

The first test of the applicability of the new IHS criteria for primary headaches on 200 clinical charts from our headache center prompted us, in these last months, to validate the new diagnostic criteria with the aid of a computerized device. In the near future, we will examine a substantial number of clinical charts, possibly by a multicenter study, to clarify some of the points which emerged from the first validation, and to search for answers to those questions already raised and those yet to be proposed.

A debate on the above topics is urgently needed for all who are trying to apply the new diagnostic criteria, both in the clinical setting and in the research field. The comments, suggestions, or explanations provided by the experts who contributed to the elaboration of the ICHD-II classification will be invaluable.

References

1. Headache Classification Committee of the International Headache Society. Classification and diagnostic criteria for headache disorders, cranial neuralgias and facial pain. *Cephalalgia* 1988; **8** (Suppl 7): 1–96.
2. Headache Classification Subcommittee of the International Headache Society. The International Classification of Headache Disorders: 2nd edition. *Cephalalgia* 2004; **24** (Suppl 1): 9–160.
3. Gallai V, Sarchielli P, Alberti A, *et al*. ICHD 2nd Edition: Some considerations on the application of criteria for primary headaches. (In press in *Cephalalgia*) 2004.

43 French survey network on headaches and facial pains

M. Lantéri-Minet, A. Autret, G. Baudesson,
M. G. Bousser, C. Creach', A. Donnet, V. Dousset,
N. Fabre, G. Giraud, E. Guégan-Massardier, N. Guy,
C. Lucas, H. Massiou, G. Mick, M. Navez,
A. Pradalier, F. Radat, D. Valade, G. Géraud,
on behalf of the Société Française d'Etudes des
Migraines et Céphalées (SFEMC)

The Société Française d'Etudes des Migraines et Céphalées (SFEMC), i.e French Headache Society, sets up a survey network on headaches and facial pains based on International Headache Society diagnostic classification. We present the main purposes of the network, the methodology, the results after one year, and prospective for 2004.

Objectives

The main goals of the network are the following: (1) constitution of a French computerized database on headaches and facial pains using the International Headache Society diagnostic criteria and (2) development of a clinical research toll.

Methods

Initially the network covered nearly two-thirds of the French territory and involved thirteen French headache centers (Fig. 43.1): 12 in tertiary-care academic hospitals (Bordeaux, Clermont-Ferrand, Lille, Marseille, Nice, Paris Colombes, Paris Lariboisière with two centers, Rouen, Saint-Etienne, Toulouse, Tours) and one in a tertiary-care general hospital (Annecy). Centers are affiliated to different departments: neurology for seven centers, pain management for three centers,

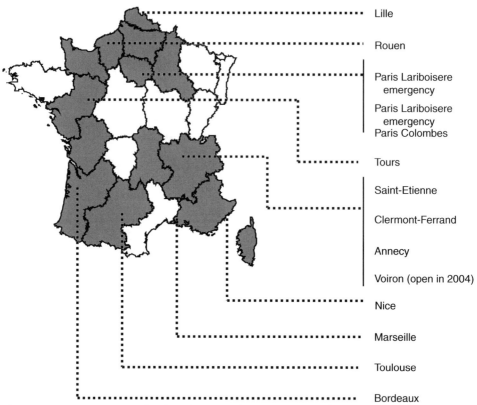

Fig. 43.1 Centers involved in the French survey network on headaches and facial pains (shaded areas: part of French territory covered by the network).

neurosurgery for one center, internal medicine for one center, and emergency for one center (Fig. 43.2).

The network is organized through common data capture software developed on behalf of the Société Française d'Etudes des Migraines et Céphalées. During the first phase (from which results are presented in this communication), the data capture software allowed the collection of socio-demographic data and diagnostic ones according to the International Headache Society classification. For the future, the software allows the capture of further data (see prospective). Paris Lariboisière I (Emergency Headache Center) includes all patients consulting for primary or secondary headache or facial pain in an emergency context. Other centers include all patients consulting in a programmed way for primary or secondary headache or facial pain. All data are then centralized on a national server via Internet.

	Care	Structure	Speciality	
Annecy	Tertiary	General hospital	Neurology	
Bordeaux	Tertiary	Academic hospital	Pain	
Clermont-Ferrand	Tertiary	Academic hospital	Neurology	
Lille	Tertiary	Academic hospital	Neurology	
Marseille	Tertiary	Academic hospital	Neurosurgery	
Nice	Tertiary	Academic hospital	Pain	
Paris Colombes	Tertiary	Academic hospital	Internal medicine	
Paris Lariboisière I	Tertiary	Academic hospital	Emergency	
Paris Lariboisière II	Tertiary	Academic hospital	Neurology	
Rouen	Tertiary	Academic hospital	Neurology	
Saint-Etienne	Tertiary	Academic hospital	Pain	
Toulouse	Tertiary	Academic hospital	Neurology	
Tours	Tertiary	Academic hospital	Neurology	
Voiron (open in 2004)	Primary	Network	Pain	

Fig. 43.2 Centers involved in the French survey on headaches and facial pains – care level, structure location, and speciality involved.

Results (from January 2003 to February 2004)

After set up from September to December 2002, 21 923 patients were included during the whole year 2003 and at the beginning of year 2004: 10 912 patients consulting in a programmed way and 11 011 patients in an emergency context (Fig. 43.3).

From January 2003 to February 2004, inclusion of patients was exhaustive for nine centers: Paris Lariboisère I (11 011 patients), Paris Lariboisère II (2626 patients), Toulouse (1425 patients), Marseille (1416 patients), Rouen (1377 patients), Nice (1184 patients), Saint-Etienne (825 patients), Paris Colombes (561 patients), and Annecy (321 patients). For initial technical difficulties (absence of compatibility with the hospital information processing system), the inclusion was not exhaustive in four centers: Lille (505), Bordeaux (260), Tours (249), and Clermont-Ferrand (163).

During the whole year of 2003, diagnostic data capture was done according to the first edition of the International Headache Society classification. From beginning of 2004, an updated version of the data capture software included the second edition of the International Headache Society classification and, in order to pool 2003 data, an algorithm allowing correspondence between first and second editions of the International Headache Society classification was developed. The development of such an algorithm was possible because the initial software allowed the capture of diagnoses not individualized in the first edition of International Headache Society like chronic migraine, triptan-overuse, short-lasting unilateral neuralgiform headache attacks with conjunctival injection and tearing (SUNCT) or hypnic headache. Nevertheless, not enough information was available by the initial software to allow the correspondence with the 13th diagnostic category (headache attributed to psychiatric disorder) of the revised classification.

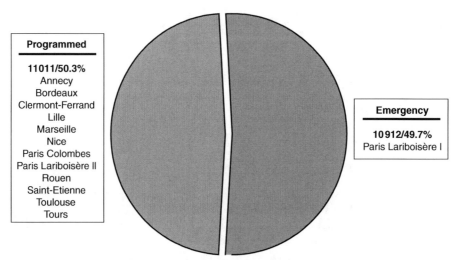

Fig. 43.3 Patients included from 01/2003 to 02/2004: patients consulting in a programmed way and patients consulting in an emergency context.

Diagnostic categories (IHS classification)	Number	%
1. Migraine	13050	59.5%
2. Tension-type headache	4486	20.5%
3. Trigeminol autonomic cephalalgias	1418	6.5%
4. Other primary headaches	358	1.6%
5. Head and/or neck trauma	327	1.5%
6. Cranialor cervical vascular disorders	325	1.5%
7. Non vascular intracranial disorders	357	1.6%
8. Substance or its withdrawal	1371	6.3%
9. Infection	202	0.9%
10. Disorders of homeostasis	82	0.4%
11. Disorders of cervical, facial, or cranial structures	672	3.1%
12. Psychiatric disorder	9	–
13. Neuralgias and central pains	658	3%
14. Unclassified headaches	151	0.7%

Fig. 43.4 Number and distribution of diagnostic categories according to IHS classification.

Diagnostic categories (IHS classification)	Number	%
1. Migraine	59.5%	44.1%
2. Tension-type headache	20.5%	23.9%
3. Trigeminoal autonomic cephalalgias	6.5%	7%
4. Other primary headaches	1.6%	1.5%
5. Head and/or neck trauma	1.5%	1.8%
6. Cranialor cervical vascular disorders	1.5%	1.3%
7. Non vascular intracranial disorders	1.6%	2.1%
8. Substance or its withdrawal	6.3%	1.7%
9. Infection	0.9%	1.7%
10. Disorders of homeostasis	0.4%	0.4%
11. Disorders of cervical, facial, or cranial structures	3.1%	4.0%
12. Psychiatric disorder	–	–
13. Neuralgias and central pains	3%	2.3%
14. Unclassified headaches	0.7%	1.2%

Fig. 43.5 Distribution of diagnostic categories according to IHS classification/all patients vs patients consulting in an emergency context.

Diagnostic categories for the patients included in the network are reported in Fig. 43.4. The majority were migraine (13 050/21 923 – 59.2%), tension-type headache (4486/21 923 – 20.4%), trigeminal autonomic cephalalgias (1418/21 923 – 6.5%) and headaches associated with substances or their withdrawal (1371/21 923 – 6.3%). Headache was unclassified in 151 patients (0.7%). Distribution of diagnostic categories was slightly different if only patients included following consulting in an emergency context were considered (Fig. 43.5).

It is interesting to consider the total number of patients suffering from rare diagnostic primary entities which were included in the network: 23 patients with SUNCT (code 3.3), 50 patients with a primary headache associated with sexual activity (code 4.4), 21 patients with hypnic headache (code IHS 4.6), and 55 patients with hemicrania continua (code 4.7).

Prospective (Year 2004)

The updated software allows the systematic collection of both psychiatric comorbidity through the HAD scale and functional impact through the HIT-6 scale.

An additional center (Voiron) joined the network, hence enlarging the survey on primary care since this center is itself organized as a regional network coordinating headache specialists with about 300 general practitioners for the optimization of the follow-up.

Finally, the use of this information as a clinical research tool will begin with the setting up online of a multicentric clinical study in an attempt to define the clinical typologies of the medication-overuse headaches, as individualized in the second edition of the International Headache Society Classification.

Conclusion

After a first year of effective development, such a network appears possible and allows the constitution of a national computerized data base being able to optimize French clinical research on headaches and facial pains.

Acknowledgment

This network was led with the financial support of GlaxoSmithKline.

44
ID Migraine™: validation and use of a three-item, self-administered questionnaire to identify migraine sufferers in a primary care population

R. B. Lipton, D. Dodick, K. Kolodner,
and J. Hettiarachchi

Introduction

Although migraine is one of the leading reasons for outpatient visits to neurologists in the United States,[1,2] migraine may not be the primary reason for a visit to a healthcare provider.[3] Recent surveys suggest that fewer than half of current migraineurs have received a medical diagnosis of migraine.[4] The availability of a brief, self-administered migraine screening tool in the primary care setting could help identify migraine sufferers who require further evaluation and possible referral for treatment. This study was designed to establish the validity and reliability of a simple, brief, self-administered screening questionnaire to help identify migraine patients in primary care settings.

Methods

To test the validity of a new migraine screening instrument (ID Migraine™) in the primary care setting, 563 men and women completed written screening questionnaires.

Criteria for enrollment included a visit to a primary care provider (PCP) for any reason, as well as two or more headaches within the past 3 months that were either disabling or prompted a wish to discuss the headache with a healthcare professional. The initial questionnaires contained nine items, eight paralleling International Headache Society (IHS) criteria[5] for migraine and one assessing disability. Headache specialists who were blinded to screener results evaluated each patient and assigned a diagnosis based on IHS criteria. To establish the validity of the screening instrument in terms of its ability to identify migraine and establish a 'gold standard' diagnosis of migraine consistent with IHS criteria, the following simple rules were utilized: (1) Migraine defined either by the physician, headache expert, or by IHS criteria (using clinical features recorded by the headache expert) was classified as migraine; (2) all other patients were assigned to the 'no migraine' category. The sensitivity and specificity of each question in the nine-item screener were evaluated statistically, using the medical diagnosis made by the headache expert as a benchmark. Logistic regression analysis was utilized to identify the three items most strongly associated with migraine diagnosis for use in the final ID Migraine™ screener.

Results

The validity and reliability studies were conducted in the United States at 27 primary care practice sites and 12 headache specialty practice sites. Of the 563 patients who met study eligibility requirements and agreed to participate, 550 were screened and referred for evaluation by a headache specialist (Fig. 44.1). Headache specialists evaluated 451/550 (80%) of these screened patients; this constituted the validation sample. The validation sample, which had a mean age of 39.3 ± 10.1 years, consisted of 341 women (75.6%) and 110 men (24.4%). A total of 312 patients (69%) were white, 105 (23%) were African-American, 13 (2.9%) were Asian, and 21 (4.7%) reported other races. Among patients who eventually received a gold standard diagnosis of migraine, 124 (28%) said they had received a previous migraine diagnosis.

There were only modest differences between the validation sample and the 99 patients who completed the screener and were referred to, but did not complete, the diagnostic evaluation by a headache expert.

Table 44.1 shows the key symptoms addressed in the nine-item screener. The sensitivity (how well the item or question identifies a patient who has migraine) and specificity (how well the item distinguishes migraine from nonmigraine sufferers) of each individual item on the nine-item migraine screener were calculated. Sensitivity was highest for severity of pain (0.94), type of pain ('pounding, pulsing, or throbbing;' 0.87) and functional impairment (0.87). Specificity was highest for nausea (0.81), photophobia (0.74), and aura (0.74). Based on an assessment of adjusted odds ratios, three of the nine questions on the screening questionnaire were the best predictors of migraine diagnosis: headache-related disability, nausea, and photophobia (Fig. 44.2). Empirical testing showed that an affirmative response to any two of these three test items would have a sensitivity of 0.81 (95% CI,

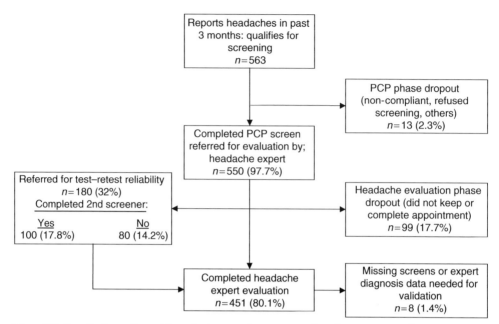

Fig. 44.1 Patient disposition during study. Reprinted with permission from Lipton RB *et al.* (2003). A self-administered screener for migraine in primary care: the ID Migraine™ validation study. *Neurology* **61**: 375–82.

Table 44.1 Sensitivity and specificity of questions on the ID Migraine screener

Survey item[a]	Sensitivity (95% CI)	Specificity (95% CI)
Pain was worse on just one side.	0.75 (0.70–0.79)	0.50 (0.39–0.61)
Pain was pounding, pulsing, or throbbing.	0.87 (0.83–0.90)	0.22 (0.14–0.33)
Pain was moderate or severe.	0.94 (0.91–0.96)	0.16 (0.09–0.25)
Pain was made worse by activities such as walking or climbing stairs.	0.67 (0.62–0.72)	0.57 (0.46–0.68)
You felt nauseated or sick to your stomach.	0.60 (0.55–0.65)	0.81 (0.71–0.89)
You saw spots, stars, zigzags, lines or gray areas for several minutes or more before or during your headaches (aura symptoms).	0.43 (0.38–0.48)	0.74 (0.63–0.83)
Light bothered you (a lot more than when you do not have headaches).	0.75 (0.71–0.80)	0.74 (0.63–0.83)
Sound bothered you (a lot more than when you do not have headaches).	0.83 (0.78–0.86)	0.56 (0.45–0.67)
You had functional impairment due to headache within the last 3 months[b].	0.87 (0.83–0.90)	0.52 (0.40–0.63)

[a]Sample size ranged from 438 to 448 due to occasional missing values.
[b]Scored positive if disability reported on any one day in the past 3 months.
Shaded areas denote items selected for three-item ID Migraine screener based on their having the highest adjusted odds ratios among all nine items in the survey.

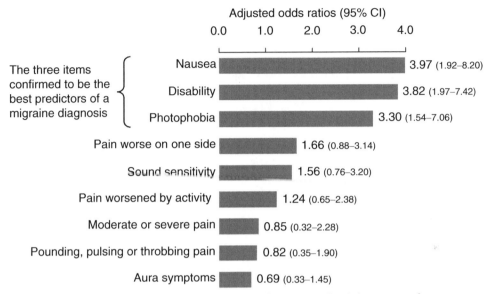

Fig. 44.2 Adjusted odds ratios: likelihood of gold-standard diagnosis of migraine.

0.77–0.85) and a specificity of 0.75 (95% CI, 0.64–0.84) for detecting migraine in the primary care setting. The sensitivity and specificity of the three-item migraine screener was similar regardless of gender, age, comorbid headaches, or previous diagnosis. The positive predictive value of the three-item screener was 93.3% (95% CI, 89.9–95.8%), which means that if the screener is positive (2/3 positive responses), there is a very high likelihood that the patient has migraine. Test–retest reliability was good, with a kappa value of 0.68 (95% CI, 0.54–0.82).

Conclusions

It may be possible to improve diagnostic rates of migraine in a primary care population utilizing just three simple, self-administered questions relating to nausea, photophobia, and headache-related disability. The simplicity, ease of use, and performance characteristics of the ID Migraine™ screener suggest that it could significantly improve migraine recognition in primary care practice.

References

1. Bekkelund SI, Albretsen C. Evaluation of referrals from general practice to a neurological department. *Fam Pract* 2002; **19**: 297–9.
2. Cockerell OC, Goodridge DM, Brodie D, *et al.* Neurological disease in a defined population: the results of a pilot study in two general practices. *Neuroepidemiology* 1996; **15**: 73–82.

3. Clouse JC, Osterhaus JT. Healthcare resource use and costs associated with migraine in a managed healthcare setting. *Ann Pharmacother* 1994; **28**: 659–64.
4. Lipton RB, Diamond S, Reed M, *et al.* Migraine diagnosis and treatment: results from the American Migraine Study II. *Headache* 2001; **41**: 638–45.
5. Headache Classification Committee of the International Headache Society Classification and Diagnostic Criteria for Headache Disorders, Cranial Neuralgias and Facial Pain. *Cephalalgia* 1988; **8** (Suppl 7): 1–96.

45 The FRAMIG III survey: first epidemiological survey in general population according to the 2004 IHS migraine criteria

C. Lucas, M. Lanteri-Minet, and M. H. Chautard

Introduction

In 1990, the first nationwide survey of migraine using the International Headache Society (IHS) criteria for the diagnosis of migraine[1] was conducted in France on a representative sample of residents aged 15 years and more. Headache sufferers were classified as IHS migraine, 'borderline' migraine, possible migraine, and non-migrainous headache. The study found an overall prevalence of HIS-migraine of 8.1%; another 4% of patients being classified as 'borderline' migraine, which we in fact considered as definite migraine.[2]

Almost ten years later, in 1999 and 2000, two large epidemiology surveys on migraine in the general population were performed in France using the IHS classification. They confirmed the 1990 data, finding a migraine prevalence of 12.45%.[3]

The aim of the present survey is to update epidemiological data on migraine in the general population in France using the recently published second edition of the IHS criteria.[4]

Methodology

A mail survey was carried out by the TNS-SOFRES statistical institute from September 26 to November 7, 2003 on a sample of 15 000 subjects aged ≥15 and representative of the French general population. Migraine was diagnosed using an algorithm based on the 2004 IHS criteria.

A deepening mail survey was secondly carried out among migraineurs and their close circle on the profile, management, and repercussion of the migraine in France using the MIDAS scores,[5] the SF-12 questionnaire,[6] and the HAD scale.[7]

Results

Population

Out of the 15 000 subjects included in the survey, 10 870 returned the questionnaire (72.5%) and 10 532 questionnaires or subjects aged ≥18 years were analysed (97%).

Prevalence rates in France

The prevalence of migraine (1.1, 1.2.1 according to the 2004 IHS classification) was 11.2% (n=1179) and the prevalence of probable migraine (1.6.1 according to the 2004 IHS classification) was 10.1% (n=1066), that is an overall prevalence or 21.3%. Furthermore, 1.7% of subjects reported experiencing a daily headache (the precise prevalence rate of chronic migraine as defined by the 2004 HIS criteria is to be published soon).

When asked if they were self-aware of being migraineurs, almost one out of two subjects with migraine, and almost three out of four subjects with probable migraine did not know they were suffering from this disease (Fig. 45.1).

Impact of migraine

Twenty-two percent of patients suffering from migraine reported a severe impairment (i.e. MIDAS score III or IV). A severe degree of impairment caused by the

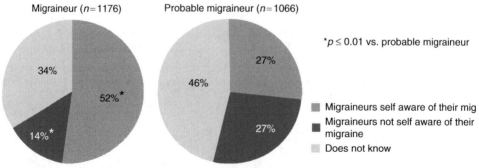

Fig. 45.1 Prevalence of migraine in France.

suffering is equally seen in subjects with probable migraine (12% with MIDAS scores III or IV).

Using the Hospital Anxiety and Depression Scale (HAD), a reliable instrument for detecting depression and anxiety, it has been shown that high levels of anxiety (anxiety subscore >8) and depression (depression subscore >8) were present in subjects with migraine (self-aware and not aware of their migraine) as well as in subjects with probable migraine ($p \leq 0.01$ vs. non-migraineurs for all groups). Moreover, levels of anxiety and depression raised significantly with the increase of migraine severity (HAD score >19 (i.e. abnormal) : 11% in subjects with MIDAS score I, 20% in MIDAS score II, $p \leq 0.01$ vs. I, 24% in MIDAS score III, $p \leq 0.01$ vs. I and 42% in MIDAS score IV, $p \leq 0.01$ vs. I and II and vs. III) (Table 45.1).

In all patients suffering from migraine, self-aware or not of their disease, overall quality of life is significantly impaired. Seven out of the eight quality of life dimensions assessed by means of the SF-12 questionnaire were altered in migraineurs vs. non-migraineurs (all items, save the 'physical activity'-item, $p \leq 0.01$) (Fig. 45.2).

Therapeutic behavior of migraineurs

In spite of the relative severity of the disease, 79% of all migraineurs have never consulted (40%) or have ceased to consult (39%) for their migraine attacks. Moreover, most of the patients did not take an adequate treatment.

Recently, the French National Agency for Accreditation and Evaluation in Health Care (ANAES) has conceived a four-item questionnaire in order to assess the migraineur's satisfaction with his treatment of migraine attacks (according to this questionnaire, a negative answer to one question out of four is sufficient to recommend the coprescription of a NSAID and a triptan at 2 h as rescue medication in case of NSAID failure.[8] Almost half of the patients having treated their last migraine attack with non-specific analgesics had answered at least once 'no' to the four-item questionnaire (most of them to the first two items, Table 45.2), needing thus a coprescription NSAID-triptan to be proposed. Results also confirm the major importance of the patient's first visit for migraine, the general practitioner being in 81% of cases the first person to see the migraineur.

Conclusions

FRAMIG III is the first epidemiological survey performed in the general population using the IHS classification. The total prevalence of migraine in France is 21.3% (migraine: 11.2% and probable migraine: 10.2%). Almost one out of two subjects with migraine are not self-aware of their disease. Twenty-two percent of patients suffering from migraine reported a severe impairment. High levels of anxiety and depression are present in subjects with migraine ($p < 0.01$ vs. non-migraineurs for all groups), levels of anxiety and depression raising significantly with the increase of migraine severity ($p < 0.05$). In patients suffering from migraine, overall quality of life is significantly impaired. Moreover, 79% of all migraineurs have never

Table 45.1 HAD global, anxiety and depression scores in migraineurs and in subjects without migraine

	No migraine (n=8287)	Migrainers (n=1179)	Probable migrainers (n=1066)	Self-aware migrainers (n=903)	Not self-aware migrainers (n=1342)
Abnormal HAD global score (>19)	9%	16%*	16%*	15%*	17%*
Abnormal HAD anxiety score (>8)	20%	37%*	37%*	36%*	37%*
Abnormal HAD depression score (>8)	11%	17%*	16%*	15%*	17%*

*$p \leq 0.01$ vs. no migraine.

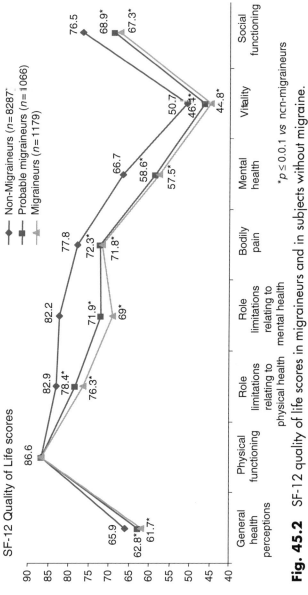

Fig. 45.2 SF-12 quality of life scores in migraineurs and in subjects without migraine.

Table 45.2 Answers to each item of the ANAES questionnaire having treated their last migraine attack with non-specific analgesics

	Answers to each item of the questionnaire (% patients)		
	NO	YES	Does not know
Significant response 2 h after the drug intake	30%	69%	1%
Only one drug intake	32%	67%	1%
Treatment well tolerated	3%	97%	<1%
Rapid normalization of daily activity	21%	78%	1%

consulted or have ceased to consult for their migraine attacks and about one in two analgesic-treated patients does not take the adequate treatment.

References

1. Headache Classification Committee of the International Headache Society. Classification and diagnostic criteria for headache disorders, cranial neuralgias and facial pain. *Cephalalgia*. 1988; **8** (Suppl 7): 1–96.
2. Henry P, Michel P, Brochet B, *et al.* A nationwide survey of migraine in France: prevalence and clinical features in adults. GRIM. *Cephalalgia* 1992; **12** (4): 229–37.
3. Lantéri-Minet M, Lucas C, Chaffaut C, *et al.* FRAMIG 2000:Medical and therapeutic management of migraine in France. Development of migraine attacks after the first treatment. *Cephalalgia* 2004 (in press).
4. Headache Classification Subcommittee of the International Headache Society. The International Classification of Headache Disorders: 2nd edition. *Cephalalgia* 2004; **24** (Suppl 1): 9–160.
5. Stewart WF, Lipton RB, Whyte J, *et al.* An international study to assess the reliability of the Migraine Disability Assessment (MIDAS) score. *Neurology* 1999; **53**: 988–94.
6. Jenkinson C, Layte R. Development and testing of the UK SF-12 (short form health survey). *J Health Serv Res Policy* 1997; **2** (1): 14–8.
7. Zigmond AS, Snaith RP. The hospital anxiety and depression scale. *Acta Psychiatr Scand* 1983; **67** (6): 361–70.
8. Agence Nationale d'Accréditation et d'Evaluation en Santé (ANAES). Recommandations pour la pratique clinique. Prise en charge diagnostique et thérapeutique de la migraine chez l'adulte et l'enfant [Recommendations for clinical practice. Diagnostic and therapeutic management of migraine in adults and children]. *Rev Neurol* 2003; **159**: 126–35.

46 Discussion summary, practical implementation and research

M. Ashina

The presentations, posters, and discussions during this session were devoted to the development of national and international simple charts or algorithms to identify and treat headache disorders, and classification research.

It was pointed out that a large number of patients in primary care do not consult about migraine headaches and a short questionnaire would be very useful in a busy general practice. However, attention was drawn to the fact that many patients with frequent migraine might have medication-overuse headache. Although a short questionnaire would identify headache as a frequent problem, it is still necessary with a comprehensive interview on headache history and symptoms and to follow patients with a headache diary that allows collecting information on frequency of migraine and amount of medication used to treat attacks. Another question is whether different ethnical groups would report disability in relation to other primary headaches than migraine, e.g. tension-type headache. It was emphasized that a friendly questionnaire was validated in the US. Such and that friendly charts require validation/evaluation in other countries before application in primary care.

Regarding national and international action plans, there was a broad agreement about the significance of developing a set of flow charts to aid diagnostic decision-making and treatment of primary headaches. This will be one of the important tasks of a joint action between World Health Organization and World Headache Alliance, International Headache Society and European Headache Federation in the Global Campaign against headache. It was suggested to produce two short versions of the IHS classification: one for headache specialists and one for general practitioners. Numbers of possible diagnostic and treatment algorithms were discussed. It would be best if the algorithms are simple and comprehensive, and include the most important/essential diagnoses such as medication-overuse headache. It was proposed using experience from other specialties. When American

Psychiatric Society had published a version of DSM IV for general practitioners, it had failed. On the other hand, the WHO version had succeeded. This was probably because management algorithms were also included. *Diagnostic and Management Guidelines for Mental Disorders in Primary Care* may thus be a good model for headache guidelines. The link to this site (search 'diagnostic cards') could be found in the WHO's homepage (*www.who.int*).

Regarding research in headache classification, a poster by an Italian group was discussed. Dr. Sarchielli and colleagues developed a computerized, structured medical record based on the ICHD classification system for primary headaches. Using this method, it is possible to identify some cases where patients might fulfill criteria for infrequent episodic tension-type headache and probable infrequent headache. The method received positive comments as a possibly important tool for identifying mistakes or inconsistencies in the IHS classification. However, it was emphasized that the method needs to be tested in clinical practice. The next step could be to diagnose, for example 200 consecutive patients in a headache center according to the computerized system. Then it would be interesting to compare the computer-based diagnosis with the clinical diagnosis in order to identify possible mistakes in classification. The French study by Lantéri-Minet and colleagues presented a French survey of headache disorders based on a computerized database. It was noticed that the study is an impressive effort to collect a headache database covering 2/3 of the French territory. Using this database, it would be possible to identify several rare headache disorders and to study pathophysiological mechanisms underlying these disorders. It would allow performing controlled drug trials in large groups of patients with rare headache disorders.

Index